Assessment and Remediation of Articulatory and Phonological Disorders

SECOND EDITION

NANCY A. CREAGHEAD
University of Cincinnati

PARLEY W. NEWMAN
Brigham Young University

WAYNE A. SECORD
Bowling Green State University

MERRILL PUBLISHING COMPANY
A Bell & Howell Information Company
Columbus   Toronto   London   Melbourne

Published by Merrill Publishing Company
A Bell & Howell Information Company
Columbus, Ohio 43216

This book was set in Times Roman

Administrative Editor: Vicki Knight
Production Coordinator: Julie Higgins
Art Coordinator: Lorraine Woost

Library of Congress Catalog Card Number: 88-63333
ISBN: 0-675-20653-7
Printed in the United States of America
1 2 3 4 5 6 7 8 9—92 91 90 89

This text is dedicated to the memory of Rolland
J. Van Hattum. Most of us knew him as
''Rollie.'' Rollie was a very special person who
gave much of his life to our profession. He saw
a great deal of humor in that life and even more
so in his own successes and failures. To him,
humor was both love and a test as often he used
that very wit to expose arrogance, smugness, and
undue pride. Rollie believed fully in the notion
that one demonstrates strength by revealing his
own vulnerability.

Preface

This text was constructed with three major goals in mind. The first was to cover in a comprehensive way the work of the past 40 years in the service of people who find intelligible speech beyond their ability to master. Thus, coverage includes traditional views toward articulation disorders and their treatment, behavioral management approaches with their greater efficiency, and, finally, current thinking and methods derived from the contributions of modern linguistics.

The second major goal was to provide a text that would emphasize treatment. Of the book's 14 chapters, 9 are fully developed discussions of remedial procedures by authors who in many cases actually developed them or who are recognized experts in the method described. This work, then, serves as a rich resource on therapy. To our knowledge, no other text fully explicates the major current approaches for remediating disorders of articulation and phonology.

Finally, the editors hoped to collect in one volume the contributions of a number of authors who have achieved national recognition for their original works. The contributors to this volume have provided extensive service to the communicatively impaired.

The text also supplies foundation material for the presentations on treatment. The first of the book's three major sections provides the bases for understanding normal articulation and phonology. Chapter 1, an opening rationale with emphasis on communication, serves as a point of departure for subsequent chapters. In chapter 2, Nancy Creaghead and Parley Newman discuss phonetics and phonology; chapter 3 by Creaghead reviews development of phonology in children. Chapter 4, by Newman and Creaghead, treats assessment of articulatory and phonologic disorders.

The second major part of the book presents an overview of remediation methods. These are intro-duced in chapter 5 by Wayne Secord, who discusses traditional articulation therapy methods. In chapter 6, Donald E. Mowrer explains how a clinician can apply the power and efficiency of behavioral methods to the remediation of disorders of articulation, and also how the clinician can write programs useful to paraprofessionals. Dr. Mowrer has achieved national recognition for his many publications and other contributions to the amelioration of speech disorders through the application of behavioral management techniques. In chapter 7, Nancy Creaghead provides an explanation of linguistic approaches to articulation therapy and phonological disorders.

Chapter 8 by Gordon M. Low, Mildred T. Ravsten, and Parley W. Newman extends our perceptions of remediating articulation and phonology through the communicative power of peer interaction. This viewpoint takes into account current pragmatic approaches to understanding and remediating disorders of language. For a quarter of a century, Dr. Low has had the vision of communication as the overarching rubric embracing disorders of speech, language, hearing, reading, and learning and has applied this vision to the treatment of disorders of communication. Professor Ravsten, a former student of Dr. Low, has been importantly involved in the clinical application of this innovative approach.

In chapter 9, Harris Winitz provides an insightful and thought-provoking refocusing on the auditory channel in treating articulatory disorders. Dr. Winitz is a distinguished scholar who is regarded as one of the truly significant contributors to the field.

Considerations for organic disorders are explained in chapter 10 by Dorothy H. Air, Ann S. Wood, and Jean R. Neils. The special assessment and remediation procedures required for individuals with motor speech disorders and cleft palate are discussed by authors who have served these clients in hospital and private-practice settings and are respected as experts by the members of their professional community.

Chapter 11 by Doris P. Bradley explains how traditional articulation treatment procedures can be applied systematically to correct multiple phoneme deficiencies simultaneously and efficiently. Dr. Bradley is well known for her many contributions to the welfare of the communicatively handicapped, not the least of which is her development of the multiphonemic approach.

In Chapter 12, Barbara W. Hodson describes the cycles approach that she and Elaine Paden presented in the book, *Targeting Intelligible Speech*. This approach embodies the concept of phonological processes in remediation as well as the principles of normal development of the phonological system. Dr. Hodson is a leader in the area of clinically relevant applications of phonological principles. The thrust of her ongoing research to determine ''what really works'' for children with severe phonological disorders.

Richard E. Shine was a student of Eugene McDonald, who pioneered the principles of sensory-motor articulation training. Dr. Shine has applied these principles extensively in working with children in a variety of clinical settings and has taught others how to apply them. He is well qualified to present information on the sensory-motor approach in chapter 13.

A current application of distinctive-feature theory to the correction of articulation disorders is presented in chapter 14 by Stephen E. Blache. Dr. Blache has distinguished himself in the current professional literature by his innovative work in analyzing distinctive features and developing methods to teach them.

The authors of the various chapters of this book, then, are the creators of the procedures presented.

These procedures represent major contemporary methods in dealing with the communication disorders of articulation and phonology. They also provide insights into the shape of the future in this field.

We take pride in bringing together the substantive works of creative scholars and clinicians in the field of speech-language pathology. We believe that what these writers have produced is not just another text on disorders of articulation and phonology, but a significant work that combines current impact with lasting value.

Nancy A. Creaghead
Parley W. Newman
Wayne A. Secord

ACKNOWLEDGMENTS

It is obvious that a project such as this cannot be accomplished without the cooperation and help of many people. First, we want to thank our 11 contributors for their fine chapters and for their cooperation in getting them to their final and polished form.

There are also a number of people from Merrill Publishing Company who have provided special support for us. We especially thank Vicki Knight, our administrative editor, for her insistence on high quality and readability for the entire text and for her patience with us. She secured for us valuable help from our reviewers Stuart Ritterman, University of South Florida; Robert A. Hull, Jr., Valdosta State College; Michael J. Moran, Auburn University; and Ronald Chambers, Wichita State University. In addition, we have received valuable help from members of the editorial staff, including our copy editor, Jean Scott Berry, and our production coordinator, Julie Higgins.

Finally, we all thank each other for time spent, support given, and an overall cooperative attitude which made difficult things easier.

Contents

CHAPTER 1 Introduction

The ability to speak is one of our most precious gifts. Speech is the most frequently used vehicle for communication and the most efficient. Not all of us, however, are able to put this gift to use in the same way. Approximately 5% to 10% of the population has some type of communication disorder involving speech, language, and/or hearing (Culton, 1986; National Center for Health Statistics, 1981; Perkins, 1977). Between 50% and 80% of these disorders are estimated to be articulatory (Fein, 1983). The mere prevalence of such problems would indicate that students and clinicians should be well versed in their clinical management.

This book is both for students in training in speech-language pathology and for practicing clinicians. It is concerned with the nature and treatment of individuals who have articulation disorders, with a focus on treatment. Although a number of approaches and methods have been commonly used in the treatment of articulation disorders, recent advances in the profession have changed our perceptions about articulation problems and have also helped to reshape our thinking. This is especially true for young children who have severe articulation disorders.

Wayne A Secord, Ph.D., is an associate professor of communication disorders at Bowling Green State University, where he serves as department chair.

The following story about a child named Sean provides background for discussion of changes in approach that have occurred in recent years. Sean was one of my first clients. The story of his treatment is a good example of the clinical approach I used 20 years ago.

About 20 years ago, I was working as a speech-language pathologist (actually, they called me a speech therapist then) at Indian Springs Elementary School in Columbus, Ohio. It was my first real professional employment. In fact, I was only 2 months out of Ohio State University. I was green, a little scared, but honestly excited about doing something for which I had trained for so long. I was even going to be paid.

It was only my third or fourth day on the job. I was screening the kindergarten class for potential speech problems when I met 5-year-old Sean. Sometimes a decision whether to pass or fail a child in screening is a close call. Unfortunately, that was not the case with Sean. I couldn't understand anything he said, nor could his teacher or any of his classmates.

I had learned in my training how important it was to conduct a thorough diagnostic work-up, and so I did just that. I gathered a complete case history, including interviews with Sean's parents and his teacher. I even talked to the teacher of his sixth-grade brother to see if she could offer any insights. I could find nothing remarkable socially, educationally, medically, or even developmentally, except that Sean did not really begin talking until about age 2½.

I then gave Sean an audiometric screening and administered several formal and informal assessments, including the Templin-Darley Tests of Articulation, Peabody Picture Vocabulary Test, Preschool Language Scale, Utah Test of Language Development, Templin Picture Sound Discrimination Test, and Boston University Speech Sound Discrimination Test. I even remember conducting a more in-depth than usual oral examination thinking there might be some organic involvement, but I found none.

I considered the possibility of a language disorder. However, Sean's receptive language was well within the norms for his age, and although his many articulation errors made evaluation of his conversational language impossible, he frequently spoke in (unintelligible) phrases and sentences. In addition, his intelligence was assessed by our school psychologist and was found to be within normal limits. After careful consideration, I finally diagnosed Sean's problem as a severe articulation disorder of no known cause. A summary of his articulation errors is given in Table 1.1.

Sean was enrolled in therapy immediately. I designed a treatment plan based on criteria I had learned in my training. In considering what sound to treat first, I weighed many factors. For example, I compared his chronological age with the age he was expected to have mastered many of his error sounds. I then examined those developmentally appropriate phonemes a step further. I considered which of them he could repeat correctly after I showed him a somewhat exaggerated model of correct production. Both of these considerations, *developmental age* and *stimulability,* are important in devising a plan of treatment. After looking at

these two factors and many others, I decided on a therapy plan. My plan was to teach the /k/ sound first. When that sound was corrected, I would move on to the /g/. When it was corrected, I would teach the /f/, and so on until Sean could say all of his error sounds correctly in conversational speech.

Notice that I made up a plan that entailed teaching one sound at a time. At the time Sean was my client, almost all clinicians taught one sound at a time. Some clinicians, however, were just beginning to try out some new procedures based on principles derived from learning theory. They were writing treatment programs for speech sounds that looked a little like those written for teaching machines and, in fact, were based on them to a large extent. But still, it was one sound at a time in therapy.

In therapy with Sean, I taught him first how to become a good listener. Before I showed him how to say a target sound, I taught him to know how his target phoneme sounded. I made sure he could identify his error sound as well as isolate it from other sounds. I bombarded him with instances of his new sound so he would develop an internal auditory model of that sound. Most of all, I made sure he could tell the difference between his new sound and his error sound. All of this work was part of what we called "ear training."

Production therapy also followed traditional methods. I always spent time establishing correct production of a new sound in isolation first. I then trained Sean to say the sound correctly in a series of increasingly more difficult stages—in syllables, in words, in phrases, in sentences, and then in conversation. I wouldn't let him move from one stage to the next unless he could say his sound correctly and consistently in the preceding stage. All of Sean's articulation errors were essentially corrected in this manner, with the process taking approximately 2 years. I somehow managed it with the help of his parents and teacher, some natural maturation, and all the state-of-the-art training I had at my command at that time.

It was not as easy as it all may sound. There were many times when I thought what I was doing was simply too difficult for Sean. My concept and his concept of a phoneme were very different, and I had him doing some rather abstract tasks at times. I never realized how difficult it could be to listen for fine differences in speech sounds. I recall asking Sean to locate a certain speech sound embedded in the middle of a multisyllabic word and his looking at me as though I were crazy. It was a look that said, "Why am I doing this? It doesn't make any sense." He sometimes gave me that same look when I'd have him say the same set of words over and over again.

My approach to Sean's articulation problem reflected my philosophy about treatment at that time. I thought then that speech sound errors were phonetic in nature and so my therapy emphasized both the auditory and articulatory properties of a phoneme. Had I the opportunity to undertake the clinical management of Sean today, I would handle his case differently. My philosophy with regard to the nature of disorders like his has changed, influenced by changes in our profession over the past 20 years. We no longer consider all articulation errors phonetic in nature. Many have been shown to be predictable occurrences in a complex phonological system. Many are based on a delayed or deviant system of rules a speaker uses. Moreover, our philosophies concerning treatment have also changed. We are no longer so rigid as to teach just one sound at a time. We now look for underlying patterns or processes that may account for a larger number of

errors and attempt to remediate them. For example, notice (Table 1.1) how Sean leaves off most final consonants. This is a pattern called *final consonant deletion* and, indeed, Sean used it regularly. If I had targeted that process instead of teaching one sound at a time, I might have substantially changed many error sounds at once. I didn't know that then. What I knew and did then, however, was effective, and similar treatment procedures (the traditional approach) are still used by many clinicians today.

The treatment approach used with Sean is explained in more detail in chapter 5. We will refer to Sean several times more in this introductory chapter as we lay the foundation for the remainder of the text.

CHANGING PERSPECTIVES

At about the same time that Sean was receiving therapy for his misarticulations, a large body of research from learning theory, linguistics, neu-

TABLE 1.1
Sean's Articulation Errors

Substitutions	
Initial:	b/f, b/v, t/θ, d/ð, d/s, t/ʃ, d/tʃ, d/dʒ, d/k, d/g, p/sp, t/sk, d/st, d/kr, t/tr, t/kl, p/fl
Medial:	b/v, s/θ, d/ð, d/s, d/z, t/ʃ, t/tʃ, d/dʒ
Final:	?/t, s/ʃ
Omissions	
Initial:	/z, h/
Medial:	none
Final:	/p, b, t, d, k, g, f, v, θ, ð, ʒ, tʃ, dʒ/
Distortions	
Initial:	/r/
Medial:	/r/
Final:	/ɚ/

rology, and communication was beginning to emerge. This research would ultimately focus our thinking along four major conceptual perspectives: articulatory, linguistic, motor speech, and communication.

The Articulatory Perspective

The case of Sean is illustrative of an articulatory approach to treatment that was heavily influenced by early practitioners who emphasized a combination of listening and speech production activities. The traditional approach targets a single speech sound at a time. Only when a client gains complete mastery of one sound is treatment initiated on another. Emphasis is placed on learning how to accurately perceive and say individual speech sounds.

The articulatory perspective was significantly influenced by concepts developed from learning theory. In the late 1960s and early 1970s, clinicians were beginning to apply behavioral principles to existing procedures. They wrote behavioral programs that served to systematize the entire treatment process. They became data keepers, program writers, and keen observers of behavior, which allowed them to harness the power and efficiency of behavioral technology. Their efforts helped make treatment more scientific and accountable. Although the behavioral era had a real impact on practice, it did not substantially alter our perception about how articulation disorders should be treated. The emphasis was still on production, typically one sound at a time, albeit a more systematic emphasis. At about the time that behavioral technology was having its greatest impact, a linguistic view of articulatory production emerged.

The Linguistic Perspective

In recent years, the profession of speech-language pathology has been influenced by contributions

from the study of linguistics. The influence of linguistic conceptions is readily apparent in relation to disorders of articulation, which may now be analyzed in terms of underlying principles or rules that govern articulatory production. The description of these principles or rules is a central aspect of *phonology,* the study of the sound system of language.

The study of phonology is concerned with the underlying system(s) that govern the use of speech sound (segments) and of stress, intonation, and pausing (suprasegments) in the production and discrimination of meaningful utterances. From the linguistic point of view (Compton, 1970; Ingram, 1976; Pollack & Rees, 1972) errors of speech sound production can be shown to be systematic, patterned, and based on underlying phonological principles. Sean omitted nearly all final consonants, reflecting a rule in his personal phonological system that is different from the rules of normal speakers. This concept (rule-based sound changes) is elaborated in a number of later chapters. Although a linguistic perspective of speech production is extremely helpful, speech production must also be considered as a motor behavior.

The Motor Speech Perspective

Speech sounds are uttered through the tongue, lips, and other parts of the articulatory mechanism. This aspect of articulation is an important consideration when treating organic disorders. If the cause of the articulation disorder is related to a neurological disturbance, structural deformity, and/or physical defect, the problem is classified as *organic* in nature. The motor speech perspective focuses attention on the physiological aspects of speech production rather than the behavioral or linguistic aspects. In the case of Sean, an organic disorder was one possibility the clinician ruled out in the assessment process. When structure, hearing, and all observable physical systems appear to be normal, the problem is termed *functional* in nature, and its origin is attributed to faulty learning (Curtis, 1956). Most articulation disorders fall into the functional category as in the case of Sean. No view of articulatory production seems complete, however, without considering the larger perspective of communication.

The Communication Perspective

One of the areas that has contributed to this broader perspective is *pragmatics,* a field that goes beyond linguistics to encompass the intentions, use, and effects of communication (Lucas, 1980; Morris, 1938, 1946; Prutting, 1982; Rees, 1978). Pragmatics requires that human communication be considered in terms of the total communicative situation. It requires consideration for communicative interactions beyond the lexical meaning of words (semantics) and the structural features of verbal utterances (syntax). The communication perspective emphasizes that remediation of faulty speech patterns occurs in and is a part of a larger communicative interaction. In the case of Sean, the treatment approach was purely articulatory in nature and placed little emphasis on the larger communicative context in which the newly learned articulation patterns were acquired.

TREATMENT OF ARTICULATION DISORDERS

The primary focus of this text is but one aspect of the total communication process—speech production. However, all of the other facets affect and interrelate with this one and must, therefore, be considered in any assessment or treatment program. Many areas of Sean's development, for example, were examined in assessing his disorder.

In order to remediate disordered articulation, it is necessary to understand certain background information, including the anatomy and physiology of articulation and the phonological rules of the language. This information is presented in chapter 2. In order to understand delayed and disordered articulation, one must also have information regarding normal development. Accurate assessment

requires thorough knowledge of normal behavior, and remediation goals and procedures are often based on the developmental process. In chapter 3 the development of adult articulation and phonological rules by the child are described.

Chapter 4 discusses assessment. Careful assessment is a necessary prerequisite to remediation. In particular, linguistic approaches require in-depth assessment procedures to analyze patterns of error. Time spent in analysis will be reflected in more effective and efficient remediation. In addition, ongoing assessment must continue throughout therapy as the clinician evaluates progress and the effectiveness of specific procedures.

This text focuses heavily on remediation procedures. Two sections are devoted to this topic. In Part II the major types of therapy are described. They include traditional approaches, behavioral approaches, and linguistic approaches. In addition, considerations for working with specific populations are discussed.

In Part III four contemporary therapy techniques are described. Each of these chapters is written by an author who has developed and used the particular approach. Each includes the author's rationale in developing the approach, his own description of the procedures, and analysis of the strengths and weaknesses.

As might be expected, considerable overlap of ideas and therapy procedures is represented. On the other hand, there may be some inconsistencies or apparent contradictions. The most important idea to be drawn from the book is that no one therapy program is best or should be used with every client. A given type of disorder or a disorder resulting from a specific etiology may be more amenable to a given therapy approach. In addition, individuals may respond differently regardless of identifiable symptoms or causes. This kind of information can be obtained only through thorough evaluation prior to and during therapy. Thus the clinician must have a large "bag of tricks" in the form of several overall approaches and a number of specific strategies. The purpose of Parts II and

III is to provide an overview of the remediation process and specific approaches so that the clinician can choose what is best for each setting and each client. Every facet of communication must be considered in making this choice.

The purpose of this book is to help clinicians become more effective in their assessment and treatment of articulatory and phonological disorders. Later chapters will expand on many of the ideas presented in this introduction.

REFERENCES

Compton, A. J. (1970). Generative studies of children's phonological disorders. *Journal of Speech and Hearing Disorders, 35,* 315–343.

Culton, G. L. (1986). Speech disorders among college freshmen: A 13-year survey. *Journal of Speech and Hearing Disorders, 51,* 3–7.

Curtis, J. F. (1956). Disorders of articulation. In W. Johnson, S. Brown, J. Curtis, C. Edney, & J. Keaster (Eds.), *Speech handicapped school children* (rev. ed). New York: Harper & Row.

Fein, D. J. (1983). The prevalence of speech and language impairments. *ASHA, 25,* 37.

Ingram, D. (1976). *Phonological disability in children.* New York: American Elsevier.

Lucas, E. V. (1980). *Semantic and pragmatic language disorders.* Rockville, MD: Aspen Systems.

Morris, C. W. (1938). Foundations of the theory of signs. In O. Nuerath, R. Carnap, & C. W. Morris (Eds.), *International encyclopedia of unified science* (Vol. 1, No. 2). Chicago: University of Chicago Press.

Morris, C. W. (1946). *Signs, language and behavior.* Englewood Cliffs, NJ: Prentice-Hall.

National Center for Health Statistics. (1981). *Prevalence of selected impairments: United States–1977* (Publication No. [PHS] 82–1562). Washington, DC: Department of Health, Education, and Welfare.

Perkins, W. H. (1977). *Speech pathology: An applied behavioral science.* St. Louis: Mosby.

Pollack, E., & Rees, N. S. (1972). Disorders of articulation: Some clinical applications of distinctive feature theory. *Journal of Speech and Hearing Disorders, 37,* 451–461.

Prutting, C. (1982). Pragmatics as social competence. *Journal of Speech and Hearing Disorders, 47,* 123–134.

Rees, N. S. (1978). Pragmatics of language: Application to normal and disordered language development. In R. L. Schiefelbusch (Ed.), *Bases of language intervention* (pp. 227–256). Baltimore: University Park Press.

PART ONE

Prerequisites for Planning Remediation

The first section of this text presents background information regarding articulation and phonology. A clinician must have such knowledge prior to remediation for several reasons. First, it is important to understand the production of speech sounds and the rules that specify their use in language production. Without a good picture of the normal system, it is not possible to evaluate adequately one that is deviant. This information is presented in chapter 2.

Second, the clinician must be well versed in the normal development process to make judgments about adequacy of a child's skills at various ages or determine if a child's delayed production is following a normal sequence. Additionally, many principles of normal development are used in planning remediation programs. Normal development is discussed in chapter 3.

Information from these two areas is used in carrying out diagnostic procedures upon which a remediation program is based. Evaluation is important not only for planning remediation, but for assessing progress and revising goals throughout the therapy process. Assessment principles and techniques are presented in chapter 4.

CHAPTER 2 Articulatory Phonetics and Phonology

Speech production is a vehicle for carrying language. Language is generally considered to consist of five sets of rules: the rules of pragmatics, semantics, morphology, syntax, and phonology. Although these sets of rules are closely interrelated, this chapter will focus only on the last set—phonology.

Phonology is the study of linguistic rules governing the sound system of the language, including speech sounds, speech sound production, and the combination of sounds in meaningful utterances. *Phonetics* is the specific branch that deals with individual speech sounds, their production, and their representation by written symbols. *Articulation* refers to the actions of the organs of speech in producing the sounds of speech.

The first part of this chapter presents basic information on articulatory phonetics. The latter portion discusses other aspects of phonology.

Nancy A. Creaghead, Ph.D., is professor and director of the Communication Disorders Program at the University of Cincinnati.
Parley W. Newman, Ph.D., is chair of the Department of Educational Psychology at Brigham Young University.

THE ARTICULATORY SYSTEM

Many parts of the human body, from the pelvis to the cranium, are involved with the process of speech production (see Figure 2.1). All of these parts form a system that operates with remarkable synergy. Within this system there are subsystems, each of which contributes to speech production. The articulatory system integrates all of the following: the breathing apparatus; the larynx, the controlling valve of airflow; the pharynx, the general passageway that connects all of the orifices and the cavities of the system; and the other parts, including the tongue, lips, teeth, mandible, hard palate, velum, oral cavity, and nasal cavity.

Each of the four major components of the system plays a specific role in sound production. First, the respiratory system provides the airflow that creates sound. Sound is created when the airstream is set into vibration by the vocal folds or the articulators. There can be no sound without vibrating air. The second component, phonation (voice), provides the sound source for vowels and voiced consonants. A periodic complex sound wave is produced by the vibration of the vocal folds at the level of the larynx. As the sound leaves the vocal folds, it enters the resonance chambers of the pharynx, oral cavity, and sometimes the nasal pas-

FIGURE 2.1
The articulatory system.
This simplified schema
identifies the major
anatomical parts of the
system. All parts with
their associated nerve
and muscle tissues work
in concert to produce the
sounds of speech.

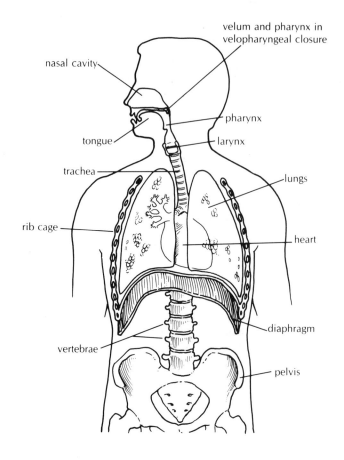

nasal cavity

velum and pharynx in
velopharyngeal closure

pharynx

tongue

larynx

trachea

lungs

rib cage

heart

diaphragm

vertebrae

pelvis

sages. These cavities create the third component of speech production, resonance, which modifies the sound waves emanating from the larynx so that different speech sounds are produced. These differing sounds result from varying the size and shape of the vocal tract. For example, each vowel results from a different vocal tract size, shape, and opening. Variations in the shape of the vocal tract are created by the movement of the articulators, primarily the tongue. Articulation is the fourth component. The movement of the articulators creates varying resonance characteristics (as already noted) and also creates other speech sounds by interfering with the flow of air through the vocal tract. When the airflow is completely interrupted and then released, or when it is restricted to create friction, characteristic speech sounds result. These two classes of speech sounds are called *stops* and *fricatives,* respectively. They are characterized

acoustically by aperiodic noise resulting from the explosion or friction.

Traditionally, the parts of the system have been thought of in a kind of linear sequence beginning with respiration, then moving on through phonation, resonance, and articulation. Actually, all of these elements are interrelated parts of the articulatory system and must be coordinated during the process of articulation. For example, within the breathing apparatus, air pressure below the glottis (opening in the larynx) is influenced not only by expiratory muscle forces but also by resistance to the airstream at the glottis or higher in the vocal tract by constrictions formed by the tongue or lips. No simple relationship exists between muscle activity and the production of syllables.

Changeover from one muscle group to another occurs during different aspects of articulation. Different types of muscle activity occur prior to and

10

following the production of syllables that are stressed or unstressed. In addition, productions of different speech sounds are accompanied by different types of breathing-muscle interplays (Draper, Ladefoged, & Whitteridge, 1959; Ladefoged, 1962). The breathing apparatus is not just a simple supplier of wind that other systems utilize. Instead, it is a dynamic, complex, interacting part of the articulatory process. Similarly, the human larynx is not simply an organ of phonation, but serves as an important and active contributor to speech articulation (Sawashima & Hirose, 1983). In the voiced-voiceless contrasts of cognate pairs such as /s/–/z/, /t/–/d/, /k/–/g/, etc., the laryngeal musculature provides the control of voicing or devoicing that is an integral part of the production of these consonants (Hirose, 1976). Coordinated actions of different combinations of laryngeal musculature activity also bring about the production of different types of stop consonants (Hirose, Lee, & Ushijima, 1974).

These findings emphasize the dynamic nature and interconnectedness of the articulatory system. The action and function of any part affects the actions and functions of the other parts, and all parts working together in different patterns produce the varieties of human noises that we call speech. The production of the sounds of speech that are the creations of this articulatory system will now be considered.

As the discussion of articulatory phonetics progresses, it is necessary to symbolize the sounds of speech using the International Phonetic Alphabet (IPA). For convenience, the IPA symbols are listed in Table 2.1. An accompanying key word is given with each symbol so that the speech sound it represents can be identified.

VOWEL ARTICULATION

Vowels are characterized in their production by an open vocal tract (see Figure 2.2). Vowels are also termed *syllabics* because each one forms the nucleus of a syllable. Some other vowel-like sounds occasionally provide this syllable-forming function. These are /m/, /n/, and /l/. When these con-

sonants serve as vowels, a short line is placed under them in transcription (/m̩/, /n̩/, /l̩/).

For general phonetic purposes, vowel production can be described by specifying the positions of the tongue, lips, and pharynx. Lips contribute to lengthening and shortening the vocal tract; rounding and protruding them lengthens the tract, as in the production of the high and mid back vowels, and retracting them shortens the vocal tract, as in production of the front vowels.

The tongue and pharyngeal cavity can be considered together. Although the elevating and constricting muscles of the pharynx influence the configuration of the pharyngeal cavity, its shape in vowel production is determined largely by the front-to-back placement of the tongue. When the tongue is carried forward the pharyngeal cavity enlarges. As the tongue moves toward the rear, the pharyngeal portion of the vocal tract diminishes in size. The changing shape of the vocal tract creates a variety of oral tract configurations, each of which has its own resonance characteristics that result in the production of the different vowels (see Figure 2.3). The vowels of English can be categorized with regard to tongue position as follows:

High front vowels: /i/ /ɪ/
Mid front vowels: /e/ /ɛ/
Low front vowels: /æ/

Mid central vowels: /ɝ/ /ʌ/ /ɚ/ /ə/

High back vowels: /u/ /ʊ/
Mid back vowels: /o/ /ɔ/
Low back vowels: /ɑ/

Vowel production is also considered on a tense–lax dimension. Vowels with more extreme tongue adjustments and longer duration are termed *tense* vowels. In general, tense vowels can appear in open syllables, as in *sew, sue, sir, see,* and *say* and in closed syllables such as *cope, coop, curt, keep,* and *cape.* The shorter vowels, which appear in closed syllables, but not in open syllables, are called *lax* vowels. Closed syllables with lax vow-

TABLE 2.1
Vowel and Consonant Symbols

Vowels (Syllabics)

Front Vowels		Central Vowels		Back Vowels	
symbol	key word	symbol	key word	symbol	key word
i	heat	ɝ	bird	u	food
ɪ	hit	ʌ	but	ʊ	wood
e	hate	ɚ	butter	o	coat
ɛ	head	ə	about	ɔ	sauce
æ	had			ɑ	hot

Contrastive Diphthongs		Noncontrastive Diphthong Examples	
symbol	key word	symbol	key word
aɪ	kite	eɪ	vacation
aʊ	cow	oʊ	low
ɔɪ	coil		

Syllabic Consonants

m̩ love 'em	n̩ more 'n more	l̩ middle

Consonants (Nonsyllabics)

Stops and Affricates		Fricatives		Nasals, Glides, Liquids		
symbol	key word	symbol	key word	symbol	type	key word
p	pin	f	file	m	nasal	come
b	bid	v	voice	n	nasal	nice
t	ten	θ	thumb	ŋ	nasal	ring
d	dog	ð	those	l**	liquid	let
k	kick	s***	see	r	liquid	red
g	go	z***	easy	j	glide	yes
ʔ	mitten	ʃ***	shoot	hw	glide	white
tʃ*	chew	ʒ***	treasure	w	glide	wet
dʒ*	jump	h	hot			

*affricates
**also termed a lateral
***also termed sibilants

els are *bit, bet, but,* and *book.* These syllables (vowels) are produced with relatively less extreme movements. Tense–lax differences can be felt to some degree by placing the thumb and forefinger on the undersurface of the lower jaw and while pressing up and in, feeling the different muscle tensions while producing /i/ followed by /ɪ/, /e/ followed by /ɛ/, and so forth.

The vocal tract assumes a relatively specific shape for each vowel, and there is a different configuration of the tract for each. Sometimes the configuration of the tract changes during vowel pro-

FIGURE 2.2
The vocal tract. The curved line from A to B travels through the vocal tract. Its length indicates the front-to-back boundaries of the tract. Velopharyngeal closure is shown also. The area of the glottis is indicated. The glottis is the opening between the vocal folds when they are abducted (open).

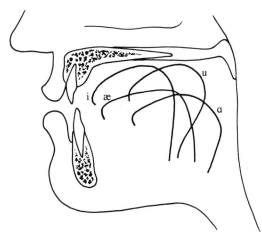

FIGURE 2.3
Approximate positions of the tongue in producing the vowels /i/, /æ/, /u/, and /ɑ/. Other vowel positions lie between and among these.

duction, which in turn alters the resonating characteristic of the tract. When this happens, a modification in resonance occurs, with a concurrent change in the quality of the vowel. This shifting of resonance and the change in vowel quality is termed *diphthongization*. Thus, in a single syllable pulse two resonances may occur, one blending into another, creating a diphthong.

Some vowels can be diphthongized without changing the meaning of the word they form, while other diphthongs contrast specific meanings. The combined vowel elements in a single diphthong are indicated by the way diphthongs are symbolized phonetically. Diphthongs that contrast meaning are: /aɪ/, /aʊ/, /ju/, and /ɔɪ/. Examples of diphthongs that do not contrast meaning are /eɪ/ and /oʊ/. For instance, the word *cake* when spoken is perceived as *cake* whether it is uttered as [kek] with a pure vowel [e] or pronounced [keɪk] with a diphthongized [eɪ]. With the contrastive diphthongs, however, the vowel /ɔ/ has an entirely different meaning from its diphthong /ɔɪ/. The word *tall* might be uttered [tɔl]. Diphthongized it becomes *toil* [tɔɪl]. Those acoustic differences that do not contrast meanings are called *phonetic* differences. Those acoustic differences that do contrast meaning are called *phonemic* differences. These will be discussed in more detail later in the chapter. When the vowels /e/ and /o/ are stressed, they tend to be diphthongized. Stressing them includes lengthening their duration, which provides time for the diphthongization to occur.

CONSONANT ARTICULATION

Vowels were described as relatively open-tract types of productions. Consonants are characterized by more constriction in the vocal tract. Some consonants temporarily require a complete closure of the tract, while others require only a partial closure at some point. Vowels are the carriers of syllables or in fact are the syllables; consonants are attached to the syllabic pulses of the vowels. Consonants may initiate syllables, terminate syllables, or both initiate and terminate syllables. The manner in which consonants are joined to vowels is sometimes referred to as *syllable shape*. The following are examples of syllable shapes. In these examples, V stands for vowel and C stands for consonant.

V shape:	oh	/oʊ/
VC shape:	oat	/oʊt/
CV shape:	toe	/toʊ/
CVC shape:	tote	/toʊt/
CCVC shape:	float	/floʊt/
CCVCC shape:	cloaks	/kloʊks/
CCCVCC shape:	strokes	/stroʊks/
CVCCCC shape:	sixths	/sɪksθs/
CCCVCCC shape:	sprints	/sprɪnts/

Note in these examples of different syllable shapes how consonants can cluster against a vowel. There is one vowel for each syllable, but there may be none or several consonants clustered in a syllable.

Some consonants are characterized by vibration of the vocal folds, while others are activated by the breath stream only; on this basis, consonants are classified as voiced or voiceless. There is great economy in the system with this voiceless–voicing contrast. The output of the system in consonant production is nearly doubled by the addition of the voicing contrast. From /p, f, θ, t, s, ʃ, tʃ, k/ the following are derived by the addition of voice: /b, v, ð, d, z, ʒ, dʒ, g/. In general, the voiceless consonants are uttered with greater physiological force than the voiced.

Consonants are named and classified by the nature of their production and also by the location of the constriction of the vocal tract. Both contribute to type and quality. The nature of the production is referred to as *manner of production*, and the location of the constriction is referred to as *place of articulation*. All consonants are classified in terms of manner and place.

The places of constriction and actual contact points are identified in Figure 2.4. In general,

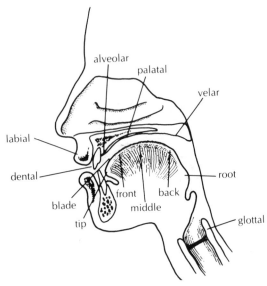

FIGURE 2.4
Places of constriction or contact in articulation: labial, dental, alveolar, palatal, velar, and glottal. Also indicated are the areas of the tongue used in articulatory contacts: tip, blade, front, middle, back, and root.

these places are the lips (bilabial), lower lip and upper front teeth (labiodental), tip of tongue and teeth (linguadental), tongue and alveolar ridge (lingua-alveolar or just alveolar), tongue and hard palate (linguapalatal or just palatal), tongue and velum (linguavelar or just velar), and glottis (glottal). For some sounds, the tongue comes into contact with the corresponding structure, actually blocking the vocal tract. For other consonants, it moves close to the part so that there is a narrowing of the tract. Both of these conditions have been referred to as constrictions in the vocal tract that make up consonant production.

The manner of production reflects the nature of the constriction. If the tract is temporarily closed off, the sound is a *stop*, indicating the temporary stoppage of sound production. Sometimes the release from the stoppage is forceful in nature, and the stop might be referred to as a *stop-plosive*. Another manner of production results from a very narrow constriction that sets up a friction type of noise. Sounds produced in this manner are termed *fricatives*. In a few cases sounds are formed as

TABLE 2.2
Classification of Consonant Phonemes by Manner and Place of Production

Manner of Articulation	Place of Articulation													
	Bilabial		Labio-Dental		Lingua-Dental		Lingua-Alveolar		Lingua-Palatal		Lingua-Velar		Glottal	
	−	+	−	+	−	+	−	+	−	+	−	+	−	+
Stop	p	b					t	d			k	g		
Fricative			f	v	θ	ð	s	z	ʃ	ʒ			h	
Affricate							tʃ	dʒ						
Nasal		m						n				ŋ		
Glide	hw	w								r, j				
Lateral								l						

− absence of voicing
+ presence of voicing

stops followed by a fricative release. These sounds are called *affricates*. Another type of sound is produced when the velum drops, coupling the nasal pharynx with the vocal tract and producing nasal resonance. These sounds, produced by the opening of the velopharyngeal port, are termed *nasals*. Some consonants are produced primarily by a movement of the tongue from one area of the oral cavity to another. Sounds produced by this transitional motion are *glides*. A narrowed tongue permitting air to pass around its sides produces a *lateral*. The consonants are depicted by manner and place of production in Table 2.2.

Stops or Plosives

In the production of stops, the oral cavity is sealed at some point. This closure for stops creates within the oral cavity a rapid growth of air pressure, which is suddenly released with the opening of the closure. There is an audible burst of air, a transient. However, in running speech, the word-final stops are often unreleased. For example, in the word *pop,* speakers release the first /p/, and the aspirate escape of air is heard, but the final /p/ may be held without the aspirate release. The buildup of

air pressure during the articulation of stops requires velopharyngeal closure during their normal production so that air does not escape through the nose.

Each of the stops occurs in a cognate pair. That is, there is a voiced and a voiceless counterpart for every English stop. The relative timing of the initiation or cessation of voicing during the transition between stop and vowel is the characteristic that distinguishes between the voiced and voiceless stops. This time element is referred to as *voice onset time* (VOT) or *voice termination time* (VTT). In English, a second characteristic differentiates voiced and voiceless stops in the initial position of syllables: voiceless stops are characterized by a greater degree of aspiration than those that are voiced.

/p/ **and** /b/. Except for the voicing component, /p/ and /b/ are formed in the same manner. The breath stream is impounded by closure of the lips. Air pressure builds up behind the seal during a moment of hold, which is followed by the release of the pressure with the parting of the lips.

/t/ **and** /d/. Except for the voicing difference, /t/ and /d/ are formed in the same manner. In forming

15

these sounds, the tongue tip and blade are in contact with the alveolar ridge behind the upper front teeth, with the sides of the tongue in contact with the upper teeth and gums, forming an airtight seal. As with all plosives, breath pressure is built up within the oral cavity, then released as the tongue moves toward the next sound.

/k/ and /g/. Again, except for the voicing distinction, these two sounds are produced in the same manner. The back of the tongue is placed in contact with the velum. Breath pressure is built up behind this closure and then released as the tongue moves toward the next sound to be articulated.

Fricatives

A variety of noises can be produced in the vocal tract by sending the voiced or voiceless breath stream through different constrictions formed in the tract. The flow of air must be sufficiently strong and the constriction sufficiently narrow to create friction noise or aperiodic sound. Because fricatives are pressure consonants, they require a firm velopharyngeal closure. Except for /h/, all fricatives have voice–voiceless cognate pairs.

/f/ and /v/. Except for the voicing distinction, /f/ and /v/ are formed in the same way. The inner border of the lower lip is raised to a close approximation with the cutting edge of the upper front teeth. The breath stream passes through this light contact, creating a disturbance in the airstream that produces the friction noise characteristic of sounds of this class.

/θ/ and /ð/. Except for the voicing distinction, /θ/ and /ð/ are formed in the same fashion. They are produced by placing the flattened tip of the tongue on, or very close to, the cutting edge of the upper front teeth. The airstream is directed through the thin but broad space between the tongue and teeth.

The lower teeth probably are in contact with the undersurface of the tongue. These two sounds are the weakest of the fricatives.

/s/ and /z/. Except for the voice-voiceless distinction, /s/ and /z/ are formed the same way. The sides of the tongue are in contact with the teeth and gums. The blade of the tongue is near but not touching the alveolar ridge. There is a narrow groove in the midline of the tongue through which the breath stream passes. The /s/ and /z/ have been called narrow-channel fricatives. This position creates turbulence in the airstream, producing the fricative quality of these sounds. The /s/ is often spoken of as a high-frequency sound. This is because there is little energy in the /s/ below 4000 Hz. There are two prominent bands of energy in the /s/, one at about 6000 Hz and the other at approximately 8000 Hz.

/ʃ/ and /ʒ/. Except for the voice-voiceless distinction, the /ʃ/ and /ʒ/ are formed in the same way. The sides of the tongue are in contact with the upper teeth and gums. The tip and blade of the tongue are raised toward, but do not touch, the alveolar ridge and front part of the palate. With the tongue in this position, the breath stream is directed against the hard palate and the alveolar ridge. The channel in the midline of the tongue is broad compared with /s/ and /z/. The /ʃ/ and /ʒ/ are broad-channel fricatives. A large portion of the body of the tongue is arched toward the palate in the production of this pair of fricatives. Also, there tends to be an everting or protrusion of the lips with their production. The intense hissing quality of the /s, z/ and /ʃ, ʒ/ has earned them a subtitle among the fricatives. They are also called *sibilants*.

/h/. The last of the fricatives to be described is /h/. It is voiceless, and the source of the turbulence that creates its fricative nature is sometimes attributed to a glottal constriction. However, the glottal constriction, if it exists, is very slight. Perhaps the more accurate way to describe the /h/ is to say that it is a voiceless onset of the following vowel.

Affricates

There are two affricates, which are a cognate pair. These sounds combine plosive and fricative characteristics.

/tʃ/ **and** /dʒ/. Except for the voicing distinction, these sounds are produced in similar fashion. They are formed by placing the blade and body of the tongue in broadly distributed contact with the hard palate, often including the alveolar ridge. The sides of the tongue are in contact with the upper teeth and gums. Air pressure is built up behind the tongue, followed by an affricate release as the tongue quickly drops and shapes itself as in production of /ʃ/ or /ʒ/.

Nasals

Most of the sounds of English are produced in a two-part tract consisting of the pharyngeal and oral cavities, extending from the lips down to the glottis. There are three exceptions: /m/, /n/, and /ŋ/. These three sounds are produced with the addition of the nasal pharynx, which is coupled to the vocal tract by the lowering of the velum. The absence of velopharyngeal closure during the production of the nasals, in effect, lengthens the vocal tract. This lengthening, along with the overall increase in area for resonance and the smaller nasal opening, changes the resonance characteristic by adding low-frequency components, which creates the nasal quality of the sound. The passage of sound through the convoluted nasal cavity also absorbs sound energy, weakening the amount of emitted energy.

/m/. In producing /m/, the lips are closed and the voiced sound travels through a tract including both oral and nasal pharyngeal resonators. The tongue position is of no consequence. It usually assumes the shape for the following vowel.

/n/. To produce /n/, the tip and blade of the tongue are placed on the alveolar ridge with the sides of the tongue in contact with the upper teeth and gums so that air cannot escape through the oral cavity. With the tongue in this position voice is produced.

/ŋ/. The /ŋ/ is produced by bringing the body of the tongue into contact with the lowered soft palate. With the tongue in this position, voiced sound is produced and is resonated primarily in the pharyngeal cavities, including the nasal pharynx. Little oral cavity resonance is possible, for it is blocked off by the tongue.

Semivowels, Glides, and Liquids

Glides are sometimes called semivowels because, like vowels, they are resonant phenomena, very similar to diphthongs. In fact, if /w/ and /j/ are spoken slowly, they sound like diphthongs. In the production of glides, the vocal tract is open as for vowels. Yet glides are considered consonants because, like consonants, they serve in initiating vowels or diphthongs. The term *semivowels* includes both the glides /j/ and /w/ and the liquids /l/ and /r/. Velopharyngeal closure accompanies the articulation of these sounds of speech. Their individual production characteristics will now be described.

/j/. The /j/ is initiated with voicing and an on-glide with the front part of the tongue raised toward the anterior part of the hard palate in the approximate position of the /i/ and /ɪ/ vowels. The glide is made as the tongue moves to the position for the following vowel of the word being spoken. Resonance change is the most distinctive characteristic of this sound.

/w/ **and** /hw/. The chief distinction between /w/ and /hw/ is presence or absence of voicing. The /w/ is articulated primarily by rounding the lips. Production of /w/ creates the most extreme position of all the lip-rounding productions. The lips are puckered to almost a point of closure, very similar to their position when whistling. In this position, voicing occurs, and the lips move quickly to the subsequent vowel position, thus producing the glide. Again, resonance change is the distinguishing characteristic of /w/. In General American speech the use of /hw/ is disappearing. It is being replaced by /w/.

/l/. The /l/ is produced with the tip of the tongue pressed against the alveolar ridge. The tongue is narrowed so that its sides do not touch the teeth toward the rear of the mouth. In this position there

are apertures on each side of the tongue that influence the resonance characteristic of the oral cavity, creating the unique quality of /l/. The tongue basically has two settings in /l/ production. In a less narrowed condition it produces the /l/ heard in words such as *let* and *love*. With a more narrowed position, it produces the variation heard in words such as *ball* and *pill,* and vowel utterances such as in *turtle*. The /l/ is a liquid, and because of the resonance chambers at the sides, it is sometimes termed the *lateral*.

/r/. The /r/ is termed a liquid, and it is also a glide. When it serves as an on-glide, initiating a vowel, the tongue moves from the /ɝ/ position (see Figure 2.5) to that of the subsequent vowel. If /r/ terminates a syllable as an off-glide, the tongue moves

FIGURE 2.5
Representative shapes of the tongue in productions of the /ɝ/ in the word *curb* by General American speakers. Note the three resonance chambers, one in front of the tongue, a second directly behind the tongue, and a third in the laryngeal pharynx. (*Source:* ''A Dialect Study of American R's by X-ray Motion Pictures'' by P. DeLattre and D.C. Freeman, 1968, *Linguistics, 44,* p. 41. Copyright 1968 by *Linguistics.* Copyright 1968 by U.S. Government.)

from a vowel position to or toward the /ɝ/ position. The essence of the sound is movement either toward or away from the /ɝ/.

Figure 2.5 illustrates the bunched tongue positions used in producing /ɝ/. The variety of tongue shapes used in producing an /ɝ/ without specific contact points in the oral cavity make it difficult to describe. The lack of articulatory points of contact and the three-chamber resonance cavities that the tongue and pharynx create perhaps account for the difficulty children have in mastering this sound in speech. The drawings in Figure 2.5 are adapted from an X-ray study of DeLattre and Freeman (1968). In the literature on /r/ productions, the retroflex tongue position is often described. In this position the tip of the tongue is turned back. However, the presence of the retroflex position was not supported by the X-ray data of DeLattre and Freeman. The tongue position for /ɝ/ can best be described as bunched with three resonance chambers, one in front of the tongue, a second directly behind the tongue, and the third in the region of the laryngeal pharynx. Ladefoged (1975) uses the term *rhotacization* to describe the quality of r-coloring. This term includes both retroflex and bunched tongue positions.

DYNAMICS OF SPEECH PRODUCTION

In the discussion thus far, speech sounds have been identified and described. It is now appropriate to consider them in the context of conversational or connected or running speech. The words printed on this page are made up of letters of the alphabet, and it is reasonable to think of the sounds of speech as being joined in a similar manner. However, this comparison between connected speech and words on a page is very misleading, for in reality speech is a continuously changing physiological and acoustic stream produced by the articulatory system. Speech sounds that we have discussed are segments, but speech is not segmented. It is a flow of syllable pulses with the articulators in constant motion except when the flow stops for pauses. The

genuine dynamic connection between the sounds of speech can be considered in light of their influence upon each other. They affect each other and alter each other. There are three aspects of sound influence: coarticulation, adaptation, and assimilation.

Coarticulation

One type of phonetic influence that occurs in connected speech is coarticulation. Strictly speaking, coarticulation means that two articulators are moving simultaneously to produce two different phones (speech sounds). This creates adaptation, in which an articulator modifies its movements due to the influence of a preceding or following phone. It also creates assimilation, in which there is an actual sound change due to a feature spreading from one phone to its neighbor. Coarticulation may result in a smear of features as found in assimilation, yet coarticulation may exist without a sound change. An example of coarticulation is when a speaker says the word *through*. In this utterance, the lips are rounded for the upcoming vowel /u/ during the production of the /θr/ cluster that precedes it. The tongue can even coarticulate with itself.

Adaptation

Phonetic adaptations are variations in the ways in which articulators move and the extent to which vocal tract configurations change shape according to preceding and following sounds. For example, the contact point for the tongue in producing /k/ is the velum. In the word *seek*, which contains a front vowel, the contact point is more forward for /k/ than it is in the word *book,* which contains a back vowel. If one repeats the two words *seek* and *book* and attends to the contact point for /k/ in these two words, the difference can be felt. In this case the preceding vowel influences the place in which /k/ is produced. In general, no sound is produced the same way twice, due to adaptation. A special case of adaptation is rapid speech. Faster rates result in the tongue's falling short of the usual target position. In summary, adaptation means that the production of a given speech sound varies according to neighboring vocal tract patterns and configurations.

Assimilation

If changes in a given sound are extensive enough, the sound may actually take on audible characteristics of its neighbor. These modifications in the way a phone sounds are called *assimilation* and will be discussed later in the chapter.

Conclusion

Coarticulation, adaptation, and assimilation are pervasive in connected speech. These processes make speech production efficient. The activities of the articulatory system are not restricted to producing one sound at a time and producing sounds in sequence; rather, movements are overlapping, and preparations for several sounds are going on simultaneously. Sounds are not produced as beads on a string with one following another, but instead phones overlap and flow into each other in a continuously changing stream of sound.

PHONOLOGICAL RULES

Phonological rules describe the sound system of a language. Some of these rules tend to be universal across languages, partly because the available set of rules is bound by the limits of the articulatory mechanism and the perceptual limitations of human beings. Other rules vary among languages.

For example, all languages have a set of both vowels and consonants, but some languages have very few different sounds whereas others have a larger set. English, for example, has approximately 17 vowels, whereas other languages like Eskimo and some dialects of Arabic have only 3—/i/, /ɑ/, and /u/ (Schane, 1973). Phonological rules describe the following parameters of a language: (a) the phonemes of the language, (b) the allophones of the phonemes and the conditions for appearance of the allophones, and (c) the allowable word positions and combinations of these phonemes.

The Phoneme

The concept of the phoneme is an idealized notion about what constitutes the discrete speech units of the language. More simply expressed, a phoneme is a family or group of sounds that are perceived as belonging to the same category. A phone is the actual speech sound uttered. Each spoken phone is classified as belonging to a particular phoneme according to its effect on meaning. For example, the difference between *pail* and *bail* is determined by the two different phonemes /p/ and /b/; however, /p/ is produced differently in each of the two sentences that follow although it is perceived as the same phoneme.

This is my pail.
This is his pail.

Similarly, /b/ is produced differently in the following sentences.

This is my bail.
This is his bail.

At any given moment in running speech, a targeted phone will differ slightly from the same phone uttered earlier (or later) due to the influence of coarticulation, adaptation, and assimilation. Under normal listening conditions, these differences are not perceived, and the listener hears the phoneme.

Any individual who is a native speaker of a given language intuitively knows the phonemes of her language. She needs no course in linguistics to know the difference between two words that differ by only one phoneme. Further, meaning is not necessary, because if a native speaker of English heard the syllables *peeb* and *beeb,* which have no meaning, she would report that they differ by the first sound. They have the potential for being different words. They might be used as names for a pet or a new detergent. Each language has a set of phonemes that are combined to form all of the words of the language. The phoneme set of all languages consists of both vowels and consonants. The number of different phonemes in a language is always balanced by two opposite forces.

1. A larger number of phonemes provides more flexibility in forming new words without making words longer. For example, if our language had only two phonemes, /p/ and /o/, we could have the words /o/, /po/, /op/, and /pop/, and then the only way to make new words would be to add syllables: /popo/, /opop/, /opopo/, /popop/, /opopop/, /popopop/, /popopopo/, etc. Very quickly, such strings of syllables would be beyond our memory capacity.
2. On the other hand, having fewer phonemes in the language places less burden on our articulatory and perceptual capabilities. If our only phonemes are /p/ and /o/, we have great latitude in production of both with the assurance that the listener will not confuse them. We could pronounce /p/ as /b/, or even as /t/, /k/, /f/, etc., and the listener would still assume the sound to be /p/ because there are no other consonant choices. In the same way, /o/ could be pronounced as a wide range of vowels with no concern for confusion. With fewer phonemes there is also less burden on the listener because she does not have to listen so carefully to be sure she heard the correct sound. If a language has two different phonemes, like /s/ and /ʃ/, that are similar except for place of articulation, then the speaker must be careful to achieve correct tongue placement so that the listener does not confuse such words as *see* and *she.* Likewise, the listener must be more alert

and often make use of context to detect the difference.

The smallest phoneme set that has been found is 5 phonemes. English has 46, which ranks with other languages having large numbers of them. The considerations just discussed influence learning the sound system of a language and affect intelligibility of children with defective articulation.

The Allophone

As already described, a phoneme is a class or category of speech sounds that have the same role in contrasting meaning. An allophone is an articulatory gesture, or phone, that is a variant of a phoneme category within the language. For example, in English, the voiceless stops have aspirated and unaspirated allophones that are determined by word position. When they initiate a stressed syllable, /p/, /t/, and /k/ are aspirated; otherwise they are not.

Therefore, although aspirated and unaspirated variants are different phones, they are not different phonemes because the difference does not change the meaning of the word. It is possible that a language could have two different words, /pil/ and /pʰil/ (with an aspirated /p/). In that case, /p/ and /pʰ/ would be two phonemes. In English, [p] and [pʰ] are allophones. Note that slashes are used to enclose phonemes. This is called *broad phonetic transcription.* Brackets are used to enclose allophones. When allophones are transcribed, it is called *close phonetic transcription.* From the example, it can be seen that the specific language being discussed may determine whether slashes or brackets are appropriate to enclose a given phone. Diacritical markings may be used to define allophones in close transcription. Examples of diacritical markings include "~" to denote nasality, as in [kæ̃n], or "⊢" to denote a lateralized production, as in a lateral lisp, e.g., [sɪt].

Other diacritical marks are shown in Table 4.3 in chapter 4.

Two observations can help us determine whether two phones are phonemes or allophones in a language:

1. If we can find two words in the language that differ only in regard to the two phones, then we have two phonemes. In English, /pæt/ and /bæt/ are different words, and therefore /p/ and /b/ are phonemes. These two words, which differ by only one phoneme, are called a *minimal pair*. If two sounds can appear in the same environment and their alternation does not produce a change in meaning, they are said to be allophones of the same phoneme and in *free variation*. For example, [hætʰ] and [hæt] are not different words. Therefore, this pair gives no evidence that [tʰ] and [t] are phonemes.

2. If the two phones always appear in complementary distribution (i.e., never appear in the same context in a word), they are not classified as different phonemes. In English, [pʰ] appears only in the syllable-initiating position of a stressed syllable ([pʰæt]); [p] appears only in syllable-final position ([hop]), as the second member of a consonant cluster ([spɪn]), or in the syllable-initiating position of an unstressed syllable ([hæpɪ]). Thus, although these /p/s are produced differently and sound different, they belong to the same phoneme category.

All of the various allophones are the direct result of the environment, or phonetic context, of the phoneme. In other words, we can say that allophones are the result of context-sensitive rules. In the above example, the use of [p] or [pʰ] is determined by the surrounding sounds—i.e., whether the /p/ is preceded or followed by a vowel, a consonant, or nothing. Context-sensitive rules describe the allophonic modifications that speakers make in rapid speech. Many of these modifications have become part of the standard production of individual words. Context-sensitive rules will be described in this chapter under "Phonological Processes."

Rules for Sound Combinations—Phonotactics

Phonological rules not only describe the set of phonemes and their allophones but they also describe the allowable syllable structures and sound combinations of a given language. All natural languages contain vowels and consonants and combine them in certain ways. The determination of what sounds and sound combinations are permissible in a language is termed *phonotactics*. Consonant-vowel (CV as in *go*), vowel-consonant (VC as in *up*), or consonant-vowel-consonant (CVC as in *cat*) syllable structures are very common across languages. In English, there are no restrictions on which vowels may occur with which consonants. All possible combinations of single vowels and single consonants are allowable. Other languages may have restrictions on consonant and vowel combinations. Japanese, for example, allows only V or CV syllable structures as seen in words like *sukiyaki* and *Tokyo*. VC or CVC syllables are not permissible.

There are in English, as well as in other languages, restrictions regarding the combination of consonants with one another. These limitations determine allowable syllable structures. In English, in addition to the CV structure, it is possible to have CCV (*true*) and CCCV (*strew*), but not CCCCV. A consonant or consonant cluster may close the syllable, as in CCCVC (*strike*). In addition to the VC syllable, we can have VCC (*oats*) and VCCC (*arms*), but not VCCCC. There are altogether 16 allowable syllable structures in English. A variety of syllable shapes was shown earlier in the chapter under "Consonant Articulation."

There are also rules specifying which consonants may be combined with one another and in what order. At the beginning of English words, we can use the consonant clusters /st/ (*stick*), /sp/ (*spoon*), /sk/ (*skate*), /sl/ (*slip*), and /sw/ (*swim*), but not /sr/, /sʃ/, /sθ/, etc. We can further have /str/ (*strike*), /spr/ (*spring*), /skr/ (*scream*), but not /slr/ or /swr/. In addition, we can say /br/ (*break*), /bl/ (*blue*), /gr/ (*great*), /gl/ (*glue*), /tr/ (*tree*), /dr/ (*drink*), but not /tl/, or /dl/. Similar but not identical rules exist for the final word position. These rules are not the same for other languages.

Morphophonemics

Earlier, the phoneme was described as the smallest unit of sound that serves to discriminate meaning. A morpheme, on the other hand, is actually the smallest unit of meaning. How are they different? /p/ and /b/ are phonemes. They do not mean anything by themselves. However, in the minimal pair /pæt/ and /bæt/ the meaning of the word depends on which of the two is present. /s/ is also a phoneme. The sequence /sæt/ has a different meaning than /pæt/ or /bæt/. But /s/ is also a morpheme. When attached to a word, it can carry other meanings: plural or possession. In the same way *ed* (pronounced /t/, /d/, or /əd/) is a morpheme, meaning past, as are *un* meaning "not," *pre* meaning "before," etc. These are bound morphemes, which means that they must be attached to another morpheme. Free morphemes such as *dog, window, truth, go, pretty,* and so forth, have meaning by themselves. Thus words are also morphemes, but what is seen as a single word may be made up of more than one morpheme as in *undeniable,* which is three morphemes, each adding to the meaning of the whole.

Morphophonemic rules govern the production of sounds in combinations of morphemes. It may be said that they relate phonological rules and syntactic rules. For example, a morphophonemic rule specifies how the past tense marker will be produced when it is attached to a specific word. It may be pronounced as /t/ (*walked*), /d/ (*played*), or /əd/ (*skated*), depending on the phonetic context. Morphophonemic rules will be discussed further under "Assimilation" and "Writing Rules."

DISTINCTIVE FEATURES

One goal of linguistics is to describe a language using the smallest number of different rules that can account for all of the possible combinations and sequences that can be generated. One attempt to describe the set of phonemes in a language is the

theory of distinctive features. A distinctive feature is an articulatory or acoustic parameter whose presence or absence defines a phoneme. Each phoneme can be thought of as a bundle of features. Most distinctive feature systems are binary systems that describe each phoneme by the presence or absence of a set of features. Some phonemes, such as /p/ and /b/, differ by the presence or absence of only one feature. These two phonemes share an identical set of features with the exception of voicing. /p/ is voiceless, whereas /b/ is voiced.

/p/	/b/
− vocalic	− vocalic
+ consonantal	+ consonantal
− high	− high
− back	− back
− low	− low
+ anterior	+ anterior
− coronal	− coronal
− voice	+ voice
− continuant	− continuant
− nasal	− nasal
− strident	− strident

On the other hand, the phonemes /u/ and /p/ have few features in common.

/u/	/p/
+ vocalic	− vocalic
− consonantal	+ consonantal
+ high	− high
+ back	− back
− low	− low
− anterior	+ anterior
− coronal	− coronal
+ round	− voice
+ tense	− continuant
	− nasal
	− strident

Strong interest in distinctive features began in the 1950s with the work of Jakobson and his colleagues, who attempted to design binary feature systems that would describe the sounds of all languages (Chomsky & Halle, 1968; Halle, 1964; Jakobson, Fant, & Halle, 1952; Jakobson & Halle,

TABLE 2.3
Distinctive Feature Composition of English Segments

	ɨ	ɪ	ū	ē	ō	ǣ	ā	ɔ̃e	ɔ̃	i	u	e	ʌ	o	æ	ɔ	y	w	ɛ	r
vocalic	+	+	+	+	+	+	+	+	+	+	+	+	+	+	+	+	−	−	−	+
consonantal	−	−	−	−	−	−	−	−	−	−	−	−	−	−	−	−	−	−	−	+
high	+	+	+	−	−	−	−	−	−	+	+	−	−	−	−	−	+	+	−	−
back	+	−	+	−	+	−	+	−	+	−	+	−	+	+	−	+	−	+	−	−
low	−	−	−	−	−	+	+	+	+	−	−	−	−	−	+	+	−	−	−	−
anterior	−	−	−	−	−	−	−	−	−	−	−	−	−	−	−	−	−	−	−	−
coronal	−	−	−	−	−	−	−	−	−	−	−	−	−	−	−	−	−	−	−	+
round	−	−	+	−	+	−	−	+	+	−	+	−	−	+	−	+	−	+	−	
tense	+	+	+	+	+	+	+	+	+	−	−	−	−	−	−	−	−	−	−	
voice																				+
continuant																				+
nasal																				−
strident																				−

Note: č = /tʃ/, ǰ = /dʒ/, š = /ʃ/, ž = /ʒ/.
Source: From *The Sound Pattern of English* by N. Chomsky and M. Halle, 1968, New York: Harper & Row. Copyright © 1982 by Harper & Row. Reprinted by permission.

1956). The goals of the researchers who designed these feature systems were (1) to design one set of features to describe all possible phonemes in all languages, (2) to design a purely binary system in which the plus or minus value of each feature could be applied to any sound, and (3) to devise the smallest number of features to accomplish goals 1 and 2. The resulting feature systems were a combination of both articulatory and acoustic features. Chomsky and Halle (1968) proposed a set of binary features that could describe all English phonemes, including both vowels and consonants. Table 2.3 shows a feature matrix for the vowels and consonants of English based on the Chomsky and Halle system. Note that some of the sound symbols used in this matrix are different from those used elsewhere in this volume. The features that Chomsky and Halle proposed are defined in Table 2.4.

Walsh (1974) describes some of the limitations of these feature systems for use in speech-language pathology. It is important to remember that the features proposed by these linguists were designed to describe an idealized linguistic system rather than actual speech production. A binary system may be appropriate for a model of the language, but it may not be useful in describing what speak-

ers do. The attempt to find a purely binary as well as an elegant system necessitated the combination of articulatory and acoustic features. Again, this combination does not reflect the physical aspects of human speech. The features and the classifications of sounds that result from their use may not reflect psychological realities. For example, the feature *coronal* creates the following two categories of consonants:

+ coronal	− coronal
/r/	
/l/	/p/
/t/	/b/
/d/	/f/
/θ/	/v/
/ð/	/m/
/n/	/k/
/s/	/g/
/z/	/ŋ/
/ʃ/	/h/
/ʒ/	
/tʃ/	
/dʒ/	

With regard to place of articulation, this feature does not seem psychologically relevant. Sounds made generally in the middle of the oral cavity are

TABLE 2.3 *(continued)*

l	p	b	f	v	m	t	d	θ	ð	n	s	z	c	č	ǰ	š	ž	k	g	x	ŋ	h	kʷ	gʷ	xʷ
+	−	−	−	−	−	−	−	−	−	−	−	−	−	−	−	−	−	−	−	−	−	−	−	−	−
+	+	+	+	+	+	+	+	+	+	+	+	+	+	+	+	+	+	+	+	+	+	−	+	+	+
−	−	−	−	−	−	−	−	−	−	−	−	−	+	+	+	+	+	+	+	+	+	−	+	+	+
−	−	−	−	−	−	−	−	−	−	−	−	−	−	−	−	−	−	+	+	+	+	−	+	+	+
−	−	−	−	−	−	−	−	−	−	−	−	−	−	−	−	−	−	−	−	−	−	+	−	−	−
+	+	+	+	+	+	+	+	+	+	+	+	+	+	−	−	−	−	−	−	−	−	−	−	−	−
+	−	−	−	−	−	+	+	+	+	+	+	+	+	+	+	+	+	−	−	−	−	−	−	−	−
																		−	−	−			+	+	+
+	−	+	−	+	+	−	+	−	+	+	−	+	−	−	+	−	+	−	+	−	+	−	−	+	−
+	−	−	+	+	−	−	−	+	+	−	+	+	−	−	−	+	+	−	−	+	−	+	−	−	+
−	−	−	−	−	+	−	−	−	−	+	−	−	−	−	−	−	−	−	−	−	+	−	−	−	−
−	−	−	+	+	−	−	−	−	−	−	+	+	+	+	+	+	+	−	−	−	−	−	−	−	−

in one group, whereas sounds made at the front (bilabials and labiodentals) and those made at the back (velars) are grouped together.

Other researchers have attempted to define feature systems that relate more closely to speech production (Miller & Nicely, 1955; Singh & Black, 1966; Singh & Polen, 1972; Singh & Singh, 1972). At least some of the feature distinctions have proved to be relevant in describing children's patterns of errors.

In actual practice, a system based on the traditional parameters of manner, place, and voicing may be more useful. The use of traditional terminology will not produce a purely binary system

TABLE 2.4
Definition of Features Used by Chomsky and Halle (1968)

Features Used in Table 2.3

Vocalic	voiced sounds that do not have a marked constriction in the vocal tract
Consonantal	sounds that have a marked constriction in the vocal tract
High	sounds made with the tongue elevated
Back	sounds made with the tongue retracted
Low	sounds made with the tongue lowered
Anterior	sounds in which the point of constriction is anterior to the point for the production of /ʃ/
Coronal	sounds made with the tongue blade raised
Round	sounds made with the lips rounded
Tense	sounds made with a relatively greater degree of muscle tension
Voice	sounds in which the vocal folds vibrate
Continuant	sounds that can be maintained in a steady state
Nasal	sounds in which the air passes through the nasal cavity
Strident	sounds in which noise is produced by forcing the airstream through a small opening

Other Features

Sonorant	sounds that allow the airstream to pass unimpeded through the oral or nasal cavity
Interrupted	sounds in which the airstream is completely blocked at some point during production
Distributed	sounds in which the constriction extends over a long part of the vocal tract
Lateral	sounds in which the midline is constricted so that the air escapes laterally

that can describe every sound with the same small set of features; however, it may better describe what the speaker of English does with his mouth. Manner, place, and voicing characteristics were described earlier in the chapter and categorized in Table 2.2. This table can be used to determine the type of articulation error in terms of natural features. One can see, for example, that a substitution of /p/ for /b/ (written p/b) constitutes a voicing error; the substitution t/k indicates a place error toward the front of the mouth; a t/s substitution reveals an error of manner.

An awareness and understanding of these feature systems is important because some research on articulation disorders and distinctive feature therapy approaches has been based on them.

Markedness Theory

Markedness theory is an attempt to account for finer details of relative articulatory and perceptual complexity within a distinctive feature system. The theory is that the presence of certain features makes a sound more difficult to produce or more difficult to discriminate from other sounds. Usually the plus value of the feature is the marked value and presumably makes the sound more difficult. In general, a sound with more plus features is considered to be more marked and thus more difficult to produce than a sound with fewer plus features. Toombs, Singh, and Hayden (1981) give the following criteria for determining the unmarked member of a consonant pair. The unmarked phoneme is the one that (a) requires less articulatory effort, (b) is less complex acoustically, (c) is less ambiguous perceptually, (d) is acquired earlier in normal development, and (e) occurs more often in the phoneme inventories of natural languages.

Table 2.5 from Toombs et al. (1981) shows the marked and unmarked values for English consonants based on Singh and Singh's (1972) feature system. From this table, it can be seen that the

voiced member of a voice-voiceless cognate pair is the marked member because voicing must be co-ordinated with the other required articulatory gestures. Comparing /t/ and /k/, it can be seen that /k/ is more marked because "back" is the marked value for the front/back feature. In later chapters, it will be seen that /t/ is a common substitution for /k/ in normal speech development and in children with articulation disorders. Other phoneme pairs can be examined in the same way to determine the more marked member of the pair. It should be noted, however, that markedness theory is a tentative hypothesis regarding a very complex issue, and its validity in explaining articulatory phenomena has not been proven (Grunwell, 1982).

The use of distinctive features for articulation therapy will be discussed in chapters 7 and 14.

PHONOLOGICAL PROCESSES

Phonological processes are patterned modifications of speech sound production. In general, processes are simplified sound productions. Some processes occur in normal adult speech. They are considered acceptable and do not interfere with intelligibility, as in assimilation of one phoneme into an adjacent phoneme in rapid speech. The nasalization of vowels that precede nasal consonants is an example ([kæ̃n]). Nasalization may occur when the velopharyngeal port is opened in preparation for the succeeding nasal sound so that the vowel also sounds nasal. Phonology includes the study of sound changes as they occur in the sequencing of ongoing speech. Phonological rules are an attempt to specify these changes. For example, the sentence *Did you eat yet?* is likely to be pronounced [dʒitjɛt] in rapid speech. The changes in this production are patterned and are predictable in other similar sequences of sounds.

The term *phonological process* generally refers to a pattern of sound change that affects a class of sounds or the overall structure of words or syllables. Nasalization of vowels, for example, is a process that generally affects all vowels in the context of nasals. A phonological rule can be written

TABLE 2.5
Markedness Values for Specific Phonemes

	Nasal-ity	Labial-ity	Voic-ing	Sono-rancy	Sibi-lancy	Contin-uancy	Front/Back
p	U	U	U	U	U	U	U
b	U	U	M	U	U	U	U
t	U	M	U	U	U	U	U
d	U	M	M	U	U	U	U
k	U	M	U	U	U	U	M
g	U	M	M	U	U	U	M
f	U	U	U	U	U	M	U
v	U	U	M	U	U	M	U
θ	U	M	U	U	U	M	U
ð	U	M	M	U	U	M	U
s	U	M	U	U	M	M	U
z	U	M	M	U	M	M	U
ʃ	U	M	U	U	M	M	M
tʃ	U	M	U	U	M	U	M
dʒ	U	M	M	U	M	U	M
w	U	U	(U)	M	U	(U)	U (flexible)
r	U	U	(U)	M	U	(U)	U
l	U	M	(U)	M	U	(U)	U
j	U	M	(U)	M	U	(U)	M
m	M	U	(U)	(U)	U	(U)	U
n	M	M	(U)	(U)	U	(U)	U
ŋ	M	M	(U)	(U)	U	(U)	M

Source: "Markedness of Features in the Articulatory Substitutions of Children" by M.S. Toombs, S. Singh, and M. E. Hayden, 1981. *Journal of Speech and Hearing Disorders, 46,* p. 186. Copyright 1981 by the American Speech-Language-Hearing Association, Rockville, MD. Reprinted by permission.

to express this same information. A phonological rule is "the (more or less formal) statement of a process" (Edwards & Shriberg, 1983, p. 91). Stampe (1969), who developed a model of "natural phonology," makes a stronger distinction. He says that processes are natural in the sense that they are innate and based on the physical characteristics of the human speech capacity. Rules, on the other hand, are not innate, but are the arbitrary characteristics of a language that must be learned. In some cases, natural processes and the rules of a language may be in opposition to each other. For this reason, simplification processes, discussed in the next section, may occur.

To the extent that phonological processes result from rules that simplify sounds and sound se-quences, the ultimate result of applying all phonological process rules would be the neutral vowel /ʌ/ or no sound at all. Because phonological processes tend to collapse sound distinctions, application of many processes would result in few sound classes. Think of the effect that the following natural processes would have on English. Weak syllable deletion would create mostly one-syllable words. Final consonant deletion would eliminate CVC syllables. Cluster reduction would eliminate all consonant clusters. Prevocalic voicing would eliminate all voiceless consonants at the beginning of words. Postvocalic devoicing would eliminate all voiced consonants at the ends of words.

These processes do affect the phonological rules in languages. As stated earlier, Japanese does not have syllable final consonants. German does not have final voiced stops or fricatives. English has limitations on the number of consonants that can occur in a cluster. The phonological rules of a language will be a compromise between the need for variety in the phonological system and the application of natural processes to facilitate production. To the extent that the language rules are in opposition to natural processes, these processes may occur in rapid speech or in the speech of individuals or dialects.

Researchers have used the term *natural processes* to describe those that occur developmentally in normal children, that seem to occur across languages, and that can be seen in historical language change (Edwards & Shriberg, 1983; Stampe, 1969). These same processes frequently persist in the speech of children with articulation disorders. Shriberg and Kwiatkowski (1980) include the following in their list of natural processes: (a) final consonant deletion (*cat*–/kæ/), (b) velar fronting (*came*–/tem/), (c) stopping (*see*–/ti/), (d) palatal fronting (*she*–/si/), (e) liquid simplification (*rope*–/wop/), (f) assimilation (*dog*–/gɔg/), (g) cluster reduction (*please*–/piz/), (h) unstressed syllable deletion (*potato*–/teto/).

Simplification Processes

In rapid conversation, speakers tend to simplify sound sequences, either by omitting phonemes or by making adjacent phonemes more similar. Some of these changes may vary from speaker to speaker or from dialect to dialect. Some occur fairly consistently across speakers of a language. In time, these become part of the standard pronunciation of words. These simplification processes cause pronunciation of the words of the language to change over time.

Simplification occurs because of the natural constraints imposed by the articulators. These constraints help in determining the allowable sound combinations in the language. Difficult sequences are less likely to be part of the language. For example, it would be difficult to have an initial cluster consisting of /zs/ because the speaker would have to be very careful to begin with voicing, turn off the voicing for /s/, and begin voicing again for the vowel. It is extremely likely that the /s/ part of the cluster would become voiced, thus reducing the cluster to the single phoneme /z/. The degree of difficulty in production of two adjacent phonemes is determined by the features that differentiate the phonemes and the kind of movement or change the articulators must make between them. Simplifications that occur in the language over time result in spellings that do not reflect the way that the word is pronounced. Following are some specific types of simplification processes.

Omission. The word *known* demonstrates the disparity between spelling and pronunciation that can occur over time. This word was probably once pronounced with both a /k/ sound and a /w/. These two phonemes were omitted over time because the word was easier to pronounce without them and because their absence did not cause that word to be confused with another. There are many English words with so-called silent letters that reflect this pattern of change: *sign, thumb, walk, sing, handkerchief.*

Assimilation. The word *sing* illustrates both omission of a phoneme and assimilation between two phonemes. Although /g/ has been omitted, its influence is seen in the remaining nasal sound. The final consonant in *sing* is not /n/, but /ŋ/—a combination of the manner of production for /n/ and the place of production for /g/. Assimilation occurs when a phoneme is changed to more nearly match another phoneme. In other words, a feature of one phone may carry over into an adjacent phone. In the example just given, the place of articulation of the lost stop influences the nasal sound. One of the most common forms of assimilation in English is the assimilation of nasality to surrounding nonnasal sounds—that is, the nasal sound influences a neighboring vowel. Pronounce *cat* and *can*. The vowels are the same with respect to the shape of the oral cavity, but they sound different because of the nasality assimilated into the /æ/ in *can*.

Further examples of the result of assimilation processes are shown in the past tense and plural markers for English verbs and nouns.

Past Tense	Plural
walked /t/	hats /s/
dragged /d/	dogs /z/
bedded /əd/	dresses /əz/
	ditches /əz/
	dishes /əz/
	judges /əz/

Can you figure out the rule? When the final phoneme is voiceless, a /t/ is added for the past tense and an /s/ for the plural. These are voiceless sounds. When the final sound is voiced, the voiced /d/ or /z/ is added. When the final phoneme is the same as the marker to be added, a vowel is inserted. In the case of the plural, this rule extends to all /s/-like sounds or sibilants. Because they never occur in the same environment, the allomorphs for the past tense and plural markers are said to be in complementary distribution.

The above examples are of voicing assimilation. As revealed in *sing*, assimilation also occurs in place of articulation. The following set of words provides another example:

imperfect	intolerable	inconceivable
improper	indiscrete	incongruous
imbalance	innumerable	incorrect
immovable	insensitive	inglorious

In the first column, the prefix is spelled and pronounced with an /m/ to match the bilabial sound at the beginning of the root word. In the second column, the /n/ matches the lingua-alveolar position of /t/, /d/, /n/, and /s/. In the final column, the prefix is spelled the same as in the second. However, many of us produce an /ŋ/ in these words, especially in rapid speech.

The examples of past tense and plural marker suffixes and the prefix meaning ''not'' illustrate morphophonemic rules. As discussed earlier, these rules govern the production of sequences of morphemes. They may be based on assimilation, which has influenced the phonological rules of the language.

Carryover of a feature from one sound to the next is called left-to-right, retentive, or progressive

assimilation. English past tense and plural markers illustrate this type of assimilation. Nasal assimilation, as in the word *can* ([kæ̃n]), is an example of right-to-left, anticipatory, or regressive assimilation.

The two sounds involved in the assimilation process may be adjacent, as in [kæ̃n], or they may be separated by other sounds in the word, as in a child saying [gɔg] for *dog*. Assimilation can take many forms. The following are the terms used for three special cases.

Coalescence, or reciprocal assimilation, occurs when the features of two sounds are combined to form a third sound as in the word *sing* described earlier.

Methathesis is the inversion of two sounds as in saying /æks/ for *ask* or /lɛrnɪks/ for *larynx*.

Epenthesis is the insertion of a sound between two others. This insertion would generally make the sequence easier to say as in /wɑrmpθ/ for *warmth*. The /p/ appears as a result of the opening of the lips during the transition from the bilabial nasal to the dental fricative.

Assimilation may occur at the single-word level; spelling will only sometimes reflect it. However, it occurs even more frequently in rapid speech and may extend across word boundaries. Unacceptable assimilation and other simplification rules may occur in the speech of individuals with articulation problems.

Vowel Reduction. A third type of simplification is vowel reduction. A tendency exists in English and other languages for unstressed vowels to become lax and centralized, thus moving toward the schwa (/ə/, the mid central vowel). Once again, spelling may reflect the original vowel as in the following words:

beautiful	button
about	butter
calorie	collar
describe	parlor

Note the variety of different vowel spellings that are pronounced as /ə/ or /ɚ/ in the unstressed syllables. This illustrates the tendency for all vowels to become schwa when unstressed. In some cases, vowel reduction may be less complete. Sometimes the vowel may become lax, but retain the tongue position so that /i/ becomes /ɪ/ (*receive*); /u/ becomes /ʊ/ (*petulant*); /e/ becomes /ɛ/ (*vacation*).

Syllable Reduction. When vowel reduction is carried even further, the vowel may be lost entirely and consequently the syllable will disappear. Pronouncing the word *probably* as /prɔblɪ/ (*probly*) is an example of syllable reduction. Words with double vowels such as *lead, motion, receive* may have originally been pronounced with the two adjoining vowels as separate syllables.

WRITING RULES

Linguists use a formal notation system for writing the rules that we have discussed in this chapter. The goal in writing a linguistic rule is to make it as general as possible so that it will cover the largest number of actual utterances while excluding those cases that do not fit the rule. The phonological rule specifies the phoneme or class of phonemes to be used and describes the context in which the phoneme or class will appear.

Rules 1 through 3 in Table 2.6 describe the use of plural endings in English discussed in an earlier section. The distinctive features from Table 2.3 are used. These three rules say that the plural marker becomes /s/, /z/, or /əz/ depending on the phoneme before it. The arrow means "becomes," the slash means "in the context of," # indicates the end of the word, and the blank indicates the position in the word of the element on the far left. In this case, the plural markers follow the context phoneme, and three rules are needed to describe what happens.

Rule 1 generates the plural marker. As stated in this rule the underlying form of the plural marker is assumed to be /s/. The rule says, "The plural marker becomes /s/ and is placed at the end of the word." Rule 2 inserts the schwa when the final sound in the word is a sibilant. This rule says, "There is no sound in this position already. This null (ø) becomes /ə/ and is placed between the sibilant at the end of the root word and the plural marker (/s/) that has been added." Rule 3 changes /s/ to /z/ when the previous phoneme is voiced. It says, "/s/ becomes /z/ when it is placed after a voiced sound at the end of the word." These rules must be ordered as shown in Table 2.6. If Rules 2 and 3 were reversed, the plural marker on *dress* would remain /s/, then it would be changed to /əs/, and finally the second rule would have to apply again to form /əz/.

In Table 2.7 the rules describe nasalization of vowels preceding nasal consonants. Rule 1 says that sounds with the feature + vowel take on the additional feature + nasal when followed by sounds with the features + consonant and + nasal. Rule 2 could also be written to show what happens in the word *can*, but it is so specific that it would not provide an adequate generalization of the language rule.

The assimilation rule for the set of words with the prefix *in-* or *im-* is shown in Table 2.8. This rule specifies that the nasal sound acquires the features + or − anterior and + or − coronal depending on the presence of those features in the following sound; i.e., if the following sound is + anterior, the nasal will be + anterior. The α and β represent this dependent relationship.

Devising formal rules implies the concepts of "underlying phonological representation" and "surface or derived representation" (Schane, 1973). The form to the left of the arrow is the *underlying form* in that it is not actually produced. The form that is derived by application of the rule (the form to the right of the arrow) is actually produced and is called the *surface form*.

The concept of underlying representation can also be applied to the difference between phonemes and allophones. Remember that phonemes are the family of sounds that listeners perceive as belonging to the same category. The allophone is the sound that is actually produced. A rule such as Rule 2 in Table 2.7 converts the phonemic or un-

TABLE 2.6
Rules for Generating Plural Markers in English

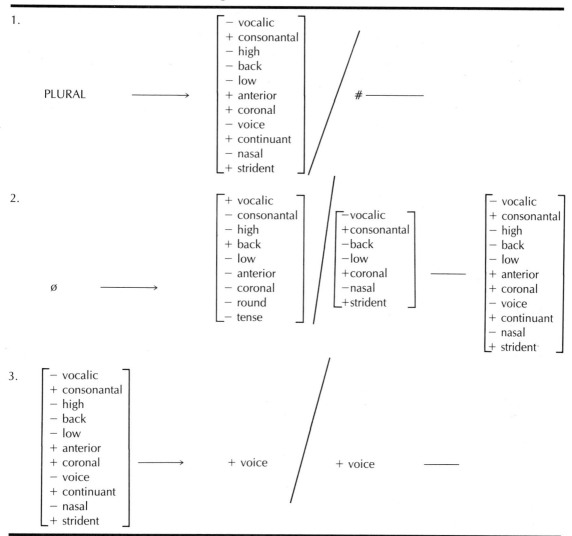

1.

$$
\text{PLURAL} \longrightarrow
\begin{bmatrix}
- \text{ vocalic} \\
+ \text{ consonantal} \\
- \text{ high} \\
- \text{ back} \\
- \text{ low} \\
+ \text{ anterior} \\
+ \text{ coronal} \\
- \text{ voice} \\
+ \text{ continuant} \\
- \text{ nasal} \\
+ \text{ strident}
\end{bmatrix}
/ \quad \# \underline{\qquad}
$$

2.

$$
\emptyset \longrightarrow
\begin{bmatrix}
+ \text{ vocalic} \\
- \text{ consonantal} \\
- \text{ high} \\
+ \text{ back} \\
- \text{ low} \\
- \text{ anterior} \\
- \text{ coronal} \\
- \text{ round} \\
- \text{ tense}
\end{bmatrix}
/
\begin{bmatrix}
- \text{vocalic} \\
+ \text{consonantal} \\
- \text{back} \\
- \text{low} \\
+ \text{coronal} \\
- \text{nasal} \\
+ \text{strident}
\end{bmatrix}
\underline{\qquad}
\begin{bmatrix}
- \text{ vocalic} \\
+ \text{ consonantal} \\
- \text{ high} \\
- \text{ back} \\
- \text{ low} \\
+ \text{ anterior} \\
+ \text{ coronal} \\
- \text{ voice} \\
+ \text{ continuant} \\
- \text{ nasal} \\
+ \text{ strident}
\end{bmatrix}
$$

3.

$$
\begin{bmatrix}
- \text{ vocalic} \\
+ \text{ consonantal} \\
- \text{ high} \\
- \text{ back} \\
- \text{ low} \\
+ \text{ anterior} \\
+ \text{ coronal} \\
- \text{ voice} \\
+ \text{ continuant} \\
- \text{ nasal} \\
+ \text{ strident}
\end{bmatrix}
\longrightarrow + \text{ voice} \quad / \quad + \text{ voice} \quad \underline{\qquad}
$$

TABLE 2.7
Rules for Describing Nasalization of Vowels Before
Nasal Consonants

1. $+ \text{ vocalic} \longrightarrow + \text{ nasal} \ / \underline{\qquad} \begin{bmatrix} + \text{ consonantal} \\ + \text{ nasal} \end{bmatrix}$

2. $æ \longrightarrow \tilde{æ} \qquad / \qquad \underline{\qquad} n$

TABLE 2.8
Rule Describing Place Assimilation of Negative Prefixes

$$
\begin{bmatrix} + \text{ consonant} \\ + \text{ nasal} \end{bmatrix}
\longrightarrow
\begin{bmatrix} \alpha \text{ anterior} \\ \beta \text{ coronal} \end{bmatrix}
/ \underline{\qquad}
\begin{bmatrix} + \text{ consonantal} \\ \alpha \text{ anterior} \\ \beta \text{ coronal} \end{bmatrix}
$$

31

derlying representation (e.g., /æ/) into the phonetic or surface representation ([æ̃]). In Table 2.8, the underlying representation is not specified. The surface form is [ɪm], [ɪn], or [ɪŋ], but which of the three is the underlying form? For cases such as this, linguists hypothesize an abstract underlying form. It may or may not be possible to determine what the underlying form actually is. Attempts are based on such factors as ability to predict all surface forms, simplicity of the solution, plausibility, spelling, and historical sound change (Edwards & Shriberg, 1983; Schane, 1973). In the example, /ɪn/ is generally considered to be the underlying form.

This type of investigative work to uncover underlying forms may be necessary in working with children with articulation problems, as will be seen in chapter 4.

SUMMARY

Information regarding the production of speech sounds and the organization of the speaker's language is imperative for the clinician who attempts to modify individual articulation errors and/or incorrect articulatory patterns. This chapter has described the production of each of the vowels and consonants of English with regard to place and manner of articulation and voicing. When these sounds are combined in running speech, their production is modified through the effects of coarticulation, adaptation, and assimilation.

Phonological rules specify the phonemes of the language and their combination into meaningful words. A distinctive feature system is one way of describing individual sounds. Changes that occur in running speech, in child language, in disordered articulation, or in the language over time can be described by phonological processes or assimilation rules. Linguists use a formal notation for writing these rules.

Information about the production of speech sounds, English phonology, and terminology for describing the rules is a necessary basis for understanding the material in later chapters.

REFERENCES

Chomsky, N., & Halle, M. (1968). *The sound pattern of English.* New York: Harper & Row.

DeLattre, P., & Freeman, D. C. (1968). A dialect study of American R's by X-ray motion pictures. *Linguistics, 44,* 29–68.

Draper, M. H., Ladefoged, P., & Whitteridge, D. (1959). Respiratory muscles in speech. *Journal of Speech and Hearing Research, 2,* 16–27.

Edwards, M. L., & Shriberg, L. D. (1983). *Phonology: Applications in communicative disorders.* San Diego: College Hill Press.

Grunwell, P. (1982). *Clinical phonology.* Rockville, MD: Aspen Systems.

Halle, M. (1964). On the bases of phonology. In J. Fodor and J. Katz (Eds.), *The structure of language: Readings in the philosophy of language* (pp. 324–333). Englewood Cliffs, NJ: Prentice-Hall.

Hirose, H. (1976). Posterior cricoarytenoid as a speech muscle. *Annals of Otology, Rhinology and Laryngology, 85,* 334–342.

Hirose, H., Lee, C. Y., & Ushijima, T. (1974). Laryngeal control in Korean stop production. *Journal of Phonetics, 2,* 145–152.

Jakobson, R., Fant, G., & Halle, M. (1952). *Preliminaries to speech analysis.* Cambridge, MA: MIT Press.

Jakobson, R., and Halle, M. (1956). *Fundamentals of language.* The Hague: Mouton.

Ladefoged, P. (1962). Sub-glottal activity during

speech. In A. Sovijarvi & P. Aalto (Eds.), *Proceedings of the Fourth International Congress of Phonetic Sciences*. The Hague: Mouton.

Ladefoged, P. (1975). *A course in phonetics*. New York: Harcourt Brace Jovanovich.

Miller, G., & Nicely, P. (1955). An analysis of perceptual confusions among some English consonants. *Journal of the Acoustical Society of America, 27*, 338–352.

Sawashima, M., & Hirose, H. (1983). Laryngeal gestures in speech production. In P. F. MacNeilage (Ed.), *The production of speech*. New York: Springer-Verlag.

Schane, S. (1973). *Generative phonology*. Englewood Cliffs, NJ: Prentice-Hall.

Shriberg, L., & Kwiatkowski, J. (1980). *Natural process analysis*. New York: Wiley.

Singh, S., & Black, J. (1966). Study of twenty-six intervocalic consonants as spoken and recognized by four language groups. *Journal of the Acoustical Society of America, 39*, 312–387.

Singh, S., & Polen, S. (1972). Use of a distinctive feature model in speech pathology. *Acta Symbolica, 3*, 17–25.

Singh, S., & Singh, K. (1972). A self-generating distinctive feature model for diagnosis, prognosis, and therapy. *Acta Symbolica, 3*, 89–99.

Stampe, D. (1969). The acquisition of phonetic representation. In R. I. Binnick, A. Davison, G. M. Greene, & J. L. Morgan (Eds.), *Papers from the Fifth Regional Meeting, Chicago Linguistic Society*. Chicago: Chicago Linguistic Society.

Toombs, M. S., Singh, S., & Hayden, M. E. (1981). Markedness of features in the articulatory substitutions of children. *Journal of Speech and Hearing Disorders, 46*, 184–191.

Walsh, H. (1974). On certain practical inadequacies of distinctive feature systems. *Journal of Speech and Hearing Disorders, 39*, 32–43.

CHAPTER 3 Development of Phonology, Articulation, and Speech Perception

How is it possible that children learn language so quickly? They are born without any knowledge of their language and without the ability to produce sounds other than crying, much less the phonemes or words of the language. Yet by the time they are 1 year old, they have learned enough to produce words, and by the age of 4, they are able to speak essentially like adults.

Articulatory-phonological acquisition requires development in two domains: cognitive and motor. Children must learn the phonological rules of the language, and they must develop the motor skills to produce not only individual speech sounds but the movements necessary for their rapid combination. These two facets are inseparable in normal development, but it is important that the speech-language pathologist be aware of both. The amount that children must learn is huge, and the learning process is fascinating.

THE OVERALL SEQUENCE OF ACQUISITION

For most children, the acquisition of the sounds of their language takes place during the first 4 years. By age 4 children know a great deal about the

This chapter was written by **Nancy A. Creaghead.**

phonological system of the language, with later development to occur primarily in the areas of morphophonology of complex word forms and metalinguistic knowledge (Ingram, 1976). Some children produce nearly all phonemes correctly in sentences by 2½ to 3 years, whereas others continue to have a few phonetic errors at age 6. Most children can be understood by strangers by 3½ years or earlier and exhibit adult-like articulation by 5 years.

At birth, the infant's only vocalization is crying. During the first year, children move through several stages while developing the ability to produce a variety of speech sounds. At this time their productions are limited to nonmeaningful cooing and babbling sounds, but they are surrounded by the meaningful speech of others. Hearing the language around them and practicing sounds prepare them for speech production. At 1 year, at least a few sounds are used in sequences that are consistent enough to be identified as words. During the next 3 years, the child's repertoire of sounds expands and correct production is stabilized. In addition, the child learns the rules for combining these sounds into the words of the language.

Locke (1983) outlined three stages in the process of phonological acquisition. During the pragmatic stage, which occurs before the onset of real words, the child begins to recognize that sounds

35

can convey information to others. The child will begin to use certain vocal movements to influence the environment. This stage, beginning some time before the first year, shows the child's knowledge of the function of speech. During the second or cognitive stage, the child begins to use "attention, storage, retrieval, and pattern matching" (p. 97) to develop a lexicon. Some of the early "words" may be similar to those of the previous period, but they will begin to be more similar to and derived from the environment. This stage generally begins at around 12 months. The third stage is called the systemic stage. This is the time during which the child's system moves toward the adult phonological system. This occurs during the rest of the preschool years.

Ingram (1976) has identified six stages of phonological development. He attempted to relate these stages to Piaget's (1962) stages of cognitive development and describe what happens phonologically at each cognitive stage. An outline of these stages follows.

Birth to about 10 or 12 months. During this stage, the child communicates through crying and gestures. Certain prerequisites for speech are also developing—speech perception, babbling or sound play, and the ability to imitate speech sounds.

12 to 18 months. The child develops a small vocabulary of perhaps 50 single words. Ingram notes that there is a qualitative difference between the phonology of these first words and those that occur after 18 months.

18 months to 4 years. During this time the child acquires most of the sounds of the language and learns to combine them into simple morphemes or words. Those simplifying phonological processes that characterize the child's earliest productions are gradually eliminated so that new classes of sounds emerge.

4 to 7 years. The phonetic inventory is completed, and the child begins to use more complex words that are derived from root words (e.g., *sign–signature*).

7 to 12 years. The child refines his or her knowledge of the morphophonemic rules of the language—e.g., the rules of tense markers and plurals and other derivational rules such as those that make nouns from adjectives (*able–ability*), nouns from verbs (*solve–solution*), and adjectives from nouns (*care–careful*). Ingram indicates that development during this period may be related to learning to read.

12 to 16 years. The advanced development of metalinguistic understanding allows the child to make conscious judgments about the phonological system, i.e., what the sounds of the language are and how they can be combined. Ingram states that this ability may be important in learning to spell.

Ingram proposes these as tentative stages and suggests research to determine their validity in describing phonological development.

THEORIES OF PHONOLOGICAL DEVELOPMENT

The theory or theories of speech sound development that a clinician subscribes to will play a large part in determining therapy procedures. Over the years a number of theories have been set forth. Some researchers have been interested in describing and explaining *how* the process of phonological development occurs in children, whereas others have directed their attention to developing theories of *why* it occurs the way it does. No one theory has been accepted as a complete account; the complexity of the system to be learned and of the organism learning it suggests that any one theory may be too simplistic an explanation.

In order to understand the development of the theories, it is important to consider how the supporting data have been obtained. Some of the research has been in the form of diary studies. Most often researchers have recorded the developing speech of their own children over a given period of time (Braine, 1974; Burling, 1959; Carlson & Anisfield, 1969; Leopold, 1947; Velten, 1943). The resulting data have been described and analyzed with regard to apparent regularities or inconsistencies in development. Some of the early diary studies have provided a wealth of data that subsequent researchers have reexamined for further interpretation, for evaluation of specific theories (Locke, 1985; Moskowitz, 1970), or for comparison with other data (Edwards & Shriberg, 1983; Ferguson & Farwell, 1975).

Large-scale cross-sectional studies of speech sound development have been an important source of normative data on which clinicians have based their decisions about adequacy of articulation in individual children. The studies of Poole (1934), Templin (1957), and Wellman, Case, Mengurt, and Bradbury (1931) have been the standards for comparison. Recently, however, new studies (Arlt & Goodban, 1976; Irwin & Wong, 1983; Olmsted, 1971; Prather, Hedrick, & Kern, 1975) have found generally younger ages for development, suggesting the possibility of discrepancies in the earlier studies or changes in the rate of development in today's children. These studies will be described in greater detail later in the chapter.

Other research has been directed toward examining the developing sound production (Gruber, 1973; Irwin, 1947a, 1947b, 1947c, 1948a, 1948b, 1948c, 1951, 1952; Irwin & Chen, 1946; Maskavinic, Cairns, Butterfield, & Weamer, 1981; Nakazima, 1975; Oller, Wieman, Doyle, & Ross, 1975; Tonkova-Yampol'skava, 1973) and speech perception (Cutting & Eimas, 1975; Eilers, 1977; Eilers, Gavin, & Wilson, 1979; Eilers & Minifie, 1975; Eilers, Wilson, & Moore, 1977; Kuhl, 1977; Miller & Morse, 1976; Williams & Golenski, 1979) of infants and the speech sound development of one or a group of children (Blasdell & Jensen, 1970; Dyson & Paden, 1983; Elbert, Dinnsen, & Weismer, 1985; Ferguson & Farwell, 1975; Ingram, Christensen, Veach, & Webster, 1980; Macken, 1980; Weir, 1966; Winitz, 1969). Many

studies have examined other specific facets of speech acquisition.

While some researchers have concentrated on describing the developmental process, others have attempted to formulate theories to explain how and/or why children learn to speak their language. As far back as 1792, Smith proposed a social-need theory for the development of speech in humans. Other theories proposed during the 1800s and early 1900s were based on the social role of speech (DeLaguna, 1927; McGeogh, 1943) and on the relationship of developing speech sounds to environmental sounds and to naturally occurring sounds produced by humans (Jespersen, 1922; Muller, 1840; Whitney, 1868). Theories have evolved as new information has become available regarding linguistics, speech production, and the developmental process in children. In some cases, new information may provide a different direction for theorizing; in most cases, the new information is reflected in expansion of already existing theories.

Ferguson and Garnica (1975) divided the modern theories into four groups: (a) behavioral theory, as illustrated by Mowrer (1952) and Olmsted (1971); (b) structuralist theory, as proposed by Jakobson (1968) and Moskowitz (1970); (c) natural phonology theory, exemplified by Stampe (1969); and (d) prosodic theory, as suggested by Waterson (1971). A fifth division is the interactionist-discovery theory of Kiparsky and Menn (1977). Although new theoretical information has become available (Edwards & Shriberg, 1983; Vihman, 1981; Yeni-Komshian, Kavanagh, & Ferguson, 1980), these general divisions still hold.

Behavioral Theory

Behavioral theories postulate that language is learned in response to the environment through the child's imitation of adult speech and reinforcement of his or her attempts. These theories are based on the principles of learning theory as described in chapter 6. They have been widely accepted because they are in accord with the explanations of the learning of other skills. However, a theory of language learning based purely on imitation presents difficulties because children will never hear all of the utterances they will produce in their early childhood, much less in their lifetime. Ferguson and Garnica (1975) point out that there is no experimental evidence to support this theory and that language learning may be different from other human behaviors.

Although a behavioral theory does not appear to be adequate to fully account for language development, learning principles play a part in normal acquisition and in teaching children with disorders. Children must have a model of the language they are learning, and they must receive some kind of reinforcement. This reinforcement is likely to be the natural reward for having communicated successfully. The clinician who accepts a behavioral account of phonological-articulation development will adhere to the learning principles described in chapter 6.

Structuralist Theory

The *structuralist theory* (Jakobson, 1968) holds that children are born with the ability to develop language and that phonological development and other aspects of language acquisition follow a universal order. Jakobson contends that there is a general order of sound development, although the exact age of acquisition may vary from child to child. He proposed that children develop their sound system by learning oppositions or contrasts of decreasing magnitude. These oppositions are expressed in terms of distinctive features (see chapter 2). The first contrast that children learn is between vowels and consonants; hence they will be likely to have a vowel and a consonant in their earliest phonetic repertoire. The consonants begin to differentiate first, with a manner distinction between oral

and nasal sounds. With regard to place, a labial sound like /b/ or /m/ is likely to appear in opposition to a dental sound like /d/ or /n/. Children are then likely to develop two or three very different vowels that form the bare essentials of the vowel triangle, such as a high front vowel like /i/, a high back vowel like /u/, and a low mid vowel like /ɑ/. The vowels will continue to differentiate in this manner until all vowels in the language have been acquired.

This universal order determines that certain groups of sounds will appear before others. For example, Jakobson states that the presence of alveolar and palatal sounds implies the presence of dental sounds. Likewise, the presence of fricatives implies stops. A given fricative will not be used until the homorganic (same place of articulation) stop has been acquired (Ingram, 1976). Based on these principles, Table 3.1 shows an outline of the possible early contrasts for a hypothetical child. It is not suggested that every child or even most children will follow this exact order of sound acquisition.

Jakobson saw this progression as beginning with the onset of meaningful speech. According to his theory, babbling is not continuous with phonemic development. During babbling the child utters a wide variety of sounds, many of which do not appear in early meaningful speech and must be learned or relearned as speech develops.

Other researchers who have adopted Jakobson's theories see more continuity between babbling and meaningful speech (Moskowitz, 1970). Moskowitz extended Jakobson's theory, but focused on the syllable as the earliest learned unit: first CV, then VC, and finally V. According to Moskowitz, children first analyze whole syllables, then phonemes. Moskowitz states that a theory of development must include both segments (individual sounds) and distinctive features. Either alone is not sufficient. Although there may be a universal set of rules that are available to children, each child uses a slightly different subset.

A structuralist or nativist theory suggests two considerations for therapy. First, because the ability to develop speech is innate, the therapy process can only provide opportunity for the child to acti-

TABLE 3.1

Possible Order of Development of Early Distinctive-Feature Contrasts in Repertoire of Hypothetical Child

First Division							
	Vowel				Consonant		
	/ɑ/				/b/		
Second Division							
				Oral		Nasal	
				/b/		/m/	
Third Division							
	High front	High back					
	/i/	/u/					
		Low mid					
		/ɑ/					
Fourth Division							
			Labial	Dental	Labial	Dental	
			/b/	/d/	/m/	/n/	
Fifth Division							
			Stop	Fricative			
			/d/	/s/			

vate his innate knowledge. Second, the clinician must be aware of the order of acquisition because the learning sequence may reflect a dependent relationship between earlier and later developing sounds.

Natural Theory

Stampe's (1969) *natural theory* of phonological development is based on the premise that the normally developing child attempts to reproduce the adult model, but because of immature motor abilities, the productions are simplified. The child's productions differ from the adult model as a result of the innate system of phonological processes that the child brings to the language-learning task. The development of adult phonology involves progressive elimination of these processes.

In general, processes simplify sound productions and produce a reduced set of phonemes. In Stampe's words, "A phonological process merges a potential phonological opposition into that member of the opposition which least tries the restrictions of the human capacity" (p. 443). The presence of a given process may cause one sound or set of sounds to be produced like another. For example, a common process in child language is stopping of stridents, which will cause sounds like /s/ and /z/ to be produced as [t] and [d] (*see*–[ti]; *zoo*–[du]). The process of fronting may cause /k/ and /g/ to be produced as [t] and [d] (*cat*–[tæt]; *go*–[do]). Thus six potential phonemes have been reduced to two.

Children's earliest productions will reflect the innate phonological system that demonstrates the full range of processes. As they move toward the adult system, children use three types of resolutions to create contrasts: (a) suppression of a process so that it becomes optional and finally nonexistent, (b) limitation of the contexts to which the process applies, and (c) ordering of the application of processes. For example, if the child demonstrates final consonant deletion and stopping, final consonant deletion must be eliminated in order for stopping to occur in the final position (Braine, 1974; Stampe, 1969). As the child eliminates processes, the set of phonemes will expand.

Stampe (1969) suggests that this theory of natural processes explains the phenomena that Jakobson (1971) described. However, Locke (1980) disagrees with this explanation and maintains that categorizing sounds by either distinctive features or phonological processes may mask some information that can be obtained by examining individual segments.

Description of phonological processes has been adopted as a model for remediating phonological disorders. The remediation task is to determine the processes that operate in the child's disordered speech and to provide opportunity to work toward eliminating them. This opportunity may be provided by allowing the child to become aware of and to practice the adult system.

Prosodic Theory

The *prosodic theory* (Waterson, 1971) holds that children initially perceive adult speech in terms of whole units of meaning rather than individual phonemes. These units of meaning may be single words, such as "milk," or groups of words, such as "get your shoes." Children first attempt to produce an overall schema of what they hear rather than a sequence of individual sounds. Ferguson (1978) agrees that the total word is the important unit in the child's early learning of phonology. According to Waterson, the earliest learned sounds are based on the input that the child receives. They will be those most frequent in adult speech or clearest to the child because of repetition, strong accent, etc. In support of this theory, Blasdell and Jensen (1970) found that 2½- to 3-year-old children imitated nonsense syllables with primary stress and those in the final position of words more often than other syllables. Both Ferguson (1978) and Weir (1966) have noted the role of intonation patterns in speech development, which provides indirect support for Waterson's theory. Children's earliest speech attempts often have very adult-like intonation patterns, even before the phonological system is correct enough to allow intelligible words (DeBoysson-Bardies, Sagart, & Durand, 1984; Oller, 1980). This suggests that the child is responding to the overall pattern of speech.

Waterson outlined five basic structure types used by young children in their first words. In each case certain prominent features characterize the utterance. The five types described by their notable features are (a) labial structures, (b) continuant structures, (c) sibilant structures, (d) stop structures, and (e) nasal structures. The adult word that the child is attempting to produce will contain some of the features that the child uses, but the sets of features will not be identical. Those features that the child latches onto are determined by the factors mentioned previously (most frequent, clearest) and by the child's perceptual and production capacities.

According to this theory, there is no set order of development. Children may vary with regard to both sequence and rate of development. One advantage of the theory, as Ferguson (1978) notes, is that it accounts for irregularities in development, which theories based on segments and rules fail to do. For example, in attempting to reproduce an adult phrase like "pat the bunny," the child might latch onto the labial aspect and produce /bæ bʌ/. In attempting to reproduce "get your shoes," one child might respond to the continuant aspect while ignoring sibilancy and thus produce /ju/, while another child might use a sibilant structure and produce /su/ or /ʃu/. Both productions recognize the saliency of "shoes," which could result from its primary stress, its final position in the phrase, and/or its concrete meaning. However, as a result of their own perceptual and production capacities, the children chose different strategies for production of that word.

If this theory is correct, it suggests that children learn the phonological system from adult speech, which contains stress patterns and word order that support meaning. This has implications for the speech models and teaching strategies to be used in therapy. Should the phonological system be taught in connected speech or divided into segments for remediation?

Interactionist-Discovery Theory

Kiparsky and Menn (1977) and Menn (1976, 1980) propose an *interactionist-discovery theory* wherein the child is an active learner who attempts to discover the structure of the adult phonological system by organizing it into manageable pieces. Like Waterson, Kiparsky and Menn suggest that children learn to produce whole words before they learn individual phonemes and phonological rules. Beginning speakers will learn a few specific words or a few types of word patterns, and from those, generalize the rules of adult speakers. Because children are creative learners, they may develop their own strategies along the way. For example, children may stick with certain familiar forms and learn new words that fit those forms. They may learn words that do not fit their current rule system, but not be ready to generalize rules from the new word to other words. Because the rules are not innate, through the process of trial and error children may develop their own temporary rules that do not fit the adult system.

Like Waterson's, this theory accounts for individual differences. It also accounts for certain strategies or phenomena that have been observed in individual children, such as progressive idioms or advanced forms (Moskowitz, 1973), overgeneralization, and selection or avoidance of sounds and words (Edwards & Shriberg, 1983).

The implication of this theory for therapy is that the child is not a passive learner upon whom the clinician can impose a new sound or phonological rule. The child must be actively involved in the learning process and make his own trial and error decisions. What the clinician must provide is a rich phonological environment from which the child can extract the rules and perhaps some guidance in making the right decisions.

THE FIRST YEAR

A major portion of the acquisition of the phonological system of the language occurs during the first year. At birth, reflexive crying is the only type of sound that infants emit. The sounds of crying are primarily nasalized vowels—sounds made with the velopharyngeal port open. Within the first few months, however, children begin to gain control over the vocal mechanism. Sounds continue to be reflexive, but they become more varied.

Oller (1976) has outlined the parameters of vocal and articulatory control that children must gain before learning speech. They include:

1. Control of phonation or voice and the vocal mechanism—Children must learn to turn voicing on and off at will.
2. Control of extremes and variations in pitch—Children first learn to make the distinction between very high sounds and very low sounds. Gradually they learn to make finer pitch variations, which are necessary for intonation patterns.
3. Control of extremes and variations in volume—As with pitch, children initially gain voluntary control over extremes in volume. Growth in volume control allows them to distinguish not only between yelling and speaking softly, but also among the fine variations needed for word and sentence stress and for adjusting volume to different listeners and speaking situations.
4. Control of resonance—Children do not make use of the full resonant characteristics of the vocal tract in their earliest utterances. They must learn to achieve the oral resonance required for appropriate voice quality and to vary the resonance characteristics for different speech needs.
5. Control of the timing aspects of alternating resonance and constriction—Children's earliest alternations between open and closed positions of the vocal tract develop into vowels and consonants. To produce syllables, they must develop the ability to make very rapid, very fine alternations.

During the first year, children move through stages of phonological development that are focused toward attainment of these five competencies. Oller (1976, 1980) has outlined the following stages of acquisition.

0–1 month: Quasi-Resonant Nucleus Stage. In this stage, children are able to produce oral sounds, but these sounds are only partially resonated because they do not open their mouths, direct the position of their tongues, or sustain the sounds. In this stage, they make large gains in the control of voice, but resonance is minimal.

2–3 months: Goo and Coo Stage. In this stage, vocalizations have greater resonance. They continue to be primarily vowel-like sounds, but some constrictions or consonant-like sounds may be introduced. Constrictions (pre-consonants) and resonances (pre-vowels) may alternate, but they do not occur in a unit as in a syllable.

4–6 months: Exploration/Expansion Stage. Alternations of resonances and constrictions appear during this stage. These alternations will later become CV or VC syllables. Vocalizations are more fully resonated, but they are not yet distinguishable as specific vowels. In the same way, specific consonants will not generally be identified. However, greater variety in constriction types occurs. During this stage, almost total constrictions that resemble /k/ or /g/, /p/ or /b/ may be heard. These will become stops. Raspberries appear, precursors of fricative sounds. Experimentation with pitch and volume extremes also occurs here. Screams and growls exemplify the extremes of pitch, while yelling and very soft vocalizations demonstrate extremes of volume.

7–10 months: Reduplicated Babbling Stage. An important step toward the production of words and sentences is the ability to combine syllables. This skill usually appears first in the form of exactly duplicated CV combinations such as *baba, dada,* etc. This demonstrates a giant step in the ability to alternate constrictions and resonances. During this stage, more definable consonant and vowel sounds appear.

11–14 months: Variegated Babbling Stage. Jargon demonstrates the child's acquisition of fine variations in pitch and volume, combined with lack of words. The child appears to be using real

sentences because the intonation (pitch) patterns and stress (loudness and timing) are well established and like those of adults. However, the child does not yet know very many of the words or grammatical rules of the language.

During the last stage, the first real words appear. When children use their first meaningful words, they must have sufficient control over the articulatory mechanism to produce at least two sounds in a consistent manner. In order for the adults in the environment to recognize the words, they must be produced in a similar fashion on several occasions. At this point children begin to acquire the phonemes of the language. Once the child has developed a small set of phonemes, this set will continue to expand, production of these sounds will become more consistent, and control over pitch and volume will become more refined.

Babbling

A number of researchers have theorized that infant babbling is random in the sense that the child produces the full range of possible human speech sounds (Jakobson, 1971; Mowrer, 1952; Velten, 1943). Between the ages of about 4 months and 10 months, the infant produces a wide variety of sounds, some of which may be recognized as resembling English phonemes, and others of which may be phonemes in other languages, but not in English. Although conclusive research does not exist (Gilbert, 1982), it has been noted that deaf and hearing children seem to begin babbling at about the same age, and their early babbling is similar (Lenneberg, 1967; Lenneberg, Rebelsky, & Nichols, 1965; Sykes, 1940). This observation lends support to the notion that initially babbling is at least partly reinforced by tactile and kinesthetic sensation in the child's mouth. Children may babble because it feels good or interesting to them. It is further theorized that this vocal play provides practice in speech sound production.

At approximately 8 months, the child begins to imitate the vocal play of adults. At this time mother can say "mama" to the child and he may repeat "mama." Children are also likely to repeat their own CV sequences. It is likely that babbling is now more directly under auditory control. Now the child may babble in response to an auditory stimulus and may continue because of the sound. Gradually the phonemes used by the adults in the child's environment will become more prevalent in the child's speech, and those not used in the language will drop out. At about this time, deaf children may fall behind hearing children in their amount of babbling.

Although children may vary greatly in their choice of babbled sounds, some generalizations can be suggested. Irwin and Chen (1946) and Irwin (1947a, 1947b, 1947c, 1948a, 1948b, 1948c, 1951, 1952) reported the results obtained from records transcribed in IPA from 95 infants recorded at 1-month intervals from 0 to 2½ years. They did not distinguish between meaningful and nonmeaningful utterances in their analysis. Irwin (1952) reported that the infants had seven phoneme types at 1 month. Irwin and Chen (1946) observed that vowels were five times more frequent than consonants at birth and that they continued to be more frequent during the first 30 months. Irwin (1948a) reported that at 2 months the most frequent vowels were /ɛ/, /ɪ/, /ʌ/. The relative percentage of these decreased with age, while the percentage of /i/, /e/, and /æ/ increased. Back vowels (ɑ/, /ɔ/, /o/, /ʊ/, /u/) began to appear at 5 to 6 months. Irwin concluded that the newborn's vowel repertoire is not like that of an adult. It begins to move toward the adult model after 5 to 6 months, but continued development occurs after 30 months.

An analysis of 18 infants showed 2 different consonants used in the initial position at 1 month (Irwin, 1951) and 11 consonants in that position at 2½ years. With regard to manner of articulation, Irwin (1947a) found that the youngest infants had only stops, /k/, /g/, /ʔ/ (glottal stop), and a fricative, /h/. Both /h/ and /ʔ/ dropped out as other stops came in. Nasals and other stops and glides came in at 5 to 6 months, semivowels and fricatives at 9 to 10 months. Glides and semivowels constituted a small percent of phonemes throughout the period studied.

Stoel-Gammon and Cooper (1984) also found fricatives to be less common, and affricates almost

nonexistent, in their subjects' babbling. CV was the predominant syllable type. Locke (1983) observed that studies of infant babbling show that the set of sounds primarily includes stops, nasals, and glides and few fricatives or liquids.

In examining sounds with respect to place of articulation, Irwin (1947b) found that during the first 2 months, velars and glottals accounted for over 90% of all consonants. At 9 to 10 months, they accounted for over 50%. Postdentals and labials became prominent by the end of the first year.

Similarly, the children recorded by Vihman, Macken, Miller, and Simmons (1981) from 9 to 16 months tended to use more labials and dentals than palatals and velars. A number of studies (DeBoysson-Bardies et al., 1984; Locke, 1983; Nakazima, 1975; Oller & Eilers, 1982; Olney & Scholnick, 1976) have shown that English and non-English infants are similar in their use of vowels and consonants during babbling.

In summary, many children seem to have front vowels and back consonants among their earliest productions. Sounds resembling /k/ and /g/ may appear very early. Often, however, these sounds drop out as the child moves toward reduplicated and imitative babbling, and a preference develops for /b/, /p/, /m/, and then /d/ and /n/. It seems likely that the preference for /p/ and /m/ as initial phonemes for the words "mother" and "father" in many languages reflects the child's early productive capabilities ("father"—*pop, papa, père, padre*; "mother"—*mama, mom, mère, madre*). Other early family names that may reflect this phenomenon include *nana, dada, baby*.

Oller et al. (1975) examined the babbling of 5 children between the ages of 6 months and 13 months in order to evaluate the theory that speech sound selection in infant babbling is random. They found that the infants showed the same speech sound preferences that are found in the meaningful speech of young children. Babbling reflected substitution and deletion processes well documented in the meaningful speech of normal and delayed children (Dyson & Paden, 1983; Hodson & Paden, 1983; Ingram, 1976; Jakobson, 1971; Shriberg & Kwiatkowski, 1980). The infants tended to use single consonants rather than consonant clusters (cluster reduction) and more initial consonants than final consonants (final consonant deletion). They used initial stops more frequently than fricatives and affricates (stopping), final fricatives more often than stops (spirantization), glides more than liquids (gliding), and front sounds more than back sounds (fronting).

Some other researchers (Locke, 1983; Stoel-Gammon, 1985; Stoel-Gammon & Cooper, 1984) have observed continuity between babbling and the sounds used in early meaningful speech. Oller et al. (1975) attributed these common phoneme preferences to the human phonological capacity. Locke (1983) also questioned the validity of some of the early assumptions about babbling. In order to shed new light on these assumptions, he reviewed a large number of studies of infants from English-speaking environments, infants from other linguistic environments, and deaf and Down syndrome infants. Like Cruttenden (1970) he did not find support for the idea that infants babble all of the sounds of English or that they babble all possible sounds, including many non-English ones, and then restrict them to English sounds. He did find that they babble a fairly small set of sounds and that English babbling is similar to non-English babbling. Based on the similarities found in cross-linguistic studies and the deaf and Down syndrome infants, Locke, like Oller et al., concluded that babbling is not primarily environmental or based on auditory input, but rather governed by the human biological and phonological capacity.

Jargon

Nonmeaningful sequences of phonemes having intonation and stress patterns that sound appropriate for meaningful speech are called *jargon*. The child exhibiting jargon sounds as though he is saying something meaningful, but it cannot be understood. Jargon develops out of babbling at about 10 months and continues after the child begins to use meaningful words. Some children produce a great deal of jargon, which may be interspersed with meaningful words. They seem to be using a gestalt strategy for producing large chunks of speech, but they do not have the meaningful words or the syntactic structure to produce sentences. Other children use very little jargon. These children tend to use single words or perhaps combinations of a few words to get their point across until they are able to put meaningful words into sentences.

Babbling and jargon can be viewed as the child's prespeech sound practice. Children produce babbling and jargon not only in interactions with adults but also when they are alone, in bed, or playing with toys. There is evidence that children may continue such practice after the development of meaningful speech (Jakobson, 1971; Weir, 1962). Weir observed the vocal play of her three children when alone in their cribs and with a sibling. Sometimes they practiced newly acquired sounds in different contexts; sometimes they practiced variable productions of a sound. While some sequences reflected articulatory practice, others seemed to be syntactic practice.

Pre-Word Transitional Forms

Children do not make a clear-cut leap from non-meaningful jargon to meaningful words. Halliday (1975) and Ferguson (1978) have noted the presence of *vocables* or *transitional forms*, which are defined as utterances produced with a phonetically consistent form (PCF) in a given context. However, these forms do not qualify as true words because they are not based on adult words. In addition, they are not generalized, but are tied to the specific context and often accompanied by a consistent gesture. These vocables may first appear during the period that Locke (1983) called the pragmatic stage. Although Ferguson stated that children will usually use about a dozen vocables, Stoel-Gammon and Dunn (1985) note that evidence (Stoel-Gammon & Cooper, 1984) indicates a much wider variation among children.

Ferguson (1978) listed four phonetic forms that are frequently used in vocables in addition to nonspeech sounds such as clicks. The phonetic types are ''(1) single or repeated vowel, (2) syllabic nasal, (3) syllabic fricative, and (4) single or repeated CV syllable, in which the C is a stop or nasal'' (p. 280).

THE DEVELOPMENT OF MEANINGFUL SPEECH

Locke (1983) suggested that there may be three mechanisms used for phonological development as the child moves from babbling to the adult system. First is *maintenance* of those sounds from the babbling repertoire that fit the adult system. The child already has some sounds that are available for producing words. The second mechanism is *learning* of new sounds to increase the repertoire, and the third is *loss* of sounds from the babbling repertoire that are not phonemic in the language.

There are two ways of examining sound development beyond babbling and jargon. One is to look at the child's phonetic repertoire, i.e., the different phones produced in attempts to communicate. The other is to examine the development of phonemes—phones used contrastively in words so that we can say they have achieved phonemic status. For example, look at the following samples from three different children:

Sample A		*Sample B*	
dog	[dɑ]	bottle	[bɑ]
	[tɑ]	baby	[bebi]
Daddy	[dæ]		[pepi]
coat	[do]	book	[pʊ]
go	[to]	puppy	[pʌpi]
two	[du]	put	[bʊ]
	[tu]		

Sample C	
dog	[dɑ]
talk	[tɑ]
door	[do]
toe	[to]
give	[dɪ]
tickle	[tɪ]

In Sample A both [t] and [d] are included in the

phonetic repertoire, but they do not appear to be different phonemes because they are used interchangeably for any lingual stop. Sample B illustrates that although the child can produce [p] and [b], they are not used consistently as two different phonemes. In some words, [b] is replaced by [p]; in others [p] is replaced by [b]. For some words, the child uses both sounds at different times. In addition, the samples do not include any minimal pairs in which the phones are used contrastively as they are in Sample C, where clear minimal pair contrasts demonstrate the phonemic value of /t/ and /d/. Unfortunately, real children do not produce samples as clear as this example, and it is often difficult to determine whether very young children are using sounds contrastively.

By the time children produce their first words, they have acquired a small set of sounds that can be recognized by the listener. Some of the words they use, however, will include phonemes they have not mastered and more sophisticated syllable structures than they are ready to produce. On the other hand, some children may tend to use only words that contain sounds that they have acquired (Vihman, 1981).

The progression to adult-like speech production does not always follow a straight line (Dyson & Paden, 1983; Edwards, 1979; Ferguson & Farwell, 1975; Ingram et al., 1980). Individual children may use sounds correctly for a period of time and then regress to incorrect production, or may alternate between correct and incorrect production at a given point in time (Ingram et al., 1980; Leonard, Rowan, Morris, and Fey, 1982). They may try out different strategies for sound production (Dyson & Paden, 1983), which may result in the use of certain processes at different points in development.

Moskowitz (1973) and Ferguson and Farwell (1975) have noted the presence of *progressive idioms*, which are defined as words that have advanced pronunciation beyond the child's current phonological system. At the same time, the child may have *regressive idioms*, where the pronunciation remains static despite the fact that the child's system has changed. These regressive idioms are likely to be often-used words or names of familiar people or pets. For example, a child whose sister's name is Cindy might call her [dɪnɪ] due to the processes of stopping, prevocalic voicing, and cluster reduction. After the child is able to produce /s/ and /nd/, he may still call her *Dinnie* because to the child that has become her name. Children may also tend to use words that contain their acquired sounds and avoid those that they cannot pronounce correctly (Ferguson & Farwell, 1975; Macken, 1980).

There is ample evidence that different children may select different strategies for learning the phonological system (Donahue, 1986; Fee & Ingram, 1982; Stoel-Gammon & Dunn, 1985; Vihman, 1981). Information about the variable progression to adult speech can be gained only by observing individual children at frequent intervals over a period of time. Cross-sectional studies like those to be described next will often mask such phenomena.

A further issue in examining speech sound development is that adults may not always perceive the changes that occur in child speech, so that gradual progress goes unnoticed. For example, Macken (1980) and Macken and Barton (1980) noted that children may make changes in distinctive features that do not fit the adult's categorical analysis. A child might acquire the correct voice onset time for prevocalic voiceless stops, but because the adult's system also requires aspiration, the sound continues to be perceived as voiced.

Acquisition of Speech Sounds

The general sequence and approximate ages of consonant acquisition in meaningful words have been documented by several cross-sectional studies that began in the 1930s. These early researchers were interested in gathering normative data based on large numbers of preschool children. Table 3.2 shows a comparison of the data obtained by Poole (1934), Templin (1957), and Wellman, Case,

Mengurt, and Bradbury (1931) and more recently by Arlt and Goodban (1976), Prather, Hedrick, and Kern (1975), and Sander (1972). These researchers asked children to name pictures or objects, answer questions, or repeat words. The studies varied in the number of children tested, the ages included, the type of stimuli, the number of sounds tested, and the criterion for mastery. These factors are outlined in Table 3.3.

A review of the normative studies by Smit (1986) suggested several generalizations regarding the procedures. First, they included children who were at least 2 years 4 months old so that sound acquisition before that age was not studied. Second, speech samples were all elicited, and the target was an individual word to represent the phoneme. In all cases, modeling was allowed, although it was used more freely in some studies. Third, the criterion for mastery was high, ranging from 75% to 100% for all studies except Sander (1972). These factors affect the nature of the results in several ways: (1) sounds that are acquired before 2 years are not represented accurately; (2) sound production in natural speech may not reflect the single word productions; and (3) a majority of children may use a given sound much earlier than the 75% criterion reflects.

There are also areas in which the studies differed. Smit (1986) noted that, although all of the studies attempted to exclude children with hearing loss or delayed language, Prather et al. were more likely to have excluded these children because they actually performed audiometric screening and obtained parent reports of language development. Some studies attempted to include all socioeconomic groups (Prather et al., 1975; Templin, 1957) while others selected only middle-class children (Poole, 1934; Wellman et al., 1931). These subject-selection factors may influence the reported age of acquisition.

An examination of the first three columns in Table 3.2 shows that the exact ages and overall sequence of mastery vary among the early studies, but only slightly, despite some differences in methodology and criteria. The discrepancy between Poole and the other two studies for /f/, /r/, and /s/ may be attributed to the more stringent

TABLE 3.2
Age Levels for Phoneme Development According to Six Studies

	Wellman (1931)	Poole (1934)	Templin (1957)	Sander (1972)	Prather (1975)	Arlt (1976)
m	3	3½	3	before 2	2	3
n	3	4½	3	before 2	2	3
h	3	3½	3	before 2	2	3
p	4	3½	3	before 2	2	3
f	3	5½	3	3	2–4	3
w	3	3½	3	before 2	2–8	3
b	3	3½	4	before 2	2–8	3
ŋ		4½	3	2	2	3
j	4	4½	3½	3	2–4	
k	4	4½	4	2	2–4	3
g	4	4½	4	2	2–4	3
l	4	6½	6	3	3–4	4
d	5	4½	4	2	2–4	3
t	5	4½	6	2	2–8	3
s	5	7½	4½	3	3	4
r	5	7½	4	3	3–4	5
tʃ	5		4½	4	3–8	4
v	5	6½	6	4	4	3½
z	5	7½	7	4	4	4
ʒ	6	6½	7	6	4	4
θ		7½	6	5	4	5
dʒ			7	4	4	4
ʃ		6½	4½	4	3–8	4½
ð		6½	7	5	4	5

TABLE 3.3
Subjects, Stimuli, and Criteria for Mastery Used in Cross-Sectional Studies of Speech Sound Development

	n	Ages	Stimuli	Number of Sounds	Criterion
Wellman et al.	204	2–6	pictures questions	133	75% 3 positions
Poole	140	2.6–8.5	pictures objects questions	23	100% 3 positions
Templin	480	3–8	pictures	176	75%
Prather et al.	147	2–4	pictures		75% 2 positions*
Arlt & Goodban	240	3–6	word repetition	79	75% 3 positions

*initial and final

criterion used by Poole. In general, it can be seen that nasal sounds are mastered early, along with stops and glides. Fricatives, affricates, and liquids tend to develop later.

Sander (1972) reinterpreted the data of Wellman et al. and Templin based on a criterion of 51% accuracy in two out of three positions. This means that 51% of the children tested at a given age level produced the sound correctly in at least two positions. He called this *the age of customary production* and compared it with the age at which 90% of the children produced the sound in at least two positions. Sander argued that the stricter criteria used by the previous researchers revealed the upper age limits for correct production, whereas the majority of children may produce the sounds correctly at an earlier age. Figure 3.1 shows the age range from the point of 51% mastery to the point of

90%. This graph shows great variability in the length of time required for acquisition by different children.

Sander's study has clinical relevance in two ways. First, by adhering to a criterion based on correct production by nearly all children, some potentially delayed children may be missed. Second, the variability shown by Sander indicates a need to examine the overall developing skills of individual children in depth rather than simply compare individual sounds against norms.

Prather, Hedrick, and Kern (1975) obtained data on 147 children for phoneme productions in the initial and final positions of words using the 75% criterion. They found earlier ages of acquisition than the previous researchers (Table 3.2), a fact that may be attributed to their inclusion of only two word positions for each consonant. When comparing the findings of Prather et al. with those of Sander, which were based on the early studies (Table 3.2), it can be seen that Sander's lower or

FIGURE 3.1

Average age estimates and upper age limits of customary consonant production. The solid bar corresponding to each sound starts at the median age of customary articulation; it stops at an age level at which 90% of all children are customarily producing the sound (from Templin, 1957; Wellman et al., 1931). (*Source*: "When Are Speech Sounds Learned?" by E. K. Sander, 1972, *Journal of Speech and Hearing Disorders, 37*, p. 62. Copyright 1972 by the American Speech-Language-Hearing Association, Rockville, Maryland. Reprinted by permission.)

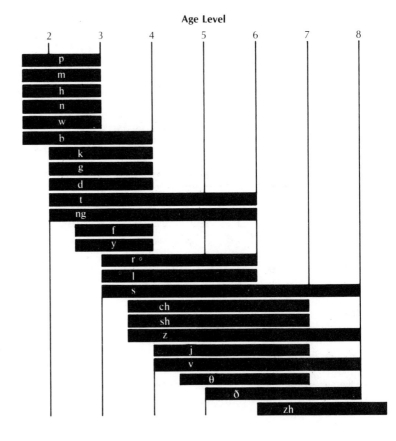

50% age limits correspond to the Prather et al. data, especially for the early-developing sounds. The upper or 90% age limits (for the early studies) tend to be much later than for the Prather et al. data.

Arlt and Goodban (1976) also found that previously established norms were inconsistent with the articulation abilities that they found in 240 children between 3 and 6. Nearly half of the phonemes tested in this investigation were produced correctly by 75% of the children from 6 months to 4½ years earlier than the Templin (1957) norms, while the other half were produced at about the same age. One third of the phonemes appeared at least 1 year earlier than would be expected from the established norms. Some sounds, including /s, z, tʃ, l, v/, were produced from 2 to 4½ years earlier than previously reported. Phonemes that were produced at the same age as the established norms included /m, n, h, ŋ, b, w/. Based on the fact that their sample and procedures were similar to the earlier studies, Arlt and Goodban suggested that children in the 1970s may be producing speech sounds at earlier ages than children of the 1930s and that normative data should be periodically updated to be clinically useful.

These studies of consonant development have shown that there is a general sequence of acquisition that can be used to help determine the adequacy of articulation development of a given child. Although there will be individual variation in specific age of acquisition and in the exact sequence of phoneme development, some generalizations can be made. Phonemes such as /p/, /b/, /m/, /w/, /t/, /d/, /n/, /k/, /g/, /h/ can be expected to develop early—before 3 years. In addition, preschoolers younger than 4 years cannot be expected to have acquired /θ/, /ð/, /z/, /v/, /ʃ/, /ʒ/, /tʃ/, /dʒ/ (Sander, 1972). Beyond these generalizations, decisions regarding articulatory adequacy will be based on number of sounds acquired and overall intelligibility.

Drawing from a variety of sources, Grunwell (1982) presented the developmental data in a different form. She used the seven stages outlined by Crystal, Fletcher, and Garman (1976) for grammatical development, and specified the sounds that might be expected at each stage. Table 3.4 shows

TABLE 3.4
Profile of Phonological Development: Phonological System

Stage	Manner	Labial	Dental	Lingual (alveolar)	Lingual (palatal)	Lingual (velar/glottal)
Stage I (0;9–1;6)	Nasal / Plosive / Fricative / Approximant					
Stage II (1;6–2;0)	Nasal	m		n		
	Plosive	p b		t d		
	Fricative					
	Approximant	w				
Stage III (2;0–2;6)	Nasal	m		n		(ŋ)
	Plosive	p b		t d		(k g)
	Fricative					
	Approximant	w				h
Stage IV (2;6–3;0) / Stage V (3;0–3;6)	Nasal	m		n		ŋ
	Plosive	p b		t d		k g
	Fricative	f		s		
	Approximant	w		(l)	j	h
Stage VI (3;6–4;0) (4;0–4;6)	Nasal	m		n		ŋ
	Plosive	p b		t d	tʃ dʒ	k g
	Fricative	f v		s z	ʃ	
	Approximant	w		l (r)	j	h
Stage VII (4;6<)	Nasal	m		n		ŋ
	Plosive	p b		t d	tʃ dʒ	k g
	Fricative	f v	θ ð	s z	ʃ ʒ	
	Approximant	w		l r	j	h

Source: Clinical Phonology (p. 98) by P. Grunwell, 1982, Rockville, MD: Aspen Systems Corporation. Copyright 1982 by Aspen Systems Corporation. Reprinted with permission of Aspen Systems Corporation.

TABLE 3.5
Olmsted's (1971) Findings Regarding Frequency of Occurrence, Percent Correct, and Variability of Correctness for Spontaneous Speech Samples of 98 Children Ages 15 to 54 Months

No.		Number of Children Attempting the Phone	Mean Percent Correct	SD of Percent Correct
1	p	91	75.5	28.4
2	t	96	52.2	26.9
3	k	96	80.4	23.6
4	b	93	90.4	14.8
5	d	97	64.9	24.4
6	g	93	75.9	31.8
7	f	76	81.9	27.9
8	v	48	46.8	43.4
9	θ	59	25.7	37.7
10	ð	89	20.3	27.2
11	s	92	61.4	30.8
12	z	88	57.6	32.2
13	ʃ	78	49.4	40.1
14	ʒ	5	20.0	44.7
15	l	95	33.5	28.3
16	m	87	81.1	24.3
17	n	95	75.3	22.4
18	ŋ	76	38.8	40.0
19	h	86	77.7	26.0
20	r	36	62.4	46.5
21	ʔ	14	69.0	46.2
22	i	97	90.6	11.8
23	ɪ	97	67.0	28.5
24	ɛ	85	58.5	35.5

the suggested phonological system of the child at each stage with sounds grouped according to manner of articulation and labial or lingual placement. Grunwell's profile begins at an earlier age (0;9) than any of the other studies. At the first stage (0;9–1;6), she indicates only features that the child includes in his productions, but at Stage II (1;6–2;0) she lists specific phonemes that occur. The age of acquisition for most sounds is earlier than found in the classical studies.

In contrast to the research described thus far, two acquisition studies have used spontaneous rather than elicited speech as data for analysis. Olmsted (1971) analyzed spontaneous speech samples of 58 girls and 42 boys who were the children

of generally highly educated parents. The children ranged in age from 15 to 54 months. Olmsted provided detailed information about individual vowels and consonants and consonant clusters at each of six age levels. The results include both number and percentage of attempts for each phoneme as well as data regarding correct production and errors in each word position. Table 3.5 provides one example of the kind of data that are included. Based on samples of 98 children, this table shows that although most phonemes were used by well over half of the children, some phonemes were not frequently used by the children. Further, there is large variation in percent of correct production, not only among the different phonemes, but also among

TABLE 3.5 *(continued)*

No.		Number of Children Attempting the Phone	Mean Percent Correct	SD of Percent Correct
25	æ	96	77.4	23.0
26	ə	39	48.4	45.0
27	ʌ	96	71.5	25.1
28	a	84	85.2	26.4
29	u	82	76.7	31.5
30	ʊ	66	66.6	40.2
31	ɔ	95	68.7	33.8
32	i̧	46	42.2	44.6
33	ɪ̧	52	36.7	41.3
34	ɛ̧	83	40.6	36.6
35	æ̧	41	42.5	46.5
36	ə̧	87	44.5	38.7
37	ʌ̧	34	20.6	39.2
38	a̧	71	33.6	39.2
39	u̧	19	43.7	45.7
40	ʊ̧	3	77.8	38.5
41	ɔ̧	79	42.9	42.1
42	ɔw	88	78.6	29.5
43	aw	71	71.2	34.5
44	ɛy	80	70.5	35.2
45	ay	91	80.2	28.0
46	ɔy	12	70.8	40.3
47	w	79	69.7	33.2
48	y	53	67.2	41.9
49	w̥	36	70.6	40.1

Source: Out of the Mouths of Babes by D. Olmsted, 1971. The Hague: Mouton. Used with permission.

children, as can be seen by the large standard deviations for each phoneme. This table is not clinically useful for comparison with individual children because it collapses age groups; it is provided to demonstrate the kind of data that can be obtained from spontaneous speech studies. Information about specific ages, phonemes, and word positions can be obtained from Olmsted's (1971) work for comparison with the performance of individual children.

Irwin and Wong and their colleagues (1983) also obtained spontaneous samples from 100 children between 18 and 72 months. The data were analyzed not only for percent of correct production of individual sounds, but also for usage and re-placement of distinctive features. Although the percent of distribution of phonemes is provided, the number of children attempting each phoneme is not given. For example, at 2 years, we find that /b/ represented 7% of all sounds produced by the children, while /f, z, ʃ, tʃ, w/ represented only 1% (Hare, 1983). However, we do not know what percentage of the children actually attempted any of these sounds. Table 3.6 shows the percent correct production for consonants at each age group studied. The authors also presented this information for vowels.

The important contribution of these studies is that they reveal children's use of sounds in spontaneous speech rather than in elicited and possibly

TABLE 3.6
Percent Correct Production for Consonants Based on Spontaneous Speech Samples at 18, 24, 36, 48, 72 Months

Phonemes	Age in Years				
	1.5	2	3	4	6
/k/	47	71	98	97	100
/g/	49	71	94	99	97
/t/	36	55	98	89	99
/d/	63	64	99	68	77
/p/	56	66	99	98	99
/b/	90	97	100	95	99
/f/	67	65	97	99	100
/v/	13	7	96	76	83
/θ/	0	2	49	81	78
/ð/	5	1	40	64	65
/s/	8	54	98	87	93
/z/	1	33	98	89	94
/ʃ/	2	43	99	95	87
/ʒ/	—	—	100	—	—
/tʃ/	22	35	97	74	100
/dʒ/	9	53	96	75	83
/m/	84	97	100	99	100
/n/	63	75	100	98	99
/ŋ/	3	74	96	46	57
/l/	4	27	93	85	95
/r/	2	20	89	81	82
/h/	68	78	100	97	91
/w/	63	94	100	99	99
/j/	71	55	99	95	98
/ʔ/	—	—	—	—	—
Total	50	63	93	88	92

Source: J. V. Irwin and S. P. Wong (Eds.), *Phonological Development in Children 18 to 72 Months.* Carbondale, IL: Southern Illinois University Press.

imitated single words. If there is a difference between the data obtained from these two sources, the spontaneous data are more representative of the child's actual sound production in communication.

It cannot be stressed too strongly that developmental norms must be interpreted with caution. The norms are averages based on evaluation of large numbers of children and as such do not reflect the performance of any given child. As Jakobson (1971) noted, the general sequence of acquisition is more stable across children than is the timetable; however, both may vary. Some children have nearly adult articulation by 2 years, while others, still within normal limits, continue to make

a few errors at 5 years. In addition, the normative studies do not provide information about the process of development of sounds or sound classes. Approximation of phonemes, phonemes that are occasionally used correctly, and sound classes that are present in the child's speech provide important information about the child's level of development.

Factors that create variability among children should be considered when comparing the performance of an individual child to the normative data. These factors may include overall maturity, overall linguistic development, medical history including middle-ear infections, psychological makeup, and environmental conditions. In addition, the child's own pattern of development should be considered, including number of correct phonemes, classes of phonemes that have been acquired, consistency, and intelligibility.

The large-scale latitudinal studies have generally examined the acquisition of individual phonemes without attention to patterns of development. Current interest in the phonological system leads to examination of patterns of acquisition rather than unrelated sounds. One way to note patterns of acquisition is to examine sound classes. Other ways include analysis of distinctive feature acquisition, elimination of phonological processes, or writing a generative grammar. These will be discussed in the next four sections.

Acquisition of Sound Classes

Nasals. Nasal sounds occur early in normal development. /m/ and /n/ are among the first sounds to develop whereas /ŋ/ has been found to develop slightly later. Other sound classes are rarely substituted for nasals, but when substitutions do occur, they are likely to be stops. Singh and Frank (1972) found that the children in their sample never substituted fricatives for nasals.

Stops. The stops are also early developing sounds with the labial stops (/p/ and /b/) being first. There is no clear-cut evidence for an order between the alveolar (/t/ and /d/) or velar stops (/k/ and /g/). Substitutions for stops will often occur within the sound class. They will usually be substitutions of voicing or place. Hare (1983) found substitutions of k/g and g/k followed by t/k and d/g to be most common at 2 years. By 4 years, Bassi (1983) found no errors on /g/ and only scattered errors on /t, d, k/.

Initially children do not produce a distinction between the voiced and unvoiced cognates. Macken and Barton (1980) indicate that the earliest production may be a voiceless unaspirated stop, which combines features of both cognates. When they first begin to make a distinction between voiced and voiceless stops, their voice onset time

(VOT) may not match that of the adult and thus the adult may not perceive the difference. Finally the child develops a VOT that resembles the adult model. Syllable position may affect correct production. Prevocalic voicing and postvocalic devoicing may result in voiced stops in the initial position and voiceless stops in the final position. This phenomenon is common across languages (Locke, 1983).

Dyson (1986) examined the acquisition of velars by 2-year-olds. She found that over the period 2;5 to 2;10, the percentage of children producing 95% to 100% correct velars increased from 50% to 70%. An interesting point is that none of the children showed deviations for 100% of the velars. She also found that final velars were acquired before initial velars. When in error, final velars were more likely to be deleted than fronted as were initial velars. This seemed to be related to a pattern of final consonant deletion for these children.

Fricatives and Affricates. The labiodental fricative /f/ frequently develops much earlier than other fricatives, but its voiced counterpart /v/ remains later. There does not appear to be a strong order for the other fricatives, although /θ/ and /ð/ are usually acquired later.

It has been observed that fricatives may be easier to produce in the postvocalic position (Edwards, 1979; Edwards & Shriberg, 1983), but Kenney and Prather (1986) did not find this to be true for /s, f, ʃ, θ/. As a matter of fact /f, ʃ, θ/ were produced more accurately in the initial position.

Incorrect production of fricatives may reflect very different error patterns. Stops and affricates may be substituted for fricatives before a child has developed the continuancy or fricative features. This has been observed not only in English but also in other languages (Locke, 1983). Ferguson (1973) also notes that liquids or glides may be substituted. However, errors made by older children are more commonly place errors shown by replacement of a fricative by another fricative. Hare (1983) found /d, t/ to be the most frequent substitutions for /s/ at 2 years; however, at 4 years /θ, z, s/ were substituted. No children in the sample substituted a stop at this age (Bassi, 1983). The late acquisition of fricatives seen in the developmental data may also reflect phonetic errors such as a distorted /s/ or /ʃ/.

Stops are also common substitutions for affricates (Olmsted, 1971). Hare (1983) and Bassi (1983) found t/tʃ and d/dʒ to be most common at 2 and 4 years.

In examining the articulation development of 2½- to 5-year-old children, Kenney and Prather (1986) found the following rank order for number of errors on voiceless fricatives and the affricate: /θ/, /ʃ/, /tʃ/, /s/, /f/. The number of errors for /ʃ, tʃ, s/ were very similar.

Glides and Liquids. The glides /w/ and /j/ are acquired early whereas the liquids /r/ and /l/ appear late. Usually a glide is substituted for a liquid before the liquid is acquired. Remember that syllable-final liquids are very different from syllable-initial forms. In the final position, liquids are usually omitted or replaced by vowels.

Most studies have found high error rates on /l, r/ during the preschool years (Irwin & Wong, 1983; Kenney & Prather, 1986; Olmsted, 1971). Clearly the most frequent substitution is /w/ in the initial position.

Clusters. Consonant clusters are usually acquired late. Olmsted (1971) found correct initial clusters to be extremely rare in his sample of children 15 to 54 months. Most often they are reduced to a single consonant, which is usually the unmarked (easier to produce) member of the pair. Consonants with three members are often reduced to one by younger children and to two members by older preschoolers (Olmsted, 1971). Olmsted also noted that some children retain the length of the cluster, but substitute for one member. These substitutions usually follow the patterns of error described for individual

sound classes. He noted that errors in place and in friction were most common with few voicing errors and almost no errors of nasality. Olmsted noted that the second member of the cluster is most often in error, no matter what the length of the cluster.

In clusters with /s/ plus stop, nasal, liquid or glide, /s/ is frequently omitted. In /sl/ clusters, /l/ may be omitted more frequently than the other second members. Catts and Kamhi (1984) observed that normal children most frequently reduced /s/ + stop clusters to the stop; however, their subjects varied regarding the voicing characteristics of the remaining stop. Clusters consisting of stops or fricatives plus liquids are most frequently reduced to the stop or fricative.

Locke (1983) observed similar patterns for children learning other languages.

Acquisition of Distinctive Features

Menyuk (1968) examined consonant development of children from a distinctive-feature viewpoint based on the Jakobson, Fant, and Halle (1963) system. Using spontaneous speech samples, she analyzed the use of the following features by preschool children: gravity, diffuseness, voicing, continuancy, stridency, nasality. She determined the percentage of sounds containing each feature that were used correctly at age levels between 2½ and 5 years for American children and 1 and 3 years for Japanese children. This feature system includes two features that were not described in chapter 2. Gravity and diffuseness both refer to articulatory position in the oral cavity. Sounds that have the + grave feature are those that are produced at the very front (/p/, /b/, /m/) or the very back (/k/, /g/, /ŋ/) of the oral cavity. Sounds that carry the + diffuse feature are those that are produced forward in the oral cavity including labials, dentals, and alveolars in comparison to palatals and velars.

Menyuk's data indicated that Japanese children acquire these features about 1½ to 2 years earlier than American children, but information regarding the universality of phonological acquisition has caused these findings to be questioned. However, the order of mastery of the features for both American and Japanese children was: nasal, grave, voiced, diffuse, continuant, strident.

Menyuk suggested that the + nasal and + voiced features may be acquired early because of their "on-off" nature—the velopharyngeal port is either open or closed for nasal and nonnasal sounds; the vocal folds either vibrate or they do not for voiced and voiceless sounds. In contrast, degree of stridency is on a continuum—/θ/ has a small degree of stridency, but is not considered to be a strident sound; /f/ contains more stridency, and is considered to be + for that feature. Another early-learned feature, + grave, carries a maximum distinction between the + and − contrasts. Those consonants that are + grave (e.g., /b/, /g/) are produced at either the front or the back of the oral cavity. This line of reasoning has also been used to account for the early appearance of these sounds in babbling.

Menyuk observed that the sequence of acquisition of the features did not correspond directly with their frequency of occurrence in adult speech, with the order of maintenance in adults' perceptual confusions, or with the order of maintenance in substitutions made by normally developing children or children with articulation problems. Maintenance of a feature means that the feature is present in both sounds when one sound is substituted for another in perception or production. It was found that the features + nasal and + voiced were well maintained in each case. This observation lends support to Menyuk's argument regarding the on-off nature of these features.

Prather et al. subjected their data from 147 children to the feature analysis used by Menyuk. As in their comparison with the Sander data, they found a similar sequence of acquisition with earlier age levels. Unlike Menyuk, Prather et al. also examined the − value of the features and found their order of acquisition to be close but not identical to the reverse order of the + features. The rank order for the three analyses is shown in Table 3.7.

TABLE 3.7
Rank Order of Feature Acquisition Found by Menyuk (1968) and by Prather, Hedrick, and Kern (1975)

Menyuk	Prather et al.	Prather et al.
+ nasal	+ nasal	− continuant
+ grave	+ grave	− strident
+ voice	+ diffuse	− diffuse
+ diffuse	+ voice	− voice
+ strident	+ continuant	− nasal
+ continuant	+ strident	− grave

Weiner and Bernthal (1976) examined the acquisition of the following features by 250 2-through 6-year-old children:

anterior	coronal	nasal
high	low	lateral
back	distributed	delayed
continuant	voice	release

They found that the features most frequently in error during production of fricative sounds were −anterior, +coronal, +high, −distributed, +continuant, and +voice. In producing stops, children had the highest number of errors on −anterior, +high, +voice, and +delayed release. There very few errors for the features +nasal and −continuant at any age. By 5 years only +coronal, −distributed, and +voice exceeded an error rate of 5%. The results for 4 of the 11 features agreed with the predictions of markedness theory (see chapter 2).

Singh (1976) applied distinctive feature analysis to a number of developmental studies (Bricker, 1967; Cairns & Williams, 1972; Irwin, 1947; Menyuk, 1968; Menyuk & Anderson, 1969; Messer, 1967; Nakazima, 1962; Poole, 1934; Prather et al., 1975; Snow, 1963; Templin, 1957; Wellman et al., 1931). Two conclusions were noteworthy: (a) based on Irwin's (1947) data, the child's priority of features is very different at 1 month from the adult's but moves between 1 and 30 months toward approximation of the adult system and (b) examination of a variety of studies with different purposes reveals similar results regarding the role of distinctive features in speech sound acquisition.

The spontaneous speech samples collected from 100 children ages 18 to 72 months by Irwin and Wong (1983) and colleagues were also analyzed for distinctive feature usage and errors. They used the Chomsky and Halle (1968) system and one developed by Irwin and Wong. They found that except for linguadental place in the Irwin and Wong system, all feature specifications in both systems were acquired by age 2.

Phonological Process Analysis of Developing Speech

As noted earlier, Stampe (1969) proposed that learning the sound system of a language involves suppressing a number of innate simplifying processes. As these processes are eliminated, the child develops an increased number of contrasts and eventually acquires the full set of sounds of the adult model. A number of authors have described the phonological processes that characterize child speech.

Ingram (1976) collected data on early child phonology from a variety of sources, including both English-speaking children and children learning other languages. He identified the probable phonetic repertoire and the processes that are common in the first words of children. Ingram holds that the child's variations from the adult model do not depend entirely on underdeveloped articulatory skills, but also result from faulty perception of the adult model. For example, the child who consistently fails to use final consonants may be able to make sense only of the CV part of the word at that point in time. The final consonant may be perceived only as meaningless noise.

In the discussion of phonological development during the first year, we presented evidence that the child learns pitch and volume variations by beginning at the extremes and gradually refining the smaller variations (Oller, 1976). Jakobson (1968) suggested the same process in the learning of individual phonemes. Examining the data of 4 children who had vocabularies of about 50 words, Ingram (1976) found the following common inventory of sounds:

Consonants			*Vowels*	
p	t		i	u
b	d			ɑ
f	s	h		

An individual child would not be likely to use all of the above sounds contrastively in his first words, but the child's set would be likely to be chosen from among them. The sounds that a given child might use would probably be maximally different from one another. This is seen most clearly in the vowel set just shown. The three vowels, high front, high back, and low mid, are extremely distinct. Following this line of reasoning, we might expect a hypothetical child to have /b/ and /h/ as a two-consonant repertoire. In fact, not all children follow the theoretical model exactly, but all do tend to use quite distinct sounds as their early phonemes.

Table 3.8 summarizes the processes that Ingram (1976) found to characterize the speech of children from 1 year 6 months to 4 years. This table provides an example of each process and suggests ages at which children are likely to use them for those cases where Ingram provides this information.

As noted in Table 3.8, certain processes are more common in normal child speech than others. Grunwell (1982) listed the following processes as being the most common in normal development: weak syllable deletion, final consonant deletion, reduplication, consonant harmony (assimilation), cluster reduction, stopping, fronting, gliding, and context-sensitive voicing. She also proposed ages at which these processes might be expected to oc-

TABLE 3.8
Summary of Phonological Processes Described by Ingram (1976)

Syllable Structure Processes

Final consonant deletion ([kæ] for *cat*). Usually eliminated by 3 years.
Unstressed syllable deletion ([nænə] for *banana*). Usually eliminated by 4 years.
Syllable reduplication ([baba] for *bottle*). Most common in the phonology of the first 50 words.
Cluster reduction, including deletion of the entire cluster ([ɪnk] for *drink*), reduction to one member ([dɪnk]), or substitution for one member ([dwɪnk]). May last for a long time during the acquisition stages.

Assimilatory Processes

Contiguous assimilation between consonants:
   Labial assimilation ([fwi] for *tree*). Probably eliminated by 4 years.
   Final consonant devoicing ([dɔk] for *dog*). Eliminated by 2 years.
Contiguous assimilation between a consonant and a vowel:
   Alveolars become velars when adjacent to back vowel ([ku] for *to*).
   Prevocalic voicing ([dæt] for *cat*). May last for only several months.
   Vowel lengthening before voiced consonant ([bæ:] for *bad*).
   Vowel nasalization ([grĩ] for *green*). Very common.
Noncontiguous assimilation between consonants:
   Back assimilation ([gɔg] for *dog*).
   Labial assimilation ([bɑp] for *stop*).
   Nasalization ([nʌ̃nə] for *another*). Not a common process.
Noncontiguous assimilation between vowels:
   Progressive assimilation ([æbæ] for *apple*).
   Regressive assimilation ([bibi] for *baby*).

Substitution Processes

Those affecting obstruents:
   Stopping of fricatives and affricates (t/s). May persist over several years.
   Fronting of palatals and velars (t/k). Most common before 3½ years.
Those affecting nasals:
   Fronting (n/ŋ). Occurs with fronting of other velars.
   Denasalization (b/m). Not a strong process.
Those affecting liquids:
   Stopping (d/r). Probably very early in development.
   Gliding (w/r). May last for some time.
   Liquid replacement (l/r). May occur late in development.
Those affecting glides:
   Frication (z/j). Not a common process.
Those affecting syllabic liquids and nasals:
   Vocalization (ə/ɚ). Very common process.
Those affecting vowels:
   Neutralization (/ə/ substituted for any vowel).
Deletion: can affect any segment. Earliest process available to child. It must be eliminated before others can occur.

cur and to be eliminated. Table 3.9 summarizes this information.

Dyson and Paden (1983) examined the elimination of five phonological processes by forty 2-year-old children. On eight occasions at 3-week intervals, they elicited 36 words to provide opportunity for the five processes to occur. At the first testing, the processes were ordered as follows with regard to frequency of occurrence: gliding, cluster reduction, fronting, stopping, and final consonant deletion. At the last testing 7 months later, the order remained the same. Final consonant deletion was almost completely eliminated; fronting and stopping were infrequent; gliding and cluster reduction, on the other hand, were still common.

Haelsig and Madison (1986) extended the phonological process analysis to fifty 3-, 4-, and 5-year-old children using the Phonological Process Analysis (Weiner, 1979). They examined the occurrence of 16 processes. They found that 3- and 3½-year-old children used the following processes: cluster reduction, weak syllable deletion, glottal replacement, labial assimilation, and gliding of liquids. Children 4½ and 5 years old used weak syllable deletion and cluster reduction. The following processes were used rarely by any age group: velar assimilation, prevocalic voicing, gliding of fricatives, affrication, and denasalization. The greatest reduction in processes occurred between 3 and 4 years with deletion of final consonants, stopping, fronting, and gliding of liquids being reduced by 50% between these ages. The authors pointed out the great individual variation in each age group.

Fronting was found by Lowe, Knutson, and Monson (1985) to be used by 6% of a sample of 1,048 preschool children between the ages of 31 and 54 months. During that age range its use dropped from 23% to 3.5%. They noted that velar fronting was more common than palatal fronting and that children did not use palatal fronting in the absence of velar fronting.

Simplification processes may be related to children's strategies for learning language. For exam-

ple, individual children may exhibit early processes such as consonant harmony (Donahue, 1986) or reduplication (Fee & Ingram, 1982; Schwartz, Leonard, Wilcox, & Folger, 1980), or include homonyms in their early words (Vihman, 1981) to varying degrees. The strategies that a child selects for producing meaningful speech can affect not only the development of the phonological system, but also the development of the lexicon and early syntax.

Phonological processes do not always occur in isolation. It is not uncommon for two or more processes to co-occur in children's speech. The following productions are examples of such co-occurrence:

| [bæt] | *bag* | fronting and final consonant devoicing |
| [taɪd] | *slide* | cluster reduction and stopping |

When processes co-occur, it becomes more difficult to determine the relationship between the realized form and the target form. What may look like random substitution is likely to be the result of the application of several processes.

The processes most common in normal children are those that are also most frequently seen at later ages in children with disordered articulation.

Generative Analysis of Developing Speech

The foregoing methods for describing child speech are based on the assumption that the child's underlying representation of phonemes, words, and sentences is like the adult underlying representation. This means that the child's attempts to say a word are attempts to reproduce the adult model that the child has heard. The inability to do this is a result of immature cognitive, perceptual, and/or physiological mechanisms. The phonological process model provides a good example of this view. The child may be attempting to match the adult word "see." This is his underlying representation of the word. However, the child produces [di] due to the stopping process.

TABLE 3.9
Chronology of Phonological Processes

	2;0–2;6	2;6–3;0	3;0–3;6	3;6–4;0	4;0–4;6	4;6–5;0	5;0—
Weak Syllable Deletion		▬▬▬	▬▬▬	▬ - -			
Final Consonant Deletion		▬▬ - -	- -				
Reduplication	▬ - - -						
Consonant Harmony	▬ - - -	- - -					
Cluster Reduction (Initial) obstruent+ approximant	▬▬▬	- - -	- - -	- -			
/s/ + consonant	▬▬▬	▬▬▬	▬▬▬	- -			
Stopping /f/	▬▬▬	▬ -					
/v/	▬▬▬	▬ - -	- -				
/θ/ /θ/ → [f]	▬▬▬	- -	▬▬▬	▬▬▬	- - -	- - -	- - -
/ð/ /ð/ → [d] or [v]	▬▬▬	▬▬▬	▬▬▬	▬▬▬	▬▬▬	- - -	- - -
/s/	▬▬ -	- -	-				
/z/	▬▬▬	- - -	- -				
/ʃ/ Fronting '[s] type'	▬▬ -	- -	▬▬▬	- - -	- -		
/tʃ, dʒ/ Fronting [ts, dz]			- - -	- - -	- - -	- -	
Fronting /k, g, ŋ/	▬▬▬	- - -	- - -	-			
Gliding /r/ → [w]	▬▬▬	- - -	- - -	- - -	- - -	- - -	- - -
Context-Sensitive Voicing	▬ - -	- - -	- -				

Source: *Clinical Phonology* (p. 183) by P. Grunwell, 1982, Rockville, MD: Aspen Systems Corporation. Copyright 1982 by Aspen Systems Corporation. Reprinted with permission of Aspen Systems Corporation.

Some researchers (Elbert, 1985; Locke, 1983, 1985; Maxwell & Rockman, 1984) have proposed that normally developing children may have unique underlying representations that change during the period of acquisition. This view would also apply to children with disordered phonology. If one concludes that the child's phonological system may be a different version rather than a deficient version of the adult system, then a method of analysis that only compares it to the adult system may not be ideal. Those who take this view might advocate a generative analysis of the child's speech.

Completing a generative phonological analysis means taking a speech sample, which ideally is spontaneous, and writing phonological rules like those described in chapter 2. These rules are based only on the data in the child's sample, not on a comparison with the adult model. Maxwell and Rockman (1984) suggest that a generative analysis should include the child's phonetic inventory, the contrasts used in his speech, a phonemic inventory and syllable structure, and occurrence restrictions. Occurrence restrictions would be written in the form of rules. Maxwell and Rockman refer to this as a "system-internal generative phonological analysis," which means that it refers only to the child's own system. There may be variations in the rules that individual children adopt in their path toward learning the phonology of the language.

METALINGUISTIC AWARENESS

As indicated by Ingram's stages as well as other information presented in this chapter, the learning of the phonological system takes place primarily during the preschool years. During the school-age years, the child learns to manipulate that system for learning to pronounce new words, for applying it to morphophonemic rules, and for learning to read (Hakes, 1980; Mattingly, 1972). Many of the activities that take place in school require metalinguistic skills—the ability to think and talk about language.

As young children learn the sound system, they do not consciously focus on sounds; their focus is on meaning. Sounds are learned as they contribute to understanding what other people say and as they are useful for communicating. The preschool child is not likely to know what a sound or even a word is, because the ability to segment into phonemes develops during the early school-age years (Fox & Routh, 1975; Leiberman, Shankweiler, Fischer, & Carter, 1974). This is important information for remediation. Some approaches may ask the child

to identify "his" sound at the beginning or end of a word. School-age children may be able to do this, but preschool children may not know that a sound is distinct from a word, or where the word begins and ends, or even what part of an utterance is actually a single word.

One of the earliest indications of metaphonological knowledge may be seen in rhyming (Calfee, Chapman, & Venezsky, 1972). Most preschool children enjoy rhymes and may begin to make rhymes themselves before they enter school. Rhyming activities are common in kindergarten because they help children begin to pay attention to the way words sound rather than what they mean. Young children may enjoy listening to rhymes just because they sound pleasant. When children can make rhymes themselves, some metaphonological awareness has developed. A second way in which metaphonological knowledge can be seen is in early jokes (Berko Gleason, 1989). Phonological or "sound-alike" jokes are among the earliest jokes that children tell. Knock-knock jokes are examples:

> Knock, knock.
> Who's there?
> Boo.
> Boo who?
> Please don't cry.

These kinds of jokes are popular with first and second graders, which indicates that they can appreciate the relationship between sound and meaning. However, children at this age would be unlikely to be able to explain why it is funny. This ability to explain the source of humor or ambiguity comes later, usually after about 12 years. It could be inferred that the ability to explain or describe a phonological rule would not develop before this time. In teaching it is important to remember this distinction between the ability to use rules and the ability to state rules.

Reading programs vary in their reliance on learning sound-letter relationships. Phonics programs may begin by teaching children to recognize the sound that a "letter makes" and by combining these sounds to form words. These programs demand metaphonological skills from the beginning.

In some schools, this approach may begin in kindergarten. Other programs start with extracting meaning from the page on the assumption that sound-symbol relationships will develop naturally or can be taught later. It is generally agreed that the ability to segment the flow of speech into words is a necessary prerequisite for reading (Calfee, Lindamood, & Lindamood, 1973; Treiman & Baron, 1981); however, recent research by Kamhi and Catts (1986) and Chabon and Prelock (1987) has questioned the exact relationship between phonemic awareness and reading ability. Spelling is another skill that requires attention to the segments that make up words. Saying a word aloud to figure out how to spell it is a metaphonological activity.

Metalinguistic ability develops primarily during the school-age years and is required for many school activities. Speech-language pathologists often rely on these skills for many of their teaching techniques for children with phonological disorders. It is important for speech-language pathologists and teachers to remember that these skills are developmental and that individual variations may exist among children.

SPEECH PERCEPTION

Research Findings

A great deal of research has recently been directed toward determining the infant's capacity for discriminating between the perceptual features that distinguish phonemes. Analysis of the responses of infants is difficult, but researchers have attempted to determine differential responses by analyzing sucking rate, heart rate, and head orientation. One typical method is to repeat the same phoneme over and over while the child sucks on an electronically wired nipple, has his heart rate measured, or gazes at a toy. The child's sucking rate or heart rate during the constant condition is measured. It is then determined if a change in response occurs when a novel stimulus is presented. For the head turn response, the child is conditioned to look at a toy when one of the phonemes is heard. Using

these methods, researchers have suggested that infants as young as 1 month are able to distinguish between /p/ and /b/, which differ only in the voicing feature (Cutting & Eimas, 1975).

Cutting and Eimas further found that 1- and 4-month-old infants perceived the difference between /p/ and /b/ on the basis of voice onset time at the same critical boundaries as did adults. Eilers and Minifie (1975) found that infants aged 4 through 17 weeks varied their sucking rate to indicate discrimination between /sɑ/ and /vɑ/ and between /sɑ/ and /ʃɑ/, but not between /sɑ/ and /zɑ/. Eilers, Wilson, and Moore (1977) found that their youngest infants (1 month) discriminated between /vɑ/ and /sɑ/ and between /sɑ/ and /ʃɑ/; their 6- to 8-month group discriminated between /sɑ/ and /zɑ/. Their oldest group (12 to 14 months) did not discriminate between /θɑ/ and /fɑ/. Eilers et al. also found that 1- to 3-month-old infants were able to discriminate voiced versus voiceless consonants in the final position of syllables when given the full set of clues that are used in production of English words, i.e., lengthening of vowels before final voiced plosives and fricatives. These syllable contrasts are /ɑt/ versus /ɑːd/ and /ɑs/ versus /ɑːz/ (where '':'' denotes vowel lengthening). Overall, they found developmental changes for certain speech contrasts. Other studies (Eilers, 1977; Kuhl, 1977, 1979; Miller & Morse, 1976) have confirmed that infants at 1 month are able to perceive certain speech contrasts and that others develop during the first year.

Research examining the perceptual abilities of children older than 12 months has indicated that speech sound discrimination abilities continue to develop during the preschool years (Barton, 1976; Edwards, 1974; Garnica, 1973; Shvachkin, 1973; Templin, 1957). Some authors have suggested a universal order of the acquisition of phonemes and phonemic distinctions (Garnica, 1973; Shvachkin, 1973), while others have questioned a strict or even general order and have noted the importance of such factors as the meaningfulness of the material, familiarity with the words, attention, and production abilities (Barton, 1976, 1980; Edwards, 1974; Strange & Broen, 1980).

Zlatkin and Koenigsknecht (1976) examined the continuing development of perception and its relationship to production in 2- and 6-year-olds. Ten children in each of these age groups and 20 adults read word pairs or named picture pairs such as *peas–bees, time–dime, coat–goat*. Using spectrographic analysis, Zlatkin and Koenigsknecht examined the distinction between voiced and voiceless consonants as measured by voice onset time. They found significant differences between the productions of 2- and 6-year-olds, but all subjects' data fell into similar regions. The adults' productions were more consistent than those of children. Another finding was that the subjects' productions tended to agree with their perceptual responses regarding the critical voice onset time for distinguishing between voiced and voiceless consonants. However, the 2-year-olds were not able to discriminate their own productions when they were played back to them, whereas the 6-year-olds were. In general, perceptual ability preceded production.

Graham and House (1971) studied the role of distinctive features in 3- to 4½-year-old girls' ability to discriminate among pairs of consonants. They found that, in general, pairs that differ by a greater number of features were more easily discriminated. The highest number of errors occurred on pairs that differed by only one feature. In addition, the high-error contrasts often reflected common substitutions. The children's performance was similar in kind to that of adults: they simply made more errors.

Strange and Broen (1980) examined the ability of 3-year-old children to discriminate among /w/, /l/, and /r/ in meaningful word pairs. They found that in a very structured task the children were able to discriminate among these consonants, which share most of the same features (approximant consonants). Further, they found that there was a relationship between perception and production in that the children who did not produce these sounds correctly made more errors in discrimination.

However, all of the children had better than chance performance.

Another area that has received attention is the effect of coarticulation on the perception of consonants (Mann, Sharlin, & Dorman, 1985; Morrongiello, Robson, Best, & Clifton, 1984; Nittrouer & Studdert-Kennedy, 1987). These studies have investigated the effects of the adjacent vowel and/or the transition into the adjacent sound on perception of consonants. Two examples of these kinds of studies involve perception of /s/ versus /ʃ/ in contexts that vary the following vowel (Mann, Sharlin, & Dorman, 1985; Nittrouer & Studdert-Kennedy, 1987) and perception of /s/ versus /st/ in contexts that vary the formant transition into the vowel. The responses of children between 3 and 7 years old have been compared to those of adults. In general, it has been found that children's responses are more variable than those of adults. Nittrouer and Studdert-Kennedy (1987) concluded that perceptual sensitivity to coarticulatory effects may be present from a very early age and that young children's perception may be based more on whole words and syllables than on individual phonemes.

Unanswered Questions

This research raises certain questions regarding the nature of speech sound discrimination. First, is there an inborn human ability to identify certain contrasts that speakers then use in language, or do children learn the contrasts that they hear around them? On the one hand, the ability of the youngest infants to make certain discriminations argues in favor of an innate device. There is, however, contradictory evidence. Eilers, Gavin, and Wilson (1979) tested 6- to 8-month-old infants from English-speaking homes and from Spanish-speaking homes. In English the difference between voiced and voiceless consonants is cued by the amount of voice onset lag time (voicing is started after the initiation of the articulation of the consonant), whereas in Spanish voice onset lead time (voicing begins before the initiation of the articulation of the consonant) is crucial. Both groups of infants were able to distinguish pairs of consonants by lag time, but only the Spanish children made the distinction on the basis of lead time. This and other data suggest that certain perceptual distinctions (such as discriminating voice-voiceless on the basis of voice onset lag time) may be innate. Other distinctions (such as discriminating on the basis of voice onset lead time as in Spanish) may be learned.

Kuhl (1980) suggests that we do not have sufficient evidence to answer this question regarding innateness. However, Aslin and Pisoni (1980) propose a compromise view called *the atunement theory*. This theory holds that infants are capable of making at least some phonetic-contrast discriminations at birth, but this ability is not fully developed. Early experience is needed to sharpen discrimination abilities. Thus, because experience does play a role, children are likely to become more attuned to contrasts important in the language they hear around them.

The innateness question may have relevance for the clinician in determining the role of perceptual training in a remediation program. If much of speech perception is innate, then it is less likely that articulation errors are a result of faulty per-

ception or, if they are, that the clinician can improve the child's ability to perceive or discriminate the correct sound. If children learn to identify contrasts, then faulty perceptual learning may affect articulation and may be improved.

A question that is important to the speech-language pathologist is the following: What is the relationship between perception and production or, more importantly, what is the role of perception in determining articulation errors and in mediating their correction? Graham and House (1971) observed that their preschool subjects tended to make discrimination errors that were similar to common substitutions. Strange and Broen (1980) found that 3-year-olds who misarticulated /l/ and /r/ had higher error rates on the discrimination task than those with correct articulation. However, the developmental data do not provide a clear answer to the perception/production question. Further information can be gained from studies involving children with articulation problems (see chapter 9).

SUMMARY

Analysis of the developing speech of normal children suggests that learning the phonological system of a language is a rule-governed process. In order to describe the acquisition process, researchers have collected data on the speech sound production of large numbers of children at a given age, or they have examined the development of one or a few children over time. Based on these data, differing theories have been proposed regarding the nature of the rules and learning strategies. These theories can be divided into the following groups: behavioral theory, structuralist theory, natural theory, prosodic theory, and interactionist-discovery theory.

Children tend to follow the same general sequence of development despite the fact that ages for acquisition vary greatly. A great deal of important learning with regard to speech perception and the basics of speech production occurs during the

first year of life, before the child begins to produce intelligible speech. We expect children to say their first consistent words at about 1 year, to be intelligible by 3 years, and to have near-perfect articulation by the time they begin school. Continued development of metalinguistic skills occurs during the school-age years.

The development of meaningful speech and the errors that children make can be described in relationship to speech sound segments, distinctive features, phonological processes, or a generative model. More often than not, children with disordered articulation will demonstrate the same kinds of errors as younger normal children. Their speech production can be described in the same ways. Therefore, information about normal development is imperative for designing effective remediation procedures.

REFERENCES

Arlt, P. B., & Goodban, M. T. (1976). A comparative study of articulation acquisition as based on a study of 240 normals, aged three to six. *Language, Speech and Hearing Services in Schools, 7,* 173–180.

Aslin, R. N., & Pisoni, D. B. (1980). Some developmental processes in speech perception. In G. H. Yeni-Komshian, J. F. Kavanagh, & C. A. Ferguson (Eds.), *Child phonology: Vol. II. Perception.* New York: Academic Press.

Barton, D. P. (1976). *The role of perception in the acquisition of phonology.* Unpublished doctoral dissertation, University of London.

Barton, D. (1980). Phonemic perception in children. In G. H. Yeni-Komshian, J. F. Kavanagh, & C. A. Ferguson (Eds.), *Child Phonology: Vol. II. Perception.* New York: Academic Press.

Bassi, C. (1983). Development at 4 years. In J. V. Irwin & S. P. Wong (Eds.), *Phonological development in children 18 to 72 months.* Carbondale, IL: Southern Illinois University Press.

Berko Gleason, J. (1989). *The development of language* (2nd ed.). Columbus, OH: Merrill.

Blasdell, R., & Jensen, P. (1970). Stress and word position as determinants of imitation in first-language learners. *Journal of Speech and Hearing Research, 13,* 193–202.

Braine, M. D. S. (1974). On what might constitute learnable phonology. *Language, 50,* 270–299.

Bricker, W. A. (1967). Errors in echoic behavior of pre-school children. *Journal of Speech and Hearing Research, 7,* 67–76.

Burling, R. (1959). Language development of a Garo and English-speaking child. *Word, 15,* 45–68.

Cairns, H. S., & Williams, F. (1972). An analysis of the substitution errors of a group of standard English-speaking children. *Journal of Speech and Hearing Research, 15,* 811–820.

Calfee, R., Chapman, R., & Venezsky, R. (1972). How a child needs to think to learn to read. In L. Gregg (Ed.), *Cognition in learning and memory.* New York: Wiley.

Calfee, R., Lindamood, P., & Lindamood, C. (1973). Acoustic phonemic skills and reading: kindergarten through twelfth grade. *Journal of Educational Psychology, 64,* 293–298.

Carlson, P., & Anisfield, M. (1969). Some observations on the linguistic competence of a 2-year-old child. *Child Development, 40,* 569–575.

Catts, H. W., & Kamhi, A. G. (1984). Simplification of /s/ + stop clusters: A developmental perspective. *Journal of Speech and Hearing Research, 27,* 556–561.

Chabon, S. S., & Prelock, P. A. (1987). Approaches used to assess phonemic awareness: There is more to an elephant than meets the eye. *Journal of Childhood Communication Disorders, 10,* 95–106.

Chomsky, N., & Halle, M. (1968). *The sound pattern of English.* New York: Harper & Row.

Cruttenden, A. (1970). A phonetic study of babbling. *British Journal of Disorders of Communication, 5,* 110–117.

Crystal, D., Fletcher, P., and Garman, M. (1976). The grammatical analysis of language disability: A procedure for assessment and remediation. London: Edward Arnold.

Cutting, J. E., & Eimas, P. D. (1975). Phonetic feature analyzers and the processing of speech in infants. In J. F. Kavanagh & J. E. Cutting (Eds.), *The role of speech in language.* Cambridge: MIT Press.

DeBoysson-Bardies, B., Sagart, L., & Durand, C. (1984). Discernible differences in the babbling of infants according to target language. *Journal of Child Language, 11,* 1–15.

DeLaguna, G. (1927). *Speech: Its function and development.* New Haven: Yale University Press.

Donahue, M. (1986). Phonological constraints on the emergence of two-word utterances. *Journal of Child Language, 13,* 209–218.

Dyson, A. T. (1986). Development of velar consonants among normal two-year-olds. *Journal of Speech and Hearing Research, 29,* 493–498.

Dyson, A., & Paden, E. (1983). Some phonological acquisition strategies by two-year-olds. *Journal of Childhood Communication Disorders, 7,* 6–18.

Edwards, M. L. (1974). Perception and production in child phonology: The testing of four hypotheses. *Journal of Child Language, 1,* 205–219.

Edwards, M. L. (1979). Phonological processes in fricative acquisition. *Papers and Reports on Child Language Development, 17,* 98–105.

Edwards, M. L., & Shriberg, L. D. (1983). *Phonology: Applications in communicative disorders.* San Diego: College Hill Press.

Eilers, R. E. (1977). Context sensitive perception of naturally produced stop and fricative consonants by infants. *Journal of the Acoustical Society of America, 61,* 1321–1336.

Eilers, R. E., Gavin, W., & Wilson, W. R. (1979). Linguistic experience and phonemic perception in infancy. *Child Development, 50,* 14–18.

Eilers, R. E., & Minifie, F. D. (1975). Fricative discrimination in early infancy. *Journal of Speech and Hearing Research, 18,* 158–167.

Eilers, R. E., Wilson, W. R., & Moore, J. M. (1977). Developmental changes in speech discrimination in infants. *Journal of Speech and Hearing Research, 20,* 766–780.

Elbert, M. (1985). Cognitive aspects of articulation learning. In *Children's phonology disorders: pathways and patterns* (pp. 9–18). Rockville, MD: American Speech-Language-Hearing Association.

Elbert, M., Dinnsen, D. A., & Weismer G. (Eds.). (1984). *Phonological theory and the misarticulating child.* Rockville, MD: American Speech-Language-Hearing Association.

Fee, J., & Ingram, D. (1982). Reduplication as a strategy of phonological development. *Journal of Child Language, 9,* 41–54.

Ferguson, C. A. (1973). Fricatives in child language acquisition. *Papers and Reports on Child Language Development* (Stanford University), *60,* 1–60.

Ferguson, C. A. (1978). Learning to pronounce: The earliest stages of phonological development in the child. In F. D. Minifie & L. L. Lloyd (Eds.), *Communicative and cognitive abilities: Early behavioral assessment.* Baltimore: University Park Press.

Ferguson, C. A., & Farwell, C. B. (1975). Words and sounds in early language acquisition. *Language, 51,* 419–439.

Ferguson, C. A., & Garnica, O. K. (1975). Theories of phonological development. In E. H. Lenneberg & E. Lenneberg (Eds.), *Foundations of language development.* New York: Academic Press.

Fox, B., & Routh, D. K. (1975). Analyzing spoken language into words, syllables, and phonemes: A developmental study. *Journal of Psycholinguistic Research, 4,* 331–342.

Garnica, O. K. (1973). The development of phonemic perception. In T. Moore (Ed.), *Cognitive development and the acquisition of language.* New York: Academic Press.

Gilbert, J. (1982). Babbling and the deaf child: A commentary on Lenneberg et al. (1965) and Lenneberg (1967). *Journal of Child Language, 9,* 511–515.

Graham, L. W., & House, A. S. (1971). Phonological oppositions in children: A perceptual study. *Journal of the Acoustical Society of America, 49,* 559–566.

Gruber, J. S. (1973). Playing with distinctive features in babbling of infants. In C. A. Ferguson & D. I. Slobin (Eds.), *Studies of child language development.* New York: Holt, Rinehart and Winston.

Grunwell, P. (1982). *Clinical phonology.* Rockville, Maryland: Aspen Systems.

Haelsig, P. C., & Madison, C. L. (1986). A study of phonological processes exhibited by 3-, 4-, and 5-year-old children. *Language, Speech, and Hearing Services in Schools, 17,* 107–114.

Hakes, D. (1980). The development of metalinguistic abilities in children. New York: Springer-Verlag.

Halliday, M. (1975). *Learning how to mean: Explorations in the development of language.* London: Edward Arnold.

Hare, G. (1983). Development at 2 years. In J. V. Irwin and S. P. Wong (Eds.), *Phonological development in children 18 to 72 months.* Carbondale, IL: Southern Illinois University Press.

Hodson, B. W., & Paden, E. P. (1983). *Targeting intelligible speech.* San Diego: College Hill Press.

Ingram, D. (1976). *Phonological disability in children.* New York: American Elsevier.

Ingram, D., Christensen, L., Veach, S., & Webster, B. (1980). The acquisition of word-initial fricatives and affricates in English by children between 2 and 6 years. In G. H. Yeni-Komshian, J. F. Kavanagh, & C. Ferguson (Eds.), *Child phonology: Vol. 1. Production.* New York: Academic Press.

Irwin, O. C. (1947a). Infant speech: Consonant sounds according to manner of articulation. *Journal of Speech Disorders, 12,* 402–404.

Irwin, O. C. (1947b). Infant speech: Consonant sounds according to place of articulation. *Journal of Speech Disorders, 12,* 397–401.

Irwin, O. C. (1947c). Infant speech: The problem of variability. *Journal of Speech Disorders, 12,* 173–176.

Irwin, O. C. (1948a). Infant speech: Development of vowel sounds. *Journal of Speech and Hearing Disorders, 13,* 31–34.

Irwin, O. C. (1948b). Infant speech: The effect of family occupational status and of age on use of sound types. *Journal of Speech and Hearing Disorders, 13,* 224–226.

Irwin, O. C. (1948c). Infant speech: The effect of family occupational status and of age on sound frequency. *Journal of Speech and Hearing Disorders, 13*, 320–323.

Irwin, O. C. (1951). Infant speech: Consonantal position. *Journal of Speech and Hearing Disorders, 16*, 159–161.

Irwin, O. C. (1952). Speech development in the young child: Some factors related to the speech development of the infant and young child. *Journal of Speech and Hearing Disorders, 17*, 269–279.

Irwin, O. C., & Chen, H. P. (1946). Infant speech: Vowel and consonant frequency. *Journal of Speech Disorders, 11*, 123–125.

Irwin, J. V., and Wong, S. P. (Eds.). (1983). *Phonological development in children 18 to 72 months*. Carbondale, IL: Southern Illinois University Press.

Jakobson, R. (1968). *Child language, aphasia and phonological universals*. The Hague: Mouton.

Jakobson, R. (1971). *Studies on child language and aphasia*. The Hague: Mouton.

Jakobson, R., Fant, G., & Halle, M. (1963). *Preliminaries to speech analysis: The distinctive features and their correlates*. Cambridge, MA: MIT Press.

Jespersen, O. (1922). *Language: Its nature, development and origin*. London: George Allen & Unwin.

Kamhi, A., & Catts, H. (1986). Toward an understanding of developmental language and reading disorders. *Journal of Speech and Hearing Disorders, 51*, 337–347.

Kenney, K. W., & Prather, E. M. (1986). Articulation development in preschool children: Consistency of productions. *Journal of Speech and Hearing Research, 29*, 29–36.

Kiparsky, P., & Menn, L. (1977). On the acquisition of phonology. In J. Macnamara, (Ed.), *Language learning and thought*. New York: Holt, Rinehart and Winston.

Kuhl, P. K. (1977). Speech perception in early infancy and perceptual constancy for the vowel categories /a/ and /ɔ/ [Abstract]. *Journal of the Acoustical Society of America, 61* (Suppl. 1), 539.

Kuhl P. (1979). The perception of speech in early infancy. In M. Lass (Ed.), *Speech and language: Advances in basic research and practice* (Vol. I). New York: Academic Press.

Kuhl, P. K. (1980). Perceptual constancy for speech-sound categories in early infancy. In G. H. Yeni-Komshian, J. F. Kavanagh, & C. A. Ferguson

(Eds.), *Child phonology: Vol. II. Perception*. New York: Academic Press.

Leiberman, I., Shankweiler, D., Fischer, W., & Carter, B. (1974). Explicit syllable and phoneme segmentation in the young child. *Journal of Experimental Child Psychology, 18*, 201–121.

Lenneberg, E. H. (1967). *Biological foundations of language*. New York: Wiley.

Lenneberg, E. H., Rebelsky, F. G., & Nichols, I. A. (1965). The vocalizations of infants born to deaf and hearing parents. *Human Development, 8*, 23–27.

Leonard, L. B., Rowan, L. E., Morris, B., & Fey, M. (1982). Intra-word phonological variability in younger children. *Journal of Child Language, 9*, 55–69.

Leopold, W. (1947). *Speech development of a bilingual child: A linguist's record*. Evanston, IL: Northwestern University Press.

Locke, J. L. (1980). Prediction of child speech errors: Implications for a theory of acquisition. In G. H. Yeni-Komshian, J. F. Kavanagh, & C. A. Ferguson (Eds.), *Child phonology: Vol. I. Production*. New York: Academic Press.

Locke, J. L. (1983). *Phonological acquisition and change*. New York: Academic Press.

Locke, J. L. (1985). Epigenetic paths to phonological disorders. In *Children's phonology disorders: pathways and patterns*. Rockville, MD: American Speech-Language-Hearing Association.

Lowe, R. J., Knutson, P. J., & Monson, M. A. (1985). Incidence of fronting in preschool children. *Language, Speech, and Hearing Services in Schools, 16*, 119–123.

Macken, M. A. (1980). Aspects of the acquisition of stop consonants: A cross-linguistic perspective. In G. H. Yeni-Komshian, J. F. Kavanagh, & C. A. Ferguson (Eds.), *Child phonology: Vol. I. Production*. New York: Academic Press.

Macken, M. A., & Barton, D. P. (1980). A longitudinal study of the acquisition of the voicing contrast in American-English word-initial stops, as measured by voice onset time. *Journal of Child Language, 7*, 41–74.

Mann, V. A., Sharlin, H. M., & Dorman, M. (1985). Children's perception of sibilants: The relation between articulation and perceptual development. *Journal of Experimental Child Psychology, 39*, 252–264.

Maskavinic, A. S., Cairns, G. F., Butterfield, E. C., & Weamer, D. K. (1981). Longitudinal observations of individual infants' vocalizations.

Mattingly, I. (1972). Reading, the linguistic process, and linguistic awareness (pp. 131–149). In J. Kavanagh & I. Mattingly (Eds.), *Language by ear and by eye.* Cambridge, MA: MIT Press.

Maxwell, E. M., & Rockman, B. K. (1984). Procedures of linguistic analysis of misarticulated speech. In M. Elbert, D. Dinnsen, & G. Weismer (Eds.), *Phonological theory and the misarticulating child* (ASHA Monograph No 22). Rockville, MD: American Speech-Language-Hearing Association.

McGeogh, J. (1943). *The psychology of human learning.* New York: Longman.

Menn, L. (1976). Evidence for an interactionist-discovery theory of child phonology. *Papers and Reports on Child Language Development, Stanford University, 12,* 169–177.

Menn, L. (1980). Phonological theory and child phonology. In G. H. Yeni-Komshian, J. F. Kavanagh, & C. A. Ferguson (Eds.), *Child phonology: Vol. I. Production.* New York: Academic Press.

Menyuk, P. (1968). The role of distinctive features in children's acquisition of phonology. *Journal of Speech and Hearing Research, 11,* 138–146.

Menyuk, P., & Anderson, S. (1969). Children's identification and reproduction of /w/, /r/, /l/. *Journal of Speech and Hearing Disorders, 12,* 39–52.

Messer, S. (1967). Implicit phonology in children. *Journal of Verbal Learning and Verbal Behavior, 6,* 609–613.

Miller, C. L., & Morse, P. A. (1976). The "heart" of categorical speech discrimination in young infants. *Journal of Speech and Hearing Research, 19,* 578–589.

Morrongiello, B. A., Robson, R. C., Best, C. T., & Clifton, R. K. (1984). Trading relations in the perception of speech by 5-year-old children. *Journal of Experimental Child Psychology, 37,* 231–250.

Moskowitz, A. I. (1970). The two-year-old stage in the acquisition of English phonology. *Language, 46,* 420–441.

Moskowitz, A. I. (1973). Acquisition of phonology and syntax: A preliminary study. In G. Hinitikka, J. Moravcsik, & P. Suppes (Eds.), *Approaches to natural language.* Dordrecht, Holland: Reidel.

Mowrer, O. H. (1952). Speech development in the young: The autism theory of speech development and some clinical applications. *Journal of Speech and Hearing Disorders, 17,* 263–268.

Muller, M. (1840). *The science of language.* New York: Longman.

Nakazima, S. A. (1962). A comparative study of the speech development of Japanese and American English in childhood. *Studies in Phonology, 2,* 17.

Nakazima, S. (1975). Phonemicization and symbolization in language development. In E. H. Lenneberg & E. Lenneberg (Eds.), *Foundations of language development.* New York: Academic Press.

Nittrouer, S., & Studdert-Kennedy, M. (1987). The role of coarticulatory effects in the perception of fricatives by children and adults. *Journal of Speech and Hearing Research, 30,* 319–329.

Oller, D. K. (1976, November). *Analysis of infant vocalizations: A linguistic and speech scientific perspective.* Miniseminar presented at the American Speech-Language-Hearing Association Annual Convention, Houston.

Oller, D. K. (1980). The emergence of speech sounds in infancy. In G. Yeni-Komshian, J. A. Kavanagh, & C. A. Ferguson (Eds.), *Child phonology: Vol. 1. Production* (pp. 93–112). New York: Academic Press.

Oller, D. K., & Eilers, R. E. (1982). Similarity of babbling in Spanish- and English-learning babies. *Journal of Child Language, 9,* 565–577.

Oller, D. K., Wieman, L. A., Doyle, W. J., & Ross, C. (1975). Infant babbling and speech. *Journal of Child Language, 2,* 1–11.

Olmsted, D. (1971). *Out of the mouths of babes.* The Hague: Mouton.

Olney, R. L., & Scholnick, E. K. (1976). Adult judgments of age and linguistic differences in infant vocalization. *Journal of Child Language, 3,* 145–155.

Piaget, J. (1962). *Play, dreams, and imitation in childhood.* New York: Norton.

Poole, E. (1934). Genetic development of articulation of consonant sounds in speech. *Elementary English Review, 11,* 159–161.

Prather, E., Hedrick, D., & Kern, C. (1975). Articulation development in children aged two to four years. *Journal of Speech and Hearing Research, 40,* 179–191.

Sander, E. (1972). When are speech sounds learned? *Journal of Speech and Hearing Disorders, 37,* 55–63.

Schwartz, R., Leonard, L. B., Wilcox, M. J., & Folger, K. (1980). Again and again: Reduplication in child phonology. *Journal of Child Language, 7,* 75–88.

Shriberg, L., & Kwiatkowski, J. (1980). *Natural process analysis*. New York: Wiley.

Shvachkin, N. K. (1973). The development of phonemic speech perception in early childhood. In C. A. Ferguson & D. I. Slobin (Eds.), *Studies of child language development*. New York: Holt, Rinehart and Winston.

Singh, S. (1976). *Distinctive features: Theory and validation*. Baltimore: University Park Press.

Singh, S., and Frank, D. C. (1972). A distinctive feature analysis of the consonantal substitutions pattern. *Language and Speech, 15,* 209–218.

Smit, A. B. (1986). Ages of speech sound acquisition: Comparisons and critiques of several normative studies. *Language, Speech, and Hearing Services in Schools, 17,* 175–186.

Smith, A. (1792). A dissertation on the origin of language. In *The theory of moral sentiments,* 7th ed. London.

Snow, K. (1963). A detailed analysis of the articulation responses of normal first grade children. *Journal of Speech and Hearing Disorders, 6,* 277–290.

Stampe, D. (1969). The acquisition of phonetic representation. In R. I. Binnick, A. Davison, G. M. Greene, & J. L. Morgan (Eds.), *Papers from the Fifth Regional Meeting, Chicago Linguistic Society*. Chicago: Chicago Linguistic Society.

Stoel-Gammon, C. (1985). Phonetic inventories. 15–24 months: A longitudinal study. *Journal of Speech and Hearing Research, 28,* 505–512.

Stoel-Gammon, C., & Cooper, J. A. (1984). Patterns of early lexical and phonological development. *Journal of Child Language, 11,* 247–271.

Stoel-Gammon, C., & Dunn, C. (1985). *Normal and disordered phonology in children*. Baltimore: University Park Press.

Strange, W., & Broen, P. A. (1980). Perception and production of approximant consonants by 3-year-olds: A first study. In G. H. Yeni-Komshian, J. F. Kavanagh, & C. A. Ferguson (Eds.), *Child phonology: Vol. II. Perception*. New York: Academic Press.

Sykes, J. L. (1940). A study of the spontaneous vocalizations of young deaf children. *Psychological Monographs, 52,* 104–123.

Templin, M. (1957). *Certain language skills in children: Their development and interrelationships*. Institute of Child Welfare, Monograph 26. Minneapolis: The University of Minnesota Press.

Tonkova-Yampol'skava, R. V. (1973). Development of speech intonation in infants during the first two years of life. In C. A. Ferguson & D. I. Slobin (Eds.), *Studies of child language development*. New York: Holt, Rinehart and Winston.

Treiman, R., & Baron, T. (1981). Segmental analysis ability. In G. E. MacKinnon & T. G. Waller (Eds.), *Reading research: Advances in theory and practice* (Vol. 3). New York: Academic Press.

Velten, H. (1943). The growth of phonemic and lexical patterns in infant language. *Language, 19,* 281–292.

Vihman, M. (1981). Phonology and the development of the lexicon: Evidence from children's errors. *Journal of Child Language, 8,* 239–264.

Vihman, M., Macken, M., Miller, R., & Simmons, H. (1981). From babbling to speech: A reassessment of the continuity issue. *Language, 61,* 397–445.

Waterson, N. (1971). Child phonology: A prosodic view. *Journal of Linguistics, 7,* 179–211.

Weiner. (1979). Phonological process analysis. Baltimore: University Park Press.

Weiner, F., & Bernthal, J. (1976). Acquisition of phonetic features in children 2–6 years old. In S. Singh (Ed.), *Distinctive feature theory and validation*. Baltimore: University Park Press.

Weir, R. H. (1962). *Language in the crib*. The Hague: Mouton.

Weir, R. H. (1966). Some questions on the child's learning of phonology. In F. Smith & G. Miller (Eds.), *The genesis of language: A psycholinguistic approach*. Cambridge, MA: MIT Press.

Wellman, B., Case, I., Mengurt, I., & Bradbury, D. (1931). Speech sounds of young children. *University of Iowa Studies in Child Welfare, 5,* (2).

Whitney, W. (1868). *Language and the study of language*. New York: Scribner's.

Williams, L., & Golenski, J. (1979). Infant behavioral state and speech sound discrimination. *Child Development, 50,* 1243–1246.

Winitz, H. (1969). *Articulatory acquisition and behavior*. Englewood Cliffs, NJ: Prentice-Hall.

Yeni-Komshian, G., Kavanagh, J., & Ferguson, C. (Eds.). (1980). *Child phonology: Vol. 1. Production*. New York: Academic Press.

Zlatkin, M. A., & Koenigsknecht, R. A. (1976). Development of the voicing contrast: A comparison of voice onset time in stop perception and production. *Journal of Speech and Hearing Research, 19,* 93–111.

CHAPTER 4 | Assessment of Articulatory and Phonological Disorders

In an articulatory or phonological assessment, a clinician's task is to evaluate the nature of the disorder by sampling the speech, analyzing it, and specifying its characteristics to provide a base for therapeutic intervention. The purpose of this chapter is to explain how to carry out the assessment. Although many of our evaluation procedures have been used for years, many others are new. The first section of this chapter explains traditional assessment procedures used in any articulatory evaluation. In the second section, a discussion of more recent linguistic rule-based procedures is presented. Knowledge of both is important in appraising the wide variety of articulatory and phonological disorders a speech-language pathologist will encounter.

TRADITIONAL METHODS OF ASSESSMENT

Obtaining Samples of Speech

Screening Tests. Screening tests identify persons whose speech may need correction. They are commonly used in preschool programs and public

This chapter was written by **Parley W. Newman** and **Nancy A. Creaghead**.

schools and may also be used as part of entrance procedures in colleges and universities. When people do not pass a screening examination, they are referred for a more formal appraisal.

For school-aged children and adults, screening examinations are relatively brief and simple. They usually consist of an inquiry of name and a simple question or two to elicit a brief sample of conversational speech. Then the person being tested might be asked to repeat a few words or sentences that contain examples of the speech sounds most frequently misarticulated. Alternatively, test sentences might be constructed so that, in one or two sentences, all of the consonant sounds of the language are included. These sentences may be read or repeated by the individual being screened. In order to pass the screening, the individual must produce all sounds within acceptable limits, i.e., in such a way that they do not call attention to themselves. A few screening tests for articulation are available commercially; they can be obtained from sources given in Appendix 4.1. In addition, instruments that are designed to screen overall speech and language skills will include articulation.

For preschool children, the screening procedures and criteria for passing may not be so clearcut. Young children may not produce an adequate spontaneous sample in response to questions, and they may be unable to repeat long sentences that contain a variety of speech sounds. In addition, holding their interest may be difficult. For these reasons, toys or pictures of objects containing the target sounds may be needed. Eliciting an adequate sample from young children may take longer than from school-aged children or adults.

For preschool children, the criteria for passing the screening will be based on developmental norms for the child's age. The clinician must evaluate the number and types of sounds in error in order to determine whether the child passes or fails. Standardized instruments for screening preschool children such as the Preschool Speech and Language Screening Test (Fluharty, 1976) base the pass/fail criterion on the number of sounds in error. Clinicians must examine the pass/fail criterion of the screening test used because this criterion may ultimately affect the children selected for further evaluation (Ritterman, Zook-Herman, Carlson, & Kinde, 1982).

Picture Inventories. For many years, speech clinicians have used pictures to obtain samples of speech from children. In general, a child names a picture of an object or event. The word spoken contains a speech sound that the examiner wishes to hear the child produce, providing the opportunity to assess the child's production of that particular sound. In a typical inventory, there are sufficient pictures so that a production of each speech sound is obtained in the initial, medial, and final positions of words. Another possibility is to ask a child simply to repeat words after the clinician. This would seem to be more efficient than having the subject name pictures on cards, but research findings suggest that the results are not the same. Although the evidence is a bit equivocal and differences are not large, it appears that if the child names pictures, the responses will be more representative of typical performance than will utterances obtained through imitation (Carter & Buck, 1958; Ham, 1958; Kresheck & Socolofsky, 1972; Paynter & Bumpas, 1977; Siegel, Winitz, & Con-

key, 1963; Smith & Ainsworth, 1967; Snow & Milisen, 1954; Templin, 1947). Another reason for using picture cards is motivation. In general, children seem to enjoy naming pictures more than repeating words after the examiner.

There are many picture inventory articulation tests on the market; sources are provided in Appendix 4.1. A clinician may also choose to make a personal set of pictures. Making up one's own set of test cards takes a little time in the beginning, but it provides opportunities for creativity and flexibility. A personal set of cards can be added to, subtracted from, or modified as needs or assessment approaches dictate. For example, the clinician may wish to supplement the main inventory with additional pictures representing the most commonly misarticulated sounds. Or additional cards may be constructed that show pictures whose names contain certain consonant clusters. If a particular stimulus item is not reliable in obtaining the desired response, then a different stimulus card can be substituted readily. In addition, there may be some words particularly suited to a specific locale. Finally, as current events, television shows, and moving pictures create new characters that capture the public imagination, a personal set of articulation cards can be adapted to heighten their interest value.

There are, however, certain disadvantages to consider in constructing one's own test. These include (a) the time required, (b) the potential lack of uniformity of the pictures, (c) the limits of the clinician's knowledge regarding test construction methods, and (d) the difficulty in obtaining a varied population for standardization.

For those who are interested, it might be helpful to describe a personal picture inventory in more detail. A test card should be of convenient size, 3 by 5 inches or 5 by 7 inches. It should contain a few pictures whose names include the phoneme under test. Test words must be appropriate to the vocabulary level of preschool children. It is often convenient to have three pictures on a card: one representing the test phoneme in the initial position of a word, one in the medial position, and one in the final position. For example, three pictures on one card designed to elicit the /s/ might be *sun* (initial), *pencil* (medial), *house* (final). On the back of the card the following information might be provided to aid test presentation and recording of data: (a) the number of the card corresponding to the item number on the test record blank, (b) the symbol of the phoneme under test, and (c) the test words, and perhaps a sentence to foster elicitation of each word. For example, for the test word *sun,* the question might be: What rises in the sky each morning and makes the night go away? With this information on the back of the card, the clinician need not see the face of the card, which is toward the child, yet all information is available to facilitate administration and recording of information. The sequence of the picture cards should correspond to the listing of items on the recording blank. Recording blanks may be obtained commercially or can be developed by the individual. Figure 4.1 gives an example of the front and back of a stimulus card.

Figure 4.2 is an example of a recording form. It is taken from a commercially available articulation test called the T-MAC Test of Minimal Articulation Competence (Secord, 1981b). Note the following information on the recording form:

1. a number to correspond with the appropriate test card
2. the symbol representing each phoneme tested
3. the test words representing the phoneme in the initial (pre), medial (inter), and final (post) positions of the test word. The terms prevocalic, intervocalic, and postvocalic refer to the relationship of the consonant to the vowel in the syllable, i.e., whether the consonant precedes the vowel, occurs between two vowels, or follows the vowel.
4. the last column in each set headed "Stim." This is an abbreviation of the word *stimulability,* which will be explained later.

Note also that in a few cases the full complement of initial, medial, and final test words is missing. These absences reflect instances in English in which some phonemes do not occur in certain po-

sitions of words. For example, in item 8, /h/ does not appear in the final position, and in item 12, /w/ does not occur in the final position. These instances reflect phonotactic constraints of the language.

There are varied sources of pictures. They may be cut out of magazines and pasted on cards, or they may be drawn if the clinician has an artistic bent. Pictures should be in color, and if the clinician draws or paints them, they should be of consistent style. It is helpful to laminate the cards so that children can handle them without fear of damage. Actual items like a button or coin make the cards somewhat difficult to handle. The more of these there are and the bulkier they are, the more unwieldy the set becomes.

Sometimes children respond to a picture by not saying the word it was intended to elicit. If the clinician then names the picture for the child, this accurate production may elicit a better than usual performance from the child. Therefore, it is wise to have prompts available for all test words in order to avoid giving the child a model to imitate. The clinician might say, "Can you give me another name for the picture?" Or the examiner might name the picture, and then say something in addition to diminish the influence of the spoken cue. For example, refer to the picture card shown in Figure 4.1. Suppose the child names the test word, *house,* as "home." The examiner is listening for the production of /s/ in the final position, and the word *home* does not satisfy the test requirement. So another name for the picture is requested. If the child says "house," then the objective is achieved. But if the child demurs or cannot think of another word, the clinician might say, "You are right. People live in homes. A place where people live is also called a *house.* Now can you tell me another word for *home*?" Responses elicited through the interjection of an utterance following the test word are called *delayed imitation.* This approach is suggested because it is reasonable to assume that the intervening words will weaken the influence of cues provided in the model. However,

Back of picture-naming card for examiner's use

12. /s/

sun

pencil

house

Sun: What rises in the sky each morning and makes the night go away?

Pencil: What do we write with?

House: What do we call a place where people live?

FIGURE 4.1
Front and back sides of articulation test card.

Consonants

Card	Phoneme	Pre	Inter	Post	Stim.	Card	Phoneme	Pre	Inter	Post	Stim.
1	p	pie	apple	cup		7	f	fire	elephant	knife	
	b	boat	baby	bathtub			v	vest	shovel	five	
2	t	table	letter	hat		8	h	house	treehouse		
	d	door	ladder	bed		9	tʃ	chair	matches	watch	
3	k	cat	turkey	book			dʒ	giraffe	pajamas	cage	
	g	gun	wagon	egg		10	m	monkey	hammer	comb	
4	s	sun	glasses	bus			n	nail	banana	bone	
	z	zipper	scissors	nose		11	ŋ		hanger	ring	
5	ʃ	shoe	dishes	fish		12	w	water	flower		
	ʒ		television	garage			j	yo-yo	yo-yo		
6	θ	thumb	toothache	teeth		13	l	lamp	balloon	ball	
	ð	that	feather	smooth			r	rabbit	carrot		

Comments:

FIGURE 4.2

Example of recording form for an articulation test. (*Source: T-MAC: Test of Minimal Articulation Competence* (p. 2) by Wayne Secord, 1981, Columbus: Merrill Publishing Co. 1986, The Psychological Corporation. Reprinted by permission.)

we do not have research evidence to support this assumption.

Other Tests. Other methods may be used for obtaining samples of speech. For example, for older children and adults who read, lists of sentences to be read aloud are often provided. Many clinicians contend that the use of pictures with these individuals is somewhat demeaning. As with the picture articulation test, a clinician can prepare a set of such sentences or they may be obtained commercially. A number of the articulation tests in Appendix 4.1 contain sentence tests in addition to their picture-naming tests.

In general, sentence tests consist of a list of sentences, each of which is designed to elicit several examples of the same phoneme. The sentences are numbered to correspond to the recording blank. As far as is possible, each sentence is created so test words provide the opportunity for the phoneme under test to appear in the initial, medial, and final positions of words.

Other procedures to obtain samples of speech are discussed later in this chapter. These other methods, in some cases, may be more valid than picture-naming procedures. Nevertheless, picture-naming tests have clinical utility, are widely used, and probably will continue to be used for the foreseeable future. Some of their limitations will be considered later in the chapter.

Although all of the tests listed in Appendix 4.1 are generally similar, certain differences may make one more appropriate than another for a given child or setting. The factors to be considered in choosing a test include: the age of the client, the time to be spent in administration, whether the test is to be used to make a diagnosis or for planning remediation, whether there is a need for a score, and finally individual clinician preferences. For example, the Goldman-Fristoe Test of Articulation (Goldman & Fristoe, 1986) has large colorful pictures of very common objects. Because more than one sound is examined in each word, the administration time is short. For these reasons, this may be an excellent choice for preschool children; however, older children or adults may find the pictures too "childish." In addition, the clinician may prefer to test only one sound per word. The Photo Articulation Test (Pendergast, Dickey, Selmar, & Soder, 1969) includes actual photographs on cards that look somewhat like playing cards. There is a different card for each sound in each word position. These materials may be more acceptable to school-aged children, and the increased number of words may provide the clinician with additional information; however, preschoolers may not know all the words or be able to finish the task. The Arizona Articulation Proficiency Scale (Fudala, 1974) gives an articulation score. This may be useful for research purposes or for justification of case selection. The clinician must be familiar with both the available instruments and the needs of the client and setting in order to make an informed choice.

Recording Responses

Several times, thus far, reference has been made to recording responses on a recording blank. What does the examiner record on these blanks? There is considerable variety in recording methods, but the following description represents common techniques. If the child produces the phoneme correctly, a check or plus mark might be made on the recording sheet. However, any type of mark might be misinterpreted later when reviewing the recording form, so the best procedure to denote a correct response is to leave the item blank. Refer again to Figure 4.2, and note there is a separate blank for the phoneme under test in the initial, medial, and final position of words. Thus an entry is made for the manner in which the phoneme is produced in at least three positions, except when the language does not allow a particular sound in a particular word position.

There are three general ways in which a speech sound is produced in error: (a) distortion, (b) substitution, and (c) omission. These types of errors are presented in this particular order to represent degrees of severity (Jordan, 1960; Milisen, 1954; Van Riper & Irwin, 1958). Distortions, which are considered the least severe type of misarticulation, offer the most difficulty in recording if the examiner is attempting to be precise. At the simplest level, the examiner could simply make some type of notation such as a capital D to indicate the error was one of distortion. That is, the sound was not omitted, neither was another sound substituted in its place, but to some degree it was produced in an unusual manner. Milisen (1954) attempted more precision in recording the nature of distortion errors by using a rating scale. A rating of 3 was given to a production interpreted to be so severe that it would attract the attention of most lay persons and frequently would make the sound difficult to recognize. A rating of 2 was given to a phoneme production mildly distorted to the degree that it would attract the attention of many lay persons, but would not make it difficult to recognize. He gave a rating of 1 to normal production.

A more precise way of considering distortions is to regard them not as distortions at all but as substitutions. That is, the so-called distorted sound actually represents a substitution of a non-English sound (Van Riper, 1972; Van Riper & Irwin, 1958; Winitz, 1975). For example, one type of lisp is referred to as a *lateral lisp*. It is produced with the tongue in position to produce an /l/, but no voicing occurs, and air is blown out of the mouth. The result is a "slushy" /s/, which might be considered a distortion of the /s/, but in some ways is like a substitution of a devoiced /l/ for an /s/. Another example is the substitution ts/tʃ, as in [tsɛr] for *chair*. This substitution, which is often recorded as a distortion, is actually another affricate that occurs in other languages (e.g., German and Russian), but not in English.

Narrow phonetic transcription can usually indicate the manner and place of a sound substitution that might be recorded as a distortion. If this type of recording is to be made, it is good practice to tape-record the child's responses so that utterances can be played back and analyzed more carefully. Thus, the difference between a substitution and a distortion is frequently based upon the transcription skills of the examiner. Does it really matter whether an error is recorded as a substitution or a distortion? The answer depends upon what is done with the information. If a distinctive-feature or phonological process analysis is going to be made, the features present in the substituted sound can contribute to the data of the analysis. Distinctive-feature and phonological process analyses are discussed later in this chapter and in chapter 14. If the error production is simply identified and the clinician plans to correct the individual phoneme, then perhaps it does not matter how the error is classified.

The preceding discussion of distortions required using the term *substitution*. However, by tradition, a *substitution* consists of replacing the intended, correct phoneme with another one from the language. Examples are common. For instance, /θ/ may be substituted for /s/ as in *think* for *sink*, /f/ for /θ/ as in *baftub* for *bathtub*, /w/ for /r/ as in *wabbit* for *rabbit*, and so forth. On the recording blank of the articulation test, common practice is simply to write in the blank the sound substituted for the target phoneme. When a recording blank is not being used, the examples just discussed are commonly written θ/s (substitution of /θ/ for /s/), f/θ (substitution of /f/ for /θ/), and w/r (substitution of /w/ for /r/).

Omissions are recorded with a minus sign (−) or a zero in the appropriate record blank. If a zero

is used, a slash should be placed in it so that it is not confused with /o/. The notation would look like this: Ø. Actually, this notation is very similar to a phonetic symbol, but its use is rare and does not create problems.

Omissions are not as simple as they first appear. Just as a so-called distortion is in reality a substitution, many omissions may also be substitutions of a more subtle nature. As Van Riper and Irwin (1958) point out, some omissions, when examined closely, are actually unvoiced articulatory gestures lacking the breath or voice of the correct sound or a substituted sound. Weismer, Dinnsen, and Elbert (1981) analyzed the acoustic signal of three children who omitted final stops. Two of the three children produced longer vowel durations that were reliably sensitive to the voicing characteristic of the omitted final stop. Smit and Bernthal (1983a) also found that "syllable reducers," children who reduced CCV or CVC syllables to CV syllables (reduction of the consonant cluster or omission of the final consonant), tended to use longer vowels on average. There were some ambiguities in the data, but in some instances the syllable reducers had significantly larger vowel duration ratios between minimal pairs with final voiced and voiceless obstruents (*bead–beet*). Again, this revealed evidence of the voicing characteristic of some word-final obstruents. Some of the syllable reducers demonstrated a second kind of contrast in production by using a glottal stop for a final voiceless target (/biʔ/ for *beet*) and a vowel glide into the last word of the carrier phrase (/bij/ for *bead* before *away*). These data clearly imply that in many instances the "omission" is actually represented by some feature or articulatory gesture. As Elbert and McReynolds (1978) and Bankson and Bernthal (1982a) put it, some children "mark" the so-called omitted sounds in their productions.

There is another type of articulation error: addition. Additions are seen much less frequently than the other error types in functional articulation disorders. An example might be the child who says [stərit] for *street*. This type of addition error is called an *intrusive schwa*. In current discussions of phonological processes it would be called epenthesis. This error may occur as an intermediate step in learning to produce consonant blends. Additions are more common in individuals who exhibit the articulation disorder known as *apraxia of speech* (described in chapter 10).

Other types of errors may not be captured on the recording form of a picture articulation test. One of these is assimilation. For example, for the test word *dog*, a child might say [gɔg]. In this case g/d might be recorded whereas further analysis might reveal that the child uses /d/ correctly in other phonetic contexts that do not elicit assimilation (i.e., words without /g/). A second example is the child who says [tɛfon] for *telephone*. Recording /l/ as an omission does not reflect the fact that the child deleted an entire syllable. These issues will be discussed in greater detail later in the chapter.

Testing for Stimulability

A logical first step in the evaluation of the articulation test results is to test for stimulability. Curtis (1956, p. 115) includes this as the last step of the articulation test. The purpose of the test of stimulability is to determine how readily a child can modify her errors when asked to imitate the examiner's correct production of them. The term *stimulability* was coined by Milisen (1954), who used three levels of stimulability: sound in isolation, syllable, and word. In Milisen's procedure, the clinician provided a model for the child to imitate and exaggerated the presentation to make the stimulus as vivid as possible. Milisen termed this energetic presentation *integral stimulation*.

The term *stimulation* and the procedure to test a client's ability to imitate misarticulated sounds correctly has been around for a long time (Travis, 1931; Van Riper, 1947). To make the distinction between this relatively common practice and Milisen's attempts at a more vivid form of modeling correct productions, the newer term was introduced. Basically, the procedure required the clinician to produce a sound, syllable, or word so that the child heard it, saw it, and perhaps felt it. Special effort was taken to make the focal point of the articulation as visible as possible. Each error phoneme identified in the articulation test was produced in this way by the clinician, and the child was asked to reproduce it. How well the child performed was, of course, recorded.

Diedrich (1983) describes stimulability testing as a measure of consistency, used to determine if there is consistency in a child's performance on two different speech tasks. The first task is the spontaneous response of the child to a picture stimulus. In the second task, the child imitates the speech model provided by the examiner. The child is consistent if similar errors are made in both tasks. The child is inconsistent to the degree that her productions on the two tasks vary. If the child is consistent, with similar errors in both tasks, the performance is regarded as showing low or poor stimulability. If there are marked differences in performance on the two tasks, the child is said to evidence high or good stimulability.

The concept of stimulability has two possible clinical applications. Both are based upon the assumption that high stimulability indicates readiness in the child to move in the direction of more normal speech. For therapeutic purposes, it would seem that error sounds that are highly stimulable would respond readily to instruction, giving the client feelings of success that would provide motivational impetus. A second implication of high stimulability is that the child may be on the verge of overcoming misarticulations without intervention and may only need more time. Thus, stimulability has been used both as a predictor of therapeutic responsiveness and as a predictor of growth and change through maturation.

Several investigators have reported that the ability of children ages 5 through 7 years to imitate syllables or words is related to the probability of their spontaneously correcting their misarticulations (Carter & Buck, 1958; Farquhar, 1961; Sommers, Leiss, Delp, Gerber, Smith, Revucky, Ellis, & Haley, 1967). Carter and Buck reported in a study of first-grade children that stimulability testing can be used for such predictive purposes. They suggested that first-grade children who correctly imitate nonsense syllables containing the error sounds 75% of the time (7 out of 9 times) are likely to correct those sounds themselves, and thus instruction is not recommended for such children. Kisatsky (1967), in an evaluation of the Carter-Buck prognostic tests, compared pretest to posttest gains over a 6-month period with no speech therapy between a group of kindergarten children identified as a high-stimulability group and a similar group of children identified as a low-stimulability group. Results indicated that significantly higher posttest articulation scores were obtained by the high-stimulability group, which showed 50% spontaneous correction. The low-stimulability group had only 10% spontaneous correction.

A thorough review of the literature on stimulability and its predictive value was published by Diedrich (1983). He concluded that precise interpretation of information from stimulability testing is not possible for any of the usual purposes of such testing, including selecting error sounds for correction; deciding upon beginning remediation at the level of isolation, syllable, word, or phrase; and selecting children who do not need therapy from among those who do. Diedrich pointed out that there is risk in postponing treatment for a child who shows high stimulability. Because stimulability data are based upon groups of children, individual variability makes prediction uncertain for any given child. His conclusions do not imply that there is not predictive power in the results of stimulability testing. All of the studies reviewed found significant positive relationships between stimulability and maturation or responsiveness to therapy, but the strength of these relationships is not great enough for accurate predictions concerning individuals. Diedrich suggested that the best evidence to foretell articulatory performance might come from a trial period of diagnostic therapy. However, this statement is more of a hypothesis to be researched than a conclusion to be drawn.

In light of the preceding, a logical question might be: Is it worthwhile to check on the stimulability of error sounds? On the one hand, the answer can be no, for the intent of the clinician is to eliminate errors regardless of their stimulability. Also, it is interesting to note a rather surprising finding in one stimulability study (Sommers et al., 1967) that children in kindergarten and first and second grades with poor stimulability scores benefited more from therapy than those with good stimulability. Nevertheless, there is a general relationship between stimulability and speech improvement. Therefore, the clinician has some reasonable assurance that speech sounds that show high stimulability have a better chance of responding readily to therapy. The clinician might just as well capitalize on that relationship to increase the probability of early progress to motivate the child. Even though it has some limitations, stimulability has potential as a clinical tool (Kisatsky, 1967; Madison, 1979; Moore, Burke, & Adams, 1976).

Orofacial Examination

A major aspect of any articulatory assessment is an appraisal of the structures and functions of the speech mechanism, particularly the orofacial structures. The intent is to determine whether both the movable and the immovable articulators are adequate for speech production. This examination is usually performed soon after all testing of articulation has been completed. In this way, the clinician can be guided in the examination by knowledge about the number and types of speech sounds that are produced in error. For example, if an individual produces a large number of alveolar sounds incorrectly, then the examiner should test carefully all structures and functions involved in alveolar articulation.

The orofacial examination is also an important part of the differential diagnostic process. A clinician gains important information not only about the factors that may have either predisposed or precipitated the present articulatory condition but also about factors presently serving to perpetuate it. The examination often allows the clinician to determine whether a disorder is *functional* or *organic* in nature. Such determinations, although sometimes misleading, usually help the clinician develop more realistic therapy goals and plan more helpful therapy experiences.

A routine orofacial examination usually involves examination of the following: (a) facial characteristics, (b) the teeth, (c) palatal and pharyngeal areas, and (d) the tongue.

To prepare for the exam, a clinician would obtain equipment such as a penlight or flashlight, examining gloves, and a tongue depressor. It should be noted that the orofacial examination procedures discussed here represent a set of general procedures that an examiner might follow in a routine orofacial exam. Naturally, what an examiner uncovers in performing the exam may require more in-depth probes of oral-mechanism functioning. For example, if routine appraisal of tongue mobility reveals sluggish side-to-side movement, then the clinician will no doubt ask the patient to perform a number of different tasks that probe tongue mobility. It is extremely important to go beyond what is "routine," departing from a set procedure, in order to secure the most accurate and detailed information possible. Further details concerning oral-mechanism examination procedures can be found in Dworkin (1978), Dworkin and Culatta (1980), Mason and Simon (1977), St. Louis and Ruscello (1981), and also in chapter 10, where articulatory considerations in organically based disorders are discussed. The orofacial exam worksheet of Mason and Simon (1977) is included in Appendix 4.2 as one example of a useful set of examination procedures.

Abnormal findings on an oral examination indicate a need for medical or dental referral for two reasons. First, additional information may be obtained that can be helpful to the clinician in planning remediation. Second, some conditions may

be amenable to medical treatment. It is surprising, but true, that the speech-language pathologist may encounter physical conditions that have been previously unnoticed or untreated.

The process of assessing the areas involved in the orofacial examination is as follows.

Facial Characteristics. In examining the facial areas, the clinician checks very general aspects such as the client's facial expression, overall appearance, coloration, facial health, size and shape of the head, and overall symmetry of the head and facial structures.

The Teeth. Some individuals, especially children, have been shown to have difficulty producing or learning certain speech sounds because of factors related directly or indirectly to either the occlusal relationship of their teeth or to the teeth themselves. On the other hand, some children compensate remarkably well and dental deviations have few if any adverse effects.

In examining the dentition, the clinician first makes a general assessment of the teeth, making sure to check for (a) overall dental health, (b) obvious structural deviations, (c) the presence of any dental appliance, and (d) supernumerary (extra) teeth. Although poor dental health will not directly affect speech production, the presence of structural deviations, dental prostheses or appliances, or extra teeth may interfere with articulation. After these preliminary procedures, an examiner will usually direct a client to close her teeth so that the back teeth come together. The purpose of this is to assess the dental occlusion. In a normal occlusion, the maxillary central incisors extend just slightly over the mandibular central incisors about one fourth of an inch. In reality, however, normality is measured by the relationship between upper and lower molars. When the lower first molars are approximately one half of a tooth ahead of the upper first molars, a normal occlusion exists. This is termed a class I normal molar occlusion. Three classes of abnormal occlusions, or *malocclusions*, are also recognized. A class I malocclusion consists of a normal molar relationship with some other minor variability in the dentition. In the class

II malocclusion, the maxillary first molar is ahead of the mandibular first molar. Finally, in a class III malocclusion, the mandibular molar is located ahead of the maxillary molar by more than one half of a tooth.

Palatal and Pharyngeal Areas. Assessing the palatal and pharyngeal areas involves examining the general integrity of component structures and functions. Of primary concern here is velopharyngeal closure and whether the oral structures involved function adequately for this purpose. Areas to be examined include the hard palate, the soft palate, and the pharyngeal area.

In examining the hard palate, a clinician is concerned primarily with its structure. Hence, inspecting for clefts or other immediately apparent structural deviations is of primary importance. Some deviations of the hard palate are not so apparent. In these instances, palatal coloration often leads the examiner to suspect a structural deformity. Anomalies such as a submucous cleft often give themselves away by the presence of a blue coloration close to the midline of the palate. An examiner can also check more closely for a submucous cleft by very gently rubbing a finger across the hard palate to feel for soft spots. Other concerns with regard to the hard palate include the presence of palatal fistulas, which are openings in the palate often caused by insufficient healing after surgery, and, to a lesser extent, the size and height of the palatal vault, which may limit the space available for tongue movement. Many clients make compensatory movements to adjust for this, whereas in others this limited space can have an adverse effect.

The soft palate, or *velum*, should be examined first for any major abnormalities, such as the presence of clefts or scar tissue. In addition, its overall size and coloration should be checked. The velum is one of the most important articulators. Its valving action is important in the control of both the dispersion of nasal resonance and the ability to build up the intraoral breath pressure that is so necessary in producing many consonant sounds. In order for the velum to valve the outgoing breath stream adequately, it must be of sufficient length. Its overall length, then, is one important consider-

ation. The velum, however, is not the only structure that works to bring about velopharyngeal closure. Other structures located in the pharyngeal area are also involved.

In discussing procedures for examining the pharyngeal area, we will again concern ourselves first with the important structures. Then, we will look at some specific procedures important in examining both velar and pharyngeal function in velopharyngeal closure.

The most important structures of the pharyngeal area, including the lateral pharyngeal walls and the posterior pharyngeal wall, cannot be examined adequately via intraoral observation. These structures, along with the velum, combine to produce the total sphincter action needed for velopharyngeal closure. Closure can be observed, however, by nasopharyngoscopy (a method of direct visualization) and by videofluoroscopy or cineradiographic studies (methods of indirect visualization).

Some general procedures that might be used in inspecting the velum and pharyngeal areas intraorally follow:

1. Make general observations first regarding the overall size, shape, and symmetry of the velar structure. Observe the general length and mobility of the velum. Have the client prolong /ɑ/ followed by repeated interrupted but sudden bursts of /ɑ/. During phonation the velum should raise symmetrically in a superior and posterior direction. It should raise to the level of the hard palate. Here, however, the examiner is cautioned that even some normal speakers may show little velar movement on these isolated productions. Look for reciprocal motion of the lateral and posterior pharyngeal walls during phonation.

2. Inspect the size, symmetry, coloration, and general appearance of the faucial pillars, the palatine tonsils, and the uvula. Some considerations here include: (a) size of the air passage and whether any obstruction

exists, (b) the possible presence of a bifid uvula or a uvula that deviates to one side, which typically indicates a paresis, and (c) the potential effects of the presence/absence of the tonsils in addition to their general appearance.

3. Check for the presence of oronasal fistulae.
4. Lightly touch the velum with a tongue depressor to elicit the gag reflex. There should be considerable movement during this reflex.
5. Look for signs of a submucous cleft in the velar area. Again, coloration differences may alert the examiner.
6. Consider the general articulatory and/or resonance characteristics generally associated with velopharyngeal incompetence, such as (a) excessive nasal resonance or hypernasal tone, (b) nasal emission of the breath stream, (c) weak or omitted consonants, and (d) compensatory articulation productions, e.g., glottal stops, pharyngeal fricatives, pharyngeal plosives, and use of nasal for oral phonemes.
7. A lack of nasal resonance on nasal consonants may indicate almost anything, from a structural deviation in the nasal cavity to something as basic as a cold.

The Tongue. The tongue is unquestionably the most important articulator. Its movement is necessary in practically all speech sounds. Its examination begins in a manner consistent with earlier procedures: First the structure itself is examined, and then its functions.

The tongue is usually checked first for the presence of obvious growths or lesions of any kind and also for its appearance. Then, its overall size is considered. Some tongues may appear to be either too small or too large, but in reality there is a rather large range of normality. It is rare that a clinician actually gets to view a congenitally small tongue (*microglossia*) or a congenitally enlarged one (*macroglossia*). In spite of substantial variability in tongue size, some individuals can compensate very well.

A second observation that can be made is how the tongue is positioned when it is at rest in the mouth. The examiner should note its symmetry, the presence of any scar tissue, and whether the tongue appears to quiver or undulate in any abnormal manner.

Next, the tongue tip should be elevated with a tongue depressor to permit inspection of the lingual frenum. A short lingual frenum can restrict tongue movement considerably. Again, many clients compensate quite well for this so that the actual number of individuals who are affected adversely is no doubt much smaller than would be expected. This will come up again in discussing the examination of tongue functioning.

Several procedures can be used to examine tongue functions. In general, they assess the movement, mobility, and general strength of the tongue. All three of these areas should be considered in a routine orofacial examination. These procedures are summarized briefly below:

1. Hold the client's lower jaw down. Ask her to elevate the tongue tip to the maxillary central incisors and then retract it backward and upward toward the alveolar ridge. This should give the clinician some idea of the upward range of movement, while also allowing observation of any effect an apparent restricted frenum might have. This would be an obviously important procedure if the individual misarticulated a number of alveolar consonants.
2. Ask the client to perform tongue exercises, among them (a) protruding the tongue out of the mouth, upward and downward, then licking the lips in a circular fashion; (b) moving the tongue up and down inside the mouth; (c) moving it from front to back at various speeds; (d) protruding it and moving it from side to side, (e) touching the tongue tip to various locations on the hard and soft palate after these areas have been stimulated by a tongue depressor; and (f)

making a clicking noise with the tongue. Many of these procedures have been used by clinicians for years in order to determine if the tongue is physically capable of performing the range and speed of movements necessary for speech production.

An examiner should consider carefully certain types of movements that are often related to organically based articulation disorders. For example, some children and adults diagnosed as developmental apraxics or as adult apraxic speakers, respectively, experience difficulty in the volitional planning of certain oral and even facial movements. Individuals with physical impairments such as these often differ substantially in their abilities to perform imitative versus volitional movements. Therefore, an examiner should consider both oral and facial movements elicited by imitative command and those called forth voluntarily (by verbal command only). These movements then must also be viewed in light of the actual movements required for speech. Much more detailed information about the nature and assessment of apraxia of speech is presented in chapter 10, along with a more in-depth presentation of orofacial examination procedures.

3. Make a quick determination of tongue strength by holding a tongue depressor vertically in front of the client's teeth and instructing her to push it away with the tongue. Alternatively, have the client close her mouth and push the tongue outward and against the cheek to make it appear as if there were a large ball of gum in her mouth. The clinician then tries to push the tongue back in the client's mouth while the client attempts to resist this motion. If there is normal and sufficient tongue strength available, the client will have little difficulty with this task.

4. Finally, assess rate of movement of the tongue by obtaining measures of *diadochokinetic rate* or maximum repetition rate

(Kent, Kent, & Rosenbek, 1987). The client is asked to repeat /pʌ/, or /pʌtʌ/, and then /pʌtʌkʌ/. Usually the clinician gives the client an opportunity to practice these phonetic groups before actually performing the measurement. Most experienced examiners are well aware of the very shocked look you get from a client, especially a young child, when you suddenly ask her to repeat /pʌtʌkʌ/ as fast and as accurately as possible. Norms for diadochokinetic rate are presented in Appendix 4.3. More detailed discussion of diadochokinesis is presented in chapter 10.

These are the general procedures followed in performing an orofacial exam, but it is important to go beyond what is considered "routine" when the results merit it. No orofacial examination should be a set of rigid procedures that prevent probes for more information. Only by getting the best and most accurate information possible can a clinician become a truly effective diagnostician.

Comparing Performance to Age Norms

In conducting the articulation assessment, each error phoneme is considered in relation to the age of the child. The previous chapter on normal development presented data on phoneme acquisition as it relates to age. In general, vowels are acquired before consonants. Normally all vowels are included in speech by the age of 3 years. Consonants take more time to be mastered. On average, the order of acquisition of consonants is something like this: 18 months–/p, m, h, n, w, b/; 2 years–/k, g, d, t, ŋ/; 30 months–/f, j/; 3 years–/r, l, s/; 42 months–/ʃ, tʃ, z/; 4 years–/dʒ, v/; 54 months–/θ/; 5 years–/ð/; 6 years–/ʒ/ (Sander, 1972). These data are summarized from chapter 3, where a more complete presentation is given.

This information should be used in making judgments about whether the child should be given more time for phoneme development to occur through maturation, or whether to intervene therapeutically. However, reason and caution should be exercised in the use of normative data. Norms are statistical averages, so that their application to the development of one child is problematic. In addition, Winitz (1975) explains that developmental tests should not be used for predictive purposes. That is, the speech clinician cannot predict, from normative data, where a given child will be in 6 months or a year in phoneme acquisition. Winitz suggests that normative data can be used for a guide in counseling parents, but if a parent is concerned about a particular child and desires professional help, then it is wise to improve the whole situation by providing the service.

Existing normative data suggest which sounds children should have developed at each age level. In addition to parental concern, at least two other factors should be considered. First, the total number of error sounds is an indicator of severity. An even more important consideration is intelligibility of the child and the degree to which communication is affected. Although these factors (age norms for sounds, number of sounds, and degree of intelligibility) are closely interrelated, each may be weighted differently in individual cases.

Olmsted (1971) reports that the course of speech-sound development consists of a mixture of successes and errors in successive attempts to produce a given phoneme, with gradual increases in the percentage of successes and decreases in the relative number of errors, and that coexistence of success and error is the most frequent pattern of developing use of the sounds of speech. Normative data conceal this pattern as well as obscuring the fact of high individual variability in mastering the phonology of adult language.

Turton (1980) points out that there are two basic problems in the use of normative data in articulation assessment. The first is that speech sound development is not normally distributed; the second is that children cannot be placed into discrete categories. He indicates a need for better assessment

procedures, more akin to those that are discussed later in this chapter. He also recommends criterion-referenced testing instead of normative-based testing. In criterion-referenced testing, the items of the test are selected from a teaching model that is determined by the goals of an instructional program. The level of performance of the person being assessed is not compared to a statistical average but rather to a predetermined performance goal (criterion). Of course, criterion-referenced testing requires knowledge on the part of the examiner of the type of behavior under study.

Contextual Testing

Contextual testing is concerned with the influence of surrounding phones on a particular phone. It is often a part of the assessment procedure. Spriestersbach and Curtis (1951) studied inconsistency in children's articulatory production of /s/ and /r/ and found that many children who misarticulated these sounds sometimes spoke them correctly in a specific context.

For example, words containing /s/ were most often produced correctly in the context /sp/, while /r/ was produced correctly more often in the context /tr/. It is well documented that adjacent sounds influence each other during speech production (Curtis & Hardy, 1959; Gallagher & Shriner, 1975a, 1975b; Hoffman, Schuckers, & Ratusnik, 1977; Zehel, Shelton, Arndt, Wright, & Elbert, 1972). Context change produces variability of speech sound production.

McDonald (1964) developed what he termed a *deep test* of articulation. Its purpose was to test each error sound in a variety of contexts to discover contexts in which the error phonemes were produced correctly. He objected to the traditional procedures of testing a sound in the initial, medial, and final position of three words. He pointed out that (a) three-position testing procedures are word oriented; however, words do not appear in speech as entities, but instead speech is composed of sequences of syllables; (b) consonants do not appear in initial, medial, and final positions in connected speech, but rather exist only as releasers and arrestors of syllables; (c) three-position testing simply provides too small a sample, preventing study of the influence of context; and (d) in speech there are four types of consonant connections: simple, double, compound, and abutting.

The simple consonant connection is the CV, VC, or CVC arrangement, as in *toe, at,* and *tote,* respectively. A double consonant is one that occurs between two vowels, such as the fricative /s/ in the word *missing,* or across word boundaries, e.g., *passsome* as in *Pass some turkey please.* A double consonant, then, is one that can perform both an arresting and a releasing function in a sequential manner. The next type is the compound consonant. It occurs in a consonant cluster where two or more consonants combine to release or arrest a syllable. The /str/ in *street* and /st/ in *wrist* are examples. The fourth type of consonant combination, abutting, is the instance where two adjacent consonants are components of two different syllables, such as the /g/ and /p/ in *magpie.* The /g/ arrests the first syllable, while the /p/ releases the second. The McDonald deep test assesses numerous abutting contexts.

A three-position test offers limited opportunities (usually two or three) to study how various contexts influence production of error phonemes. The deep test, however, is composed of picture stimuli designed to examine production of one phoneme at a time in a variety of phonetic contexts. A consonant such as /s/, for example, can both release and arrest a syllable in English. It is tested systematically as an abutting releaser and arrester in several different phonetic contexts. The McDonald deep test is referenced with the list of published articulation tests given at the end of the chapter.

Some researchers have considered even broader contexts than did McDonald. Zehel et al. (1972) studied the influence of broad and immediate context on /s/ production. *Immediate context* refers to those sounds immediately adjacent to the speech sound that is under study. *Broad context* refers to speech sounds that are part of the larger contextual environment. For example, note the location of the /s/ in the word *history.* Its immediate context is /ɪ/ and /t/, and the broader context includes /h/ and /r/.

Zehel et al. found that, although broad contexts had little influence on the articulation of /s/, immediate contexts were influential in some cases. Though subjects produced significantly more satisfactory /s/ phones in some immediate contexts than in others, it is difficult to generalize from these data to treatment of the individual. Zehel et al. indicate that the clinician who wishes to begin articulation training in contexts in which a sound is produced correctly must find contexts suitable for the individual. This implies that clinicians probably should develop contextual tests of the more commonly misarticulated phonemes that provide an even greater number of items than the McDonald deep test. These might consist of lists of words or phrases with a specific phoneme in a variety of contexts. These could be spoken by the clinician for the child to imitate. Any context in which the misarticulated phoneme is uttered correctly would be noted and used as a facilitative context for the initiation of therapy. Zehel et al. also conjecture that for those children who easily modify their articulations in response to stimulation (highly stimulable), context is relatively unimportant in articulation remediation. More investigations (Elbert & McReynolds, 1978; Moore, Burke, & Adams, 1976) support this conclusion.

Still other research supports the notion of facilitating contexts. Gallagher and Shriner (1975a, 1975b) studied the spontaneous speech of 3-year-old children and analyzed sound sequences for contextual variables related to correct and incorrect productions. They found that the correctness of /s/ and /z/ was not affected by the position of the sounds in words or the phonological acceptability of the sequences. However, more correct productions were observed in CCV contexts than in CV contexts. Also, /s/ and /z/ were produced correctly more often when followed by stop plosives, specifically /t/ and /k/, than when preceded by consonants or vowels. Their findings suggest that speech clinicians could increase assessment information by analyzing spontaneous speech samples using a VC_nV syllabic segmentation procedure. C_n represents any arrangement of consonants occurring between vowels. Within the consonantal portion of the syllable, contextual patterns that are systematically related to correct and incorrect productions should be identified. These contextual patterns could be incorporated into remediation.

Hoffman, Schuckers, and Ratusnik (1977) studied the influence of context on /r/ misarticulations. The specific contexts analyzed were: (a) lexically constrained /r/, e.g., He has *pr*ide; (b) nonlexically constrained /r/, e.g., The jee*p r*ide was fun; and (c) nonlexically constrained /ɚ/, e.g., The kick*er* kicked the ball. The context that brought about the greatest number of accurate productions was the nonlexically constrained /ɚ/, the next most effective context in eliciting correct productions was the lexically constrained /r/, and the context that produced the least number of correct productions was the nonlexically constrained /r/. These differences were significant and provide the kind of helpful information that tests of context can be based upon. Similarly, in connection with contextual influences on /r/ productions, Curtis and Hardy

(1959) found the most facilitative context to be C/r/ as in *pr*esent and *tr*ain. The second most facilitative context was C/ɚ/ as in wat*er* and riv*er*.

The McDonald deep test and C-PAC: Clinical Probes of Articulation Consistency (Secord, 1981a) are the only commercially available instruments to assess use of context. The deep test is limited in the number of contexts provided. Hoffman et al. (1977) discuss some of its limitations. They note in particular its semantic and syntactic ill-formedness and recommend the use of short sentences for contextual testing because the effects of coarticulation transcend multiphonetic and lexical boundaries. Though stimulability may be more important in articulation remediation than the influence of context, there still is value in studying contextual influences. It is recommended that the testing go beyond that provided by the McDonald deep test, even though this requires the clinician to develop some contextual testing materials.

More recently, Secord (1981a) introduced an instrument to assess the production of any phoneme in a variety of phonetic contexts. The C-PAC: Clinical Probes of Articulation Consistency provides an alternative to traditional picture-based deep testing. The C-PAC is a comprehensive set of

TABLE 4.1
Phonetic Contexts Assessed by C-PAC Consonant Probes

Type	*Definition*
Prevocalic	Occurring before a vowel to release a one-syllable word
Postvocalic	Occurring after a vowel to arrest a one-syllable word
Intervocalic	Occurring between two vowels in a two-syllable word, acting to release and/or arrest the first, second, or both syllables
Initial cluster	Occurring in combination with another consonant to release a one-syllable word
Final cluster	Occurring in combination with another consonant to arrest a one-syllable word
Medial cluster	1. Preceding another consonant in the middle of a two-syllable word, acting to arrest the first syllable
	2. Following another consonant in the middle of a two-syllable word, acting to release the second syllable
Word boundary cluster	1. Occurring postvocalically in a word followed by a prevocalic consonant in another word
	2. Occurring prevocalically in a word preceded by a postvocalic consonant in another word

Source: C-PAC: Clinical Probes of Articulation Consistency (p. 5) by Wayne Secord, 1981, Columbus: Merrill Publishing Co. 1986, The Psychological Corporation. Reprinted by permission.

articulation probes that can be used with subjects from preschool to adulthood. Each C-PAC probe assesses articulatory production in (a) pre- and postvocalic position of words, (b) initial, medial, final, and word-boundary clusters, (c) sentences, and (d) conversation (storytelling). These probes can be used both to measure consistency and to identify contexts that can be used as beginning

points in therapy. The types of phonetic contexts assessed by C-PAC are summarized in Table 4.1. A sample C-PAC probe for the /s/ phoneme is shown in Figure 4.3. The C-PAC is also referenced in Appendix 4.1.

FIGURE 4.3
C-PAC probe for the /s/ phoneme. (*Source: C-PAC: Clinical Probes of Articulation Consistency* (p. 137) by Wayne Secord, 1981, Columbus: Merrill Publishing Co. 1986, The Psychological Corporation. Reprinted by permission.)

Testing Auditory Discrimination

The ability to distinguish between speech sounds is termed *auditory discrimination*. Speech-language pathologists have been interested in this phenomenon for many years. In 1931, Travis and Rasmus published a study reporting that normal speakers were superior to people with functional articulation disorders in making discriminations between speech sounds. That study spawned many investigations of the subject. Testing speech sound discrimination ability became part of the speech clinician's assessment battery. Several tests of speech sound discrimination have been published. Three frequently used tests are the Wepman Auditory Discrimination Test (Wepman, 1973), the Templin Test of Auditory Discrimination (Templin, 1957), and the Goldman-Fristoe-Woodcock Test of Auditory Discrimination (Goldman, Fristoe, & Woodcock, 1970).

Although poor auditory discrimination has been thought to be a significant factor in functional articulation disorders and although testing auditory discrimination ability has been given a place in assessment procedures, the empirical base for these beliefs and procedures is not strong. Powers (1957, p. 742), after reviewing the findings of research on the topic, wrote that results of studies on speech sound discrimination and its relation to articulation skill were conflicting and inconclusive. She also pointed out that the great weight of evidence was against there being a systematic inferiority in persons with functional misarticulations in ability to discriminate speech sounds. A decade later, as he viewed the general acceptance within the profession of the still-possible relation between speech sound discrimination ability and articulation disorders, Weiner (1967) conducted a critical review of the existing literature. His review concluded that auditory discrimination shows a developmental progression. The ceiling of this development seems to be reached at about the eighth year. The most important conclusion was that the evidence does support a link between auditory dis-

crimination and articulation. This relationship holds until about 8 or 9 years of age. Beyond that age there does not seem to be a relationship. Strong positive findings are noted in groups with severe articulation disorders, but the relationship appears negligible when errors are few. Thus age seems to be the primary influence in studies on auditory discrimination, and number of sounds misarticulated seems to play a secondary but still important role.

The key issue in speech sound discrimination testing hinges on the nature of the stimulus material presented to the subject for a discriminating response. In general, there are two types of discriminative stimuli. The first of these consists of pairs of words or syllables that include a wide range of stimulus sounds. For example, in the Wepman Auditory Discrimination Test, the subject is presented with 40 pairs of similar-sounding words. Examples are *tub–tug, web–wed, lag–lack, gum–dumb, coast–toast*. The examiner utters a pair, and the client responds by saying ''same'' if the pair are perceived as the same, or ''different'' if they are perceived as different. Bernthal and Bankson (1981) term this type of test a *general test of auditory discrimination*, meaning this type of test compares a wide variety of sounds. The three frequently used published tests mentioned earlier (Wepman, Templin, and Goldman-Fristoe-Woodcock) are all general discrimination tests.

The second type of auditory discrimination test requires the client to make discriminations between the correct form of his error sound and other sounds, including the incorrect form. This type of test is phoneme specific and is called a *test of internal discrimination*.

The research of Aungst and Frick (1964) highlights important issues in the area of speech sound discrimination testing. They included in their design an idea expressed by Van Riper and Irwin (1958, p. 25) that perhaps a discrimination test will yet be devised that will match the speaker's own error against the correct utterance presented either simultaneously or successively. Aungst and Frick selected 27 children between 8 and 10 years of age, all of whom misarticulated the /r/. Four difconsistency score was obtained for each subject on a deep test of articulation. Three of the discrimination tests were created especially for the study; the fourth was a traditional test of discrimination, consisting of 50 pairs of syllables to which the subject responded ''same'' or ''different'' following presentation of each syllable pair (Templin, 1957). The three new tests were constructed to determine the subject's ability to judge her own speech productions in these situations: (a) when compared to the audio-tape-recorded productions of another speaker, called the *Test of Comparison*; (b) immediately after her own production, the *Test of Instantaneous Judgment*; and (c) when self-productions were played back from a tape recording, the *Test of Delayed Judgment.*

Their results showed that the three new auditory discrimination tests were measuring the same ability. They also showed that some relationship exists between articulation ability and the ability to judge the correctness of one's own speech. Correlations among their three new tests of sound discrimination ranged between .93 and .95. However, correlations with the traditional test were low and nonsignificant, ranging from $-.21$ to $-.26$. The correlations between the three new tests and the articulation test were .69, .59, and .66, respectively. But again, the relationship between the traditional sound discrimination test and the articulation test was only $-.03$. The difference between the three new tests and the traditional test apparently was in the distinction between the judgments of one's own speech and the discrimination between pairs of general stimulus items spoken by someone else.

This study by Aungst and Frick has been reported in some detail because it suggests the kinds of tests that need to be developed. It seems reasonable to conclude from their results that traditional tests that are external to a client's specific misarticulations have limited utility. It appears more desirable to develop phoneme-specific tests of internal discrimination that have relevance for specific children. Aungst and Frick's internal discrimination test (the Test of Instantaneous Judg-

ment), combined with a measure of articulatory consistency, might yield more accurate information. Unfortunately, work by other researchers has only brought about more debate.

The controversy over the efficacy of auditory discrimination testing was heightened by the 1971 work of Woolf and Pilberg. In a study similar to that of Aungst and Frick, in which children who misarticulated /r/ also served as subjects, results indicated that articulation ability is not related to speech sound discrimination skill. Interestingly, these findings are not in agreement with those of Aungst and Frick. Also, in an attempt to replicate part of the Aungst and Frick study, Shelton (1978) reported administering a similar test of delayed judgment to /r/- and /s/-misarticulating children before and after a period of ''articulation change.'' Shelton could obtain a correlation no higher than .35 between any discrimination and articulation measures. Shelton stated his disagreement with those who focus efforts on the child's self-discrimination, and concluded that no one has yet demonstrated that discrimination measures account for a significant percentage of articulation variance.

The preceding has explained that the efficacy of general auditory discrimination testing as a standard component of articulation assessment has not been demonstrated. Indeed, it appears that the most fruitful type of discrimination testing would be that of internal monitoring of error sound productions. It is particularly important that the client be able to discriminate errors in her own speech, though this skill is difficult to measure (Bernthal & Bankson, 1981). Thus, it appears that if the clinician is going to assess speech sound discrimination ability, the nature of the testing instrument used will follow models suggested by the work of Aungst and Frick or Woolf and Pilberg, in which the clinician will need to create tests using the subjects' error phonemes and correct articulatory targets as the material for discrimination testing. The general commercial tests simply do not measure relevant skills.

Before concluding the discussion of speech sound discrimination, it seems appropriate to suggest future directions these procedures may take. They are perhaps suggested in a study conducted by Monnin and Huntington (1974). In this investigation, the basic task for the children who served as subjects was to identify phonemes, as opposed to making comparative judgments as required in discrimination tasks. In comparing two phonemes in a discrimination task, the child may perceive them as two allophones of the same phoneme because the child's acceptable range for a given phoneme may be different from that of adults. Phoneme identification, therefore, may be presumed to be more pertinent than the discrimination of allophonic or other differences. An appropriate response to an identification task implies an appropriate selection of phoneme categories. Conversely, an inappropriate response to an identification task implies an inappropriate choice of phoneme categories, which may be due to defects of discrimination or inappropriate labeling or both.

In their study, Monnin and Huntington included identification of two types of phonemes: (a) those related to the misarticulations of the experimental group, who misarticulated /r/, and (b) phonemes distant from /r/ in place and manner of production. Vowel identification was also studied. Basically, the child's task was to point to a picture of an object whose name was presented from a tape recording. There were four sets of test words, and these were presented under seven conditions, representing a continuum of distortion of the speech signal ranging from no distortion in the first condition to maximum distortion in the seventh. As expected, the more the speech signal was distorted, the greater the number of errors made by the subjects. The experimental group (/r/-misarticulating children) made significantly more errors in the identification tasks, and errors were specific to misarticulated phonemes, indicating a positive relationship between production and identification ability.

Hoffman, Stager, and Daniloff (1983) also studied discrimination of error-specific contrasts. They recorded the speech of 12 children who consistently misarticulated /r/ and 5 children who correctly articulated /r/. All of the children were asked to identify the recorded productions by pointing to pictures that represented possible interpretations of /r/–/w/ contrasts such as "They run the race" versus "They won the race" or "The clock is round" versus "The clock is wound." The two groups were about the same in their ability to identify /w/ productions. A similar result was obtained for perception of correctly produced /r/. However, the performance of the two groups differed when the children were asked to identify misarticulated /r/. Those who correctly articulated /r/ were only able to identify 35% of the misarticulated /r/ productions as members of the phoneme /r/. Apparently, children who do not misarticulate /r/ classify the misarticulated /r/ as a member of the /w/ phoneme class. The misarticulating children were apparently confused by error productions, assigning nearly 50% to each phoneme category. This guessing strategy did not apply to misarticulating children's intended productions of /w/. Misarticulating children identified 65% of these correctly. Essentially, these data suggest that children who misarticulate /r/ differ from those who do not only in regard to their perceptions of /r/ error productions. In particular, children who misarticulate adopt a guessing strategy that assigns approximately half of the error productions to the /w/ phoneme and half to the /r/ phoneme. An additional finding was a wide range of self-perception ability among the misarticulating children.

Results of the above two studies underline the need for more discrete types of analyses. These probably will consist of identification tasks as opposed to discrimination tasks. In addition, the stimuli used in the testing will probably be well-controlled synthetic stimuli. Tests using synthetic stimuli are yet to come from the speech science laboratories. In the meantime, the interested clinician might follow the kinds of procedures discussed by Locke (1980a, 1980b). Locke provides a thoughtful rationale for discrimination testing and explains the inadequacies of general tests of auditory discrimination. He also highlights the error potential in asking children to make same–different judgments. As Bernstein (1978) explains, young children interpret the word *different* to mean "same." As they mature, *different* comes to mean "similar," then finally, children acquire the adult meaning for the term. This is another justification for identification tasks as opposed to discrimination tasks. In Locke's procedure the child replies "yes" or "no" to a sequence of stimulus questions. For example, suppose the child substitutes /f/ for /θ/. The examiner extends a thumb or shows a picture of a thumb and asks, "Is this thumb?", "Is this /fʌm/?", or "Is this /sʌm/?" using a perceptually similar control phoneme. For each error phoneme, Locke elicits 18 yes or no responses from the child, using in the names of six objects or pictures (a) the correctly articulated target phoneme, (b) a perceptually similar control phoneme, and (c) the phoneme substituted by the child. This last part can be difficult in the case of substitutions that lie outside the perceptual boundaries of the phonological system of the examiner. The order of presentation is randomized to avoid establishing a pattern of response based upon order of presentation.

The place of auditory discrimination in management of articulation disorders will be discussed further in chapter 9.

Summary

The first section of this chapter has described traditional approaches to assessment of articulation disorders. These approaches generally involve elicitation of a single-word sample that includes all consonant phonemes of English and completion of an error analysis including distortions, substitutions, omissions, and additions. Testing for stimulability, the orofacial examination, testing sounds in context, and evaluating auditory discrimination provide clinicians with additional information about the severity and etiology of the articulation problem and prognosis for improvement.

The next section will describe assessment approaches that are based on assessment of the client's phonological system.

PHONOLOGICAL ANALYSIS

Obtaining the Sample

Current linguistic approaches to analyzing children's speech and/or language are based on an examination of the child's habitual rule system as revealed by single words (Hodson, 1980; Khan & Lewis, 1986; Weiner, 1979), phrases (Weiner, 1979) and/or conversation (Grunwell, 1985; Ingram, 1981; Shriberg & Kwiatkowski, 1980). The optimal sample should (a) reflect the child's production in actual communicative situations, (b) reveal both inconsistencies and consistent patterns, and (c) contain the full set of English phonemes. Ideally, the sample should include conversational speech.

Information regarding imitation, single-word production, and coarticulation has suggested several issues regarding the adequacy of various types of speech samples.

1. As noted earlier in this chapter, the child's imitated production may not reflect her spontaneous production.
2. The child's production of single words may not reflect conversational production. Sounds may be produced correctly in single words but be misarticulated in conversation (Dubois & Bernthal, 1978; Faircloth & Faircloth, 1970; Johnson, Winney, & Pederson, 1980), or different processes may be exhibited in a single-word articulation test and in a spontaneous speech sample (Shriberg & Kwiatkowski, 1980).
3. The child may not produce a given phoneme the same way in all phonetic contexts. Coarticulation of the surrounding

phonemes may influence production of a target phoneme (Curtis & Hardy, 1959; Grunwell, 1985; Hoffman, Schuckers, & Ratusnik, 1977; Johnson, Winney, & Pederson, 1980; McDonald, 1964).

4. Despite the arguments for a spontaneous sample, analysis of such a sample may not be possible for severely unintelligible children because the clinician is unable to understand and gloss the child's utterances (i.e., write down the intended words). More structured samples may need to be considered because, as Grunwell (1985) notes, these unintelligible children are precisely the ones for whom we need phonological analysis.

With this set of considerations in mind, the clinician must determine what type of sample will be adequate to evaluate the phonological system of a given child.

One conclusion the clinician may draw is that a spontaneous sample of continuous speech should be obtained in order to tap the child's production in real communication and to provide for the influence of coarticulation. Dubois and Bernthal (1978) used three methods to obtain samples from children with articulation errors: (a) continuous speech in response to pictures, (b) modeled continuous speech in response to a story told by the examiner (with the story being modeled and told back in six parts), and (c) spontaneous picture naming. The children exhibited errors in spontaneous speech that they did not demonstrate by the other two methods. They also had errors on the modeled sample that they did not show in single words.

Hence, it appears that a single-word sample or even a modeled sample may not tap all of the child's errors. Shriberg and Kwiatkowski (1980) compared the canonical forms (word structures) of the words from five currently used articulation tests with the words found in speech samples of language-delayed children. They found a higher percentage of complex canonical forms on the ar-

ticulation tests than in the delayed-speech samples. The articulation tests contain multisyllabic words like *telephone, Santa Claus*, and *Christmas tree*, whereas the children used words with only one and two syllables. They hypothesized that, "for young children with delayed speech, the complexity of some articulation test items may trigger simplification processes" (p. 6). Further, they found that sounds such as fricatives, affricates, and liquids that are most likely to be in error are often tested in the more complex canonical forms (*Christmas tree, Santa Claus*). This means that the likelihood of simplification is increased (p. 7).

Despite the importance of obtaining a spontaneous speech sample, simply allowing the child to talk may not elicit a sufficiently large variety of phonemes and contexts. Therefore, it is important to design materials that will encourage the child to produce variety. With very young children, a variety of toys with different phonemes in their names may be useful. For older children, action pictures can be used to elicit descriptions. Asking the child to tell a story is a useful way to elicit connected speech with somewhat controlled content. Of course, picture-naming is the most commonly used method for eliciting the total set of phonemes.

Shriberg and Kwiatkowski (1985) compared five conditions for sampling the spontaneous speech of children with articulation problems. The degree of examiner control over the sample ranged from a free situation where the type of continuous speech and the content were uncontrolled to a scripted interview in which both type of speech and content were controlled. The story, routines, and interview represented intervening levels of control. The authors found few differences in the samples elicited by the five methods. They concluded that (1) examiners should be flexible in using materials and strategies to keep children talking; (2) increased control over the content of the child's utterances can help intelligibility for unintelligible children; (3) the examiner should monitor the child's output for variety, and change materials and prompts as necessary to assure variety of phonemes and contexts; and (4) the clinician should monitor the child's cognitive and affective states during sampling because change in state can affect articulatory performance. For example, a child may articulate more precisely in a "test" situation or less precisely if excited.

The ideal sample may be one that includes all of these suggestions. A model for obtaining a well-rounded sample might consist of the following procedures.

Procedures for Preschool Children. Part of a sample may be obtained by providing a set of toys for the child to play with and talk about. Included might be:

Doll	*Dishes*	*House*
hat	plate	chair
dress	cup	couch
socks	fork	table
shoes	spoon	kitchen
shirt	knife	living room
pants	pan	bedroom
zipper		bed
	Garage	bathtub
	trucks	rug
	cars	lamp
	fire truck	mother
	police car	father
	dump truck	baby
	bus	
	train	

With the four sets of toys, including about 35 items, nearly all phonemes can be represented in two positions. Engaging the child in play with the toys can elicit their names in conversation. It must be remembered, however, that asking the child to name the toys will not produce the desired results. This is a separate task, which can be used to elicit words not produced in conversation. However, these should then be recorded as single-word productions. With some very young or developmentally delayed children, it may be necessary to resort to imitated naming responses. Such responses should be attempted when spontaneous utterances cannot be obtained. However, it should be noted that they were imitated.

A second procedure is to ask the child to retell a story. It is possible to create stories that contain

key words representing a variety of phonemes. These are available commercially or can be written by the clinician. Telling the entire story to the child and asking her to retell it may produce a more accurate picture of spontaneous speech; however, key words may be lost by this method. In order to obtain a more accurate retelling, the clinician may want to tell the story in segments for the child to repeat. The Sounds in Sentences Subtest of the Goldman-Fristoe Test of Articulation (Goldman & Fristoe, 1969) presents two stories that can be used for this purpose.

Procedures for School-Aged Children. Part of the sample may be obtained by holding a conversation about the child's interests. With some talkative children, it may be possible to hold the most natural sort of conversation—discussion of interests and experiences. Such a conversation can provide good information about the child's habitual speech patterns. However, with unintelligible children, the clinician may have greater difficulty in transcribing the sample because of the lack of context to help in determining what the child has said.

A second procedure is to ask the child to describe action pictures. As with toys, the content of the pictures should be controlled so that a variety of phonemes will be represented in the descriptions.

Third, the clinician may use standard picture-naming tests of articulation. An articulation test can be used to supplement the connected-speech data in order to assure that all phonemes are represented in the sample. Bankson and Bernthal (1983) have made a strong case for continued use of the traditional articulation test battery to identify phonological patterns that affect syllable shape or several sounds within a sound class.

Finally, the clinician can ask the child to retell a story. Stories can be used in the same way that they are used with preschool children.

Use of these procedures should provide a sample that adequately represents the child's spontaneous speech and also yields the complete set of

English phonemes. The goal should be to elicit as many phonemes as possible spontaneously, but failing in that, to elicit them through naming pictures or imitation.

Recording the Sample

Recording a sample of spontaneous speech is more complicated than recording picture-naming responses or imitations of single-word utterances. Grunwell (1982) states that the sample should "be recorded in such a way as to facilitate a detailed and comprehensive phonological analysis, whose validity can be checked by another analyst" (p. 198). The clinician needs to use more than one means of getting an accurate recording. All samples should be tape-recorded to permit repeated listenings for accurate transcription. However, even high-quality tape recordings have limitations. Two problems can occur in attempting to transcribe samples from the tape recorder: (a) Missing acoustic and visual clues may prevent accurate phonetic transcription and (b) missing contextual clues may interfere with the examiner's comprehension of the situation and thereby prevent accurate transcription. For these reasons, it is important to record as much on-the-spot information as possible to supplement the tape recording.

It may be more convenient to reduce the spontaneous sample to a list of single words, but the words should be kept in order so that information regarding the effect of phonetic environment across word boundaries is not lost. Table 4.2 shows a possible abbreviated sample for a preschool child. The analysis of the sample will be discussed later in the chapter.

Phonetic Transcription

Although phonetic transcription is necessary for administering articulation tests and was discussed earlier in this regard, there are special consider-

ations in regard to transcription of spontaneous samples for phonological analysis. The beginning clinician will need to give careful attention to the transcription of the sample. In normal communicative situations, listeners do not attend to individual phoneme production, but integrate sounds into meaningful units of words and phrases. This means that the clinician may overlook distortions of the signal, perceiving them as units that make the message meaningful. We do this frequently in noise. When a part of the message is not heard, we "fill in" what makes sense in the context.

In transcribing a client's articulation, it is important to extract meaning from partially unintelligible speech, but at the same time the clinician must attend to details of utterances. For example, it is important to avoid assuming that the client said "bed" when the actual production was [bɛ]. Careful listening and practice are necessary.

In order to be able to examine generalizations in the child's system, it is important to have a close phonetic transcription. In some cases, the client may substitute phones that are not English phonemes. These are more difficult for the English-speaking clinician to perceive and transcribe, but they may indicate important generalizations, errors, or approximations in the client's speech. Two examples will illustrate this fact. First, imagine a child who substitutes ʃ/s and ʒ/z. A broad transcription reveals /ʃ/ and /ʒ/ to be produced correctly or marked only as distorted. However, a closer transcription reveals x/ʃ and ɣ/ʒ, i.e., that velar fricatives are substituted for palatal fricatives (see Table 4.3). We now see that all four sibilants are produced with a tongue position further back in the mouth than for normal speakers. We can make the generalization that sibilants are "backed."

As a second example, another child produces the following words: *thumb*—[fʌ̃], *ran*—[ræ̃], *ring*—[rĩ], all with nasalized vowels; *bad*—[bæː], *bed*—[bɛː], *car*—[kɑˠ], *ball*—[bɔˠ], all with lengthened vowels. The clinician might record these words as /fʌ/, /ræ/, /rɪ/, /bæ/, /bɛ/, /kɑ/, /bɔ/. This transcription would indicate that the child omits final consonants; however, a closer transcription reveals that the child is aware of final nasal sounds because the nasality is assimilated in the vowel. Awareness of final voiced stops is also revealed by the lengthening of the vowel. In the same way, the beginnings of final glides are exhibited by the addition of a brief schwa (*ball*—[bɔ°]). These observations indicate that the child may be in a transition stage of developing final consonants. Thus it can be seen that careful observation and analysis yield much meaningful information.

The accurate application of phonological process analysis to be described later requires close attention to precise transcription. Table 4.3 provides a listing of phonetic symbols according to place and manner of articulation and additional diacritical markings for nasalization, syllable lengthening, etc. The student may not need to memorize the non-English symbols, but should use such a chart when transcribing samples.

Analyzing the Sample

Grunwell (1982) lists five criteria that the analysis of a speech sample should satisfy. It should (a) describe the patterns used by the speaker, (b) identify the ways in which these patterns differ from those used by normal speakers, (c) determine the implications of these disordered patterns for effective communication, (d) provide the necessary information for developing treatment goals and guidelines, and (e) provide a basis for assessing changes during treatment (p. 198).

A variety of assessment strategies have been devised in attempts to meet these kinds of goals. Distinctive-feature approaches and phonological process analysis are the two most common; however, a number of different kinds of analysis may be suggested in order to provide a complete picture of the child's phonological system and to plan treatment goals. These strategies will be described in the following sections.

Distinctive-Feature Approaches. Distinctive-feature theory, which initially gave impetus to the development of multiphonemic therapy approaches, is one attempt to meet these criteria. As explained in chapter 2, distinctive-feature theory

groups sounds into classes according to the common features that define them. For example, according to the system used by Singh and Polen (1972), the following phonemes share the features +continuant, − sonorant, − nasal: /f, v, θ, ð, s, z, ʃ, ʒ/. If for all of these phonemes the child substitutes sounds that change one of the features, it might be assumed that the child has difficulty with the group of sounds that are characterized by that feature. Rather than treat the problem as if there were eight separate errors, it might be more economical to try to establish the missing feature. The child might then learn to produce all eight phonemes.

If the child made the substitutions noted in Table 4.2, there would be evidence that the feature +continuant did not appear in conjunction with − sonorant, − nasal sounds; e.g., the child substitutes p/f, d/θ, d/ð, d/s, d/z, d/ʃ. Based on this observation, it seems reasonable that teaching the child to produce continuancy might result in correction of all eight phonemes. In order to plan remediation in this way, it is necessary to complete a distinctive feature analysis. An analysis of these errors is shown in Table 4.4.

Speech-language pathologists may find the use of distinctive features unwieldy for analyzing children's articulation. One criticism is that the features proposed by Chomsky and Halle (1968) or Jakobson, Fant, and Halle (1963) were designed as a theoretical model to describe the language, not the language user (Parker, 1976; Walsh, 1974). Chomsky (1968) has maintained that the generative-transformational grammar model is not a production model. Therefore, the features may not be meaningful in describing a child's errors.

The features used in Table 4.5 (Singh & Polen, 1972) represent one of many feature systems proposed by linguists and speech scientists. It is abbreviated compared to Chomsky and Halle's (1968) or Jakobson, Fant, and Halle's (1963) feature systems, but it is practical in that it is closely related to speech production and speech perception.

TABLE 4.2
Abbreviated Speech Sample for a Preschool Child

Gloss	Transcription	Canonical Form	Substitutions I	Substitutions F	Omissions I	Omissions F	Distortions
I. Spontaneous Speech Playing with Toys							
put	pʊ	CV				t	
the	ə	V			ð		
bed	bɛ	CV				d	
in	ĩ	V				n	
bedroom	bɛʊ	CVV			r	d,m	
mommy	mɑmɪ	CVCV					
in	ĩ	V				n	
the	ə	V			ð		
kitchen	tɪə	CVV	t/k		tʃ	n	
they	de	CV	d/ð				
gonna	dʌnə	CVCV	d/g				
eat	i	V				t	
II. Retelling a Story							
Jerry	dɛwɪ	CVCV	d/dʒ,w/r				
playing	peĩ	CVV	p/pl			ŋ	
with	wɪ	CV				θ	
his	hɪ	CV				z	
drum	dʌ̃	CV	d/dr			m	
his	hɪ	CV				z	
ball	bɔə	CVV		ə/l			
his	hɪ	CV				z	
wagon	wædə̃	CVCV	d/g			n	
III. Picture Naming							
lamp	wæ̃	CV	w/l			mp	
house	haʊ	CV				s	
cup	tʌ	CV	t/k			p	
wagon	wædə̃	CVCV	d/g			n	
wheel	wiᵊ	CVV		ə/l			
telephone	tɛpõ	CVCV	p/f			n	
rabbit	wæbɪ	CVCV	w/r			t	
car	tɑᵊ*imitated	CVV	t/k	ə/r			
chicken	tɪtɪ	CVCV	t/tʃ,t/k			n	
church	tʌᵊ	CVV	t/tʃ	ʌᵊ/ɝ		tʃ	
stove	do	CV	d/st			v	
airplane	eəpẽ	VVCV	p/pl	ə/r		n	
knife	naɪ	CV				f	
thumb	dʌ̃	CV	d/θ			m	
finger	pĩə	CVV	p/f	ə/ɚ	g	ŋ	
zipper	dɪpə	CVCV	d/z	ə/ɚ			
shoe	du	CV	d/ʃ				
ring	wĩ	CV	w/r			ŋ	
Santa Claus	dætɔ	CVCV	d/s,t/kl			n,z	

TABLE 4.2 *(continued)*
Abbreviated Speech Sample for a Preschool Child

Gloss	Transcription	Canonical Form	Substitutions I	Substitutions F	Omissions I	Omissions F	Distortions
Christmas tree	dımə dı	CVCVCV	d/kr,d/tr			s,s	
sleep	di	CV	d/sl			p	
carrot	tɛwə	CVCV	t/k,w/r			t	
duck	dʌ	CV				k	
yellow	wɛo	CVV	w/j		l		
bathtub	bætʌ	CVCV				θ,b	
bath	bæ	CV				θ	
jump rope	dʌwo	CVCV	d/dʒ,w/r			mp,p	

Summary Word Structures	Substitutions I	Substitutions F	Omissions I	Omissions F	Distortions
V	p/f	ə/l	ð	p	
CV	d/θ	ə/r	l	b	
CVV	d/ð	ə/ɚ	r	m	
CVCV	d/s	ʌ²/ɝ	tʃ	f	
CVCVCV	d/z		g	v	
VVCV	w/l			θ	
	t/tʃ			t	
	d/dʒ			d	
	d/ʃ			n	
	w/r			s	
	w/j			z	
	t/k			l	
	d/g			tʃ	
	p/pl			k	
	d/tr			ŋ	
	d/dr			mp	
	d/st				
	t/kl				
	d/kr				
	d/tr				

Phonemic Repertoire
1. Always used correctly: w, h
2. Used correctly in some context: p, b, m, w, t, d, n, h
3. Appearing; not used correctly: none
4. Not represented in sample words: ʒ

Processes
1. Final consonant deletion—all phonemes
2. Stopping
3. Liquid simplification
4. Vocalization
5. Cluster reduction
6. Fronting

TABLE 4.3
The International Phonetic Alphabet

THE INTERNATIONAL PHONETIC ALPHABET

(Revised to 1979)

	Bilabial	Labiodental	Dental, Alveolar, or Post-alveolar	Retroflex	Palato-alveolar	Palatal	Velar	Uvular	Labial-Palatal	Labial-Velar	Pharyngeal	Glottal
Nasal	m	ɱ	n	ɳ		ɲ	ŋ	N				
Plosive	p b		t d	ʈ ɖ		c ɟ	k g	q ɢ		k͡p g͡b		ʔ
(Median) Fricative	ɸ β	f v	θ ð s z	ʂ ʐ	ʃ ʒ	ç ʝ	x ɣ	χ ʁ		ʍ	ħ ʕ	h ɦ
(Median) Approximant		ʋ	ɹ	ɻ		j	ɰ		ɥ	w		
Lateral Fricative			ɬ ɮ									
Lateral (Approximant)			l	ɭ		ʎ	ʟ					
Trill			r					ʀ				
Tap or Flap			ɾ	ɽ				ʀ				
Ejective	p'		t'				k'					
Implosive	ɓ		ɗ				ɠ					
(Median) Click	ʘ		ǀ									
Lateral Click			ǁ									

(pulmonic air-stream mechanism)
(non-pulmonic air-stream)
C O N S O N A N T S

VOWELS

	Front	Back
Close	i ɨ / y ʉ	ɯ u
Half-close	e ø / ɘ ɵ	ɤ o
Half-open	ɛ œ / ɜ	ʌ ɔ
Open	æ / a ɶ	ɑ ɒ

Front — Back (Unrounded — Rounded)

OTHER SYMBOLS

ɕ, ʑ Alveolo-palatal fricatives
ʎ̥, ʝ Palatalized ʃ, ʒ
ɺ Alveolar fricative trill
ɺ Alveolar lateral flap
ɧ Simultaneous ʃ and x
ʦ Variety of ʃ resembling s, etc.
ɪ = ɩ
ʊ = ɷ
ɜ = Variety of ə
ɚ = r-coloured ə

DIACRITICS

˳ Voiceless n̥ d̥
ˬ Voiced s̬ t̬
ʰ Aspirated tʰ
.. Breathy-voiced b̤ a̤
. Dental t̪
ₒ Labialized t̫
ⱼ Palatalized tʲ
˞ Velarized or Pharyngealized ɫ, ɫ̵
˳ Syllabic n̩ l̩
˘ or ⌣ Simultaneous ʃf (but see also under the heading Affricates)
. or , Raised e̝, ẹ, e̞ w
. or . Lowered e̞, ẹ, e̞ ɤ
+ or . Advanced u̟, ...
- or . Retracted i̠, ı̠-, ...
" Centralized ë
˜ Nasalized ã
ɹ, ɻ, ʀ r-coloured a˞
: Long aː
. Half-long aˑ
˘ Non-syllabic ŭ
˒ More rounded ɔ˒
˓ Less rounded y˓

STRESS, TONE (PITCH)

ˈ stress, placed at beginning of stressed syllable: ˌ secondary stress: ˉ high level pitch, high tone: ´ high rising: ˊ low level: ˋ low rising: ˆ high falling: ˇ low falling: ^ rise-fall: ˇ fall-rise.

AFFRICATES can be written as digraphs, as ligatures, or with slur marks; thus ts, tʃ, dʒ: ʦ tʃ ʤ ʣ. c, ɟ may occasionally be used for tʃ, dʒ.

Source: International Phonetic Association, London. Reproduced with permission.

96

TABLE 4.4
Distinctive Feature Analysis of a Preschool Child's Substitutions for Fricatives

Substitutions	Similar Features in Target and Substituted Sounds	Different Features in Target and Substituted Sounds	
		Target	Substituted
p/f	−voice −nasal −sibilant +front −sonorant +labial	+continuant	−continuant
d/θ	−nasal −sibilant +front −sonorant −labial	+continuant −voice	−continuant +voice
d/ð	+voice −nasal −sibilant +front −sonorant −labial	+continuant	−continuant
d/s	−nasal +front −sonorant −labial	+continuant +sibilant −voice	−continuant −sibilant +voice
d/z	+voice −nasal +front −sonorant −labial	+continuant +sibilant	−continuant −sibilant
d/ʃ	−nasal −sonorant −labial	+continuant +sibilant −front −voice	−continuant −sibilant +front +voice

Maintained features shared by all target phonemes
−nasal
−sonorant
Error feature for all target phonemes
+continuant

97

TABLE 4.5
Distinctive Feature System

0 1	Front Back	Nonlabial Labial	Nonsonorant Sonorant	Nonnasal Nasal	Stop Continuant	Nonsibilant Sibilant	Voiceless Voiced
p	0	1	(0)	(0)	0	(0)	0
b	0	1	0	0	0	(0)	1
t	0	0	(0)	(0)	0	(0)	0
d	0	0	0	0	0	(0)	1
k	1	(0)	(0)	(0)	0	(0)	0
g	1	(0)	0	0	0	(0)	1
f	0	1	(0)	(0)	1	0	0
v	0	1	0	0	1	0	1
θ	0	0	(0)	(0)	1	0	0
ð	0	0	0	0	1	0	1
s	0	0	(0)	(0)	1	1	0
z	0	0	0	0	1	1	1
ʃ	1	(0)	(0)	(0)	1	1	0
tʃ	1	(0)	(0)	(0)	0	1	0
dʒ	1	(0)	0	0	0	1	1
j	1	(0)	1	0	(1)	(0)	(1)
r	1	(0)	1	0	(1)	(0)	(1)
l	0	0	1	0	(1)	(0)	(1)
w	1	1	1	0	(1)	(0)	(1)
m	0	1	1	1	(1)	(0)	(1)
n	0	(0)	1	1	(1)	(0)	(1)
h	1	(0)	(0)	(0)	1	0	(0)

Source: "Use of a Distinctive Feature Model in Speech Pathology" by S. Singh and S. Polen, 1972, *Acta Symbolica, III*, p. 22. Copyright 1972 by *Acta Symbolica*. Reprinted by permission.

The features used in this system are defined by Costello (1975, p. 66) as follows:

□ *front/back:* articulated in front of or against the alveolar ridge versus behind the alveolar ridge

□ *nonlabial/labial:* articulated without the lips as the place of articulation versus with the lips

□ *nonsonorant/sonorant:* articulated with a restricted airflow versus with an unrestricted airflow and spontaneous voicing

□ *nonnasal/nasal:* presence of oral versus nasal resonance

□ *stop/continuant:* articulated by abrupt termination of airflow versus continuous airflow

□ *nonsibilant/sibilant:* frictionless airflow versus presence of high-frequency friction

□ *voiceless/voiced:* absence versus presence of voicing

Costello (1975) used this sytem for distinctive feature analysis in preparation for remediation. She advocated sampling the child's articulation by administering the following measures: (a) Fisher-Logemann Test of Articulation Competence (Fisher & Logemann, 1971), (b) Goldman-Fristoe Test of Articulation Sounds in Words Subtest, Stimulability Subtest, and Sounds in Sentences Subtest (Goldman & Fristoe, 1969), (c) a spontaneous speech sample, (d) the McDonald Deep Test of Articulation (McDonald, 1964), and (e) the Sound Production Tasks (Elbert, Shelton, & Arndt, 1967). After plotting the resulting data, the most common substitution for each error phoneme is determined and used as the basis for distinctive

TABLE 4.6

Distinctive Feature Analysis of Substitutions Using Singh and Polen's (1972) Model as Described by Costello (1975)

ERROR 0 1	Front Back	Nonlabial Labial	Nonsonorant Sonorant	Nonnasal Nasal	Stop Continuant	Nonsibilant Sibilant	Voiceless Voiced
p/f	0–0	1–1	0–0	0–0	(0–1)	0–0	0–0
d/θ	0–0	0–0	0–0	0–0	(0–1)	0–0	(1–0)
d/ð	0–0	0–0	0–0	0–0	(0–1)	0–0	1–1
d/s	0–0	0–0	0–0	0–0	(0–1)	(0–1)	(1–0)
d/z	0–0	0–0	0–0	0–0	(0–1)	(0–1)	1–1
d/ʃ	(0–1)	0–0	0–0	0–0	(0–1)	(0–1)	(1–0)

Source: "Articulation Instruction Based on Distinctive Features Therapy" by J. Costello, 1975, *Language, Speech and Hearing Services in Schools, 6,* p. 68. Copyright 1975 by the American Speech-Language-Hearing Association. Adapted by permission.

feature analysis. Table 4.6 shows this analysis re-using part of the data in Table 4.2. Those features that account for the largest number of errors can easily be examined by noting the circles on the matrix. The results are the same as shown by the distinctive feature analysis in Table 4.4. Again, failure to use continuancy is the primary error shown.

Although the traditional phonetic description terms do not provide a neat binary model, they can be used to analyze generalizations in much the same way as distinctive features, and they may more adequately describe the process of articulation.

Grunwell (1985) suggests that a child's feature contrasts be examined using a model derived from Ladefoged (1975) that is shown in Table 4.7. Singh and Frank (1979) used such a model to analyze the substitutions in children's speech. Table 4.8 shows the consonants of English described in traditional terms. Analysis of the substitutions of the child described earlier can be charted as in Table 4.9. Examination of this table shows that many substitutions occur in the fricative row and

TABLE 4.7

Articulatory Features Described by Grunwell (1985) Based on Ladefoged (1975)

Nasal (stop)	–	Oral (stop/plosive)	m n ŋ – p b t d k g
Stricture:		stop	m n ŋ p b t d k g
		fricative	f v θ ð s z ʃ ʒ
		affricate	tʃ dʒ
		approximant	w r l j
Place:		labial	m p b f v w
		lingual:	
		dental	θ ð
		alveolar	n t d s z r l
		postalveolar/palatal	tʃ dʒ ʃ ʒ j
		velar	ŋ k g
Voiced	–	Voiceless	b d g dʒ v ð z ʒ – p t k tʃ f θ s ʃ
Median approx.	–	Lateral approx.	r – l

Source: Phonological Analysis of Child Speech by Pamela Grunwell, 1985, San Diego: College Hill Press. Used by permission.

TABLE 4.8
Traditional Description of Consonants

Manner of Articulation	Place of Articulation						
	Bilabial	Labiodental	Dental	Alveolar	Palatal	Velar	Glottal
Stop	p b			t d		k g	
Fricative		f v	θ ð	s z	ʃ ʒ		h
Affricate					tʃ dʒ		
Glide	w				j		
Liquid				l	r		
Nasal	m			n		ŋ	

TABLE 4.9
Correct Sounds and Substitutions Described by Place and Manner of Articulation of the Target Sound

Manner of Articulation	Place of Articulation						
	Bilabial	Labiodental	Dental	Alveolar	Palatal	Velar	Glottal
Stop	p b			t d		t/k d/g	
Fricative		p/f	d/θ d/ð	d/s d/z	d/ʃ		h
Affricate					t/tʃ d/dʒ		
Glide	w				w/j		
Liquid				w/l	w/r		
Nasal	m			n			

change the manner of production to the stop category. Place of articulation is maintained as nearly as possible. As with the distinctive feature analysis, we find that the child is making one type of error that accounts for all fricative misarticulations.

In chapter 14, Blache describes another distinctive feature model for clinical analysis. He examines the development of the child's existing phoneme system according to the following classes of sounds: stops and nasals, semivowels, continuants, and sibilants. These classes represent a developmental order from earlier to later devleoping sounds. Further distinctive feature contrasts determine the acquisition of sounds within each class. These features are: nasal/nonnasal, voiced/voiceless, labial/lingual, front/back lingual (tongue position), retroflex/nonretroflex, continuant/interrupted, and strident/mellow. The use of these feature contrasts for analysis and training is described in chapter 14.

Although there is variation in the exact list of features used in each of the models described in this section, the goal of each is to describe patterns of error based on common features. As seen in the examples given, similar results will be obtained by all of them.

Phonological Process Analysis. Another method for describing immature patterns in the speech of normal children developing language and of individuals with multiple articulation errors is the phonological process analysis. Phonological processes simplify groups of sounds and eliminate sound contrasts. Young children exhibit processes on the way to developing adult articulation. The processes most frequently used by normal children have been described by Ingram (1976) and are discussed in chapter 2. Shriberg and Kwiatkowski (1980) refer to those processes that commonly occur during the period of normal language acquisition and occur across many languages as *natural processes*. These also tend to be most common in the speech of individuals with articulatory disorders. A number of authors (Grunwell, 1985; Hodson, 1980, 1986a; Ingram, 1981; Khan & Lewis, 1986; Lund & Duchan, 1983; Shriberg & Kwiatkowski, 1980; Weiner, 1979) have proposed methods for analyzing phonological processes and have outlined the processes to be examined. Compton and Hutton (1978) have devised a test that results, not in phonological processes, but in generative rules as described in chapter 2. Elbert and Gierut (1986) have devised a strategy for assessing what they call the child's productive phonological knowledge. Each of these methods will be described briefly.

Compton-Hutton Phonological Assessment. In 1978 Compton and Hutton devised a 50-item

picture-naming test that provides a kind of bridge between traditional error analysis and current pattern analyses. It is not a process analysis, but an attempt to provide a generative rule analysis. Forms are provided for recording responses to the test words, examining error patterns, and identifying phonological rules. For the error pattern analysis, phonemes are grouped according to word position and manner classes: stops, nasals, frictions (fricatives), affricates, liquids, glides, vocalics, final clusters, and initial blends. After marking the errors for each of these classes of sounds, the clinician circles phonological rules that apply for each class. The rules are expressed in the form:

$$\begin{bmatrix} b \\ d \\ g \end{bmatrix} \rightarrow \begin{bmatrix} p \\ t \\ k \end{bmatrix}$$

The Compton-Hutton model does not discuss the phonological analysis in terms of processes. Although the information obtained is basically the same, process analyses may provide greater generalization in some cases. For example, the rules

$$\begin{bmatrix} k \\ g \end{bmatrix} \rightarrow \begin{bmatrix} t \\ d \end{bmatrix}$$

$$\begin{bmatrix} \int \\ 3 \end{bmatrix} \rightarrow \begin{bmatrix} s \\ z \end{bmatrix}$$

$$\begin{bmatrix} l \\ r \end{bmatrix} \rightarrow w$$

indicate a general pattern of fronting, but because these rules are examined under three separate manner classes, that generalization might be lost.

The testing format for this analysis can be criticized because it includes only single-word productions. However, the authors do note the value of transcribing and analyzing any spontaneous speech or nontest words that may occur during testing in order to observe any inconsistencies between single-word and connected-speech productions.

Procedures for the Analysis of Children's Language. Ingram (1976) listed the following processes as common in the developing speech of normal children:

syllable structure processes
    final consonant deletion
    unstressed syllable deletion
    reduplication
    cluster reduction
assimilatory processes
substitution processes
    stopping
    fronting
    gliding of liquids
    frication
    vocalization
    deletion

Ingram's (1981) analysis examines a number of aspects of the individual's rule system. The phonological process analysis is one of these. The following are the components of Ingram's analysis:

1. The *phonetic analysis* determines the total number of sounds that the child uses and the frequency of use of phonemes in the initial, medial, and final position of words. Ingram provides a formula for determining a criterion of frequency in order to say that a given phoneme is included in the child's repertoire. The formula is based on the number of different words in the sample and the number of different phonemes the child uses in producing these words. For example, in a given sample, it might be necessary for the child to produce a phoneme four times in order to consider it as having been acquired. Also analyzed in this component are the child's syllable structures and word structures. The child's two most frequent syllable structures are noted, and the percentages of monosyllables and closed syllables (syllables with final consonants) are obtained. A large phonetic repertoire and a variety of syllable and word structures should mean greater intelligibility.

2. The *homonymy analysis* examines forms that sound alike but have different meanings. A percentage of homonymous forms is obtained, which plays a large part in determining the degree of intelligibility. The extent of homonymy is largely determined by the number of different phonemes in the child's repertoire. If a very limited number of phonemes are used, then many words sound the same. For example, if the child used only the consonants /b, p, m/, the following productions might result:

ball	/bɔ/	pie	/pa/	me	/mi/
gone	/bɔ/	tie	/pa/	knee	/mi/
dog	/bɔ/	kite	/pa/		

This is an example of a high percentage of homonymy.

3. The *substitution analysis* identifies the types of substitutions for adult forms and their frequency of occurrence.

4. The *phonological process analysis* calculates the percentage of use of 27 different phonological processes. The analysis also allows for the inclusion of other less common processes.

Ingram states that his method is designed to be applicable for both clinical and research purposes. His procedure is meant to meet five goals. It is (a) complete, (b) flexible regarding sample type and size, (c) adaptable for different children (the entire analysis does not have to be completed for each child), (d) cumulative in that the analysis provides new information at each step, and (e) normative for comparing results.

Ingram's workbook includes eight recording forms to aid in making the analysis. The major strength of the format is its completeness. However, the practicing clinician may criticize the amount of paperwork required.

Phonological Assessment of Child Speech. Grunwell (1985) suggests the use of a sample of at least 100 different words and preferably 200 to 250 words. Ideally, the sample should be spontaneous, but single words can be used if necessary. The sample should include the range of targets in the adult system and more than one example of the child's production of each. She recommends narrow phonetic transcription of consonants.

This analysis is similar to Ingram's in its thoroughness. Like Ingram, Grunwell describes several different types of analysis, but it is not always necessary to complete all of them for a given child. The major facets of the analysis are as follows:

1. The *Phonetic Analysis* describes the child's repertoire of consonants and their distribution according to syllable and word position as well as the occurrence of consonant clusters. Consonants in the inventory are classified according to the traditional categories of place and manner. This analysis is not optional.

2. The *Contrastive Analysis* and *Assessment* determines those phones, clusters, and syllable structures that are used contrastively to signal differences in meaning in the child's speech. These contrasts are compared with the adult phonemic system to predict inadequacies in the child's system and subsequently treatment goals that will improve communication. Contrastive phones are analyzed separately for three positions: syllable initial/word initial, syllable initial within a word, syllable final-/word final. A matrix is used to determine the child's phonotactic potential, i.e., those syllable and word structures that the child uses and how they differ from the adult targets.

3. The *Phonological Process Analysis* is an alternative to the Contrastive Analysis although both can be completed to provide additional data about the child's system. Similar information will be obtained from both, although in different form. Grunwell divides the processes into the two categories, *structural* and *systemic,* and further according to whether they are developmental or unusual. The classifications are shown in Table 4.10. Following the phonological process analysis, the results are examined to determine the existence of the

following patterns of usage characteristic of disordered phonological development: persisting normal processes, chronological mismatch, unusual/idiosyncratic processes, variable use of processes, or systemic sound preference.

Grunwell suggests other factors to consider in more detailed evaluation of the analysis for therapy planning.

The advantage of this method is its thoroughness and the direct relationship between the analysis and therapeutic strategies. Much information about the child's communication adequacy is obtained. The disadvantage is its length and the high volume of paperwork, despite the fact that all parts of the analysis are not required. The time required is not feasible for most clinical situations; however, as with Ingram's analysis, thorough knowledge of the principles and procedures can be helpful to the clinician who chooses to complete a more informal analysis.

Phonological Assessment: A Multifaceted Approach. Like Ingram, Lund and Duchan (1978, 1983) advocate the analysis of a variety of aspects of the child's phonological system. They call their procedure a *multifaceted approach* because they propose to discover more than just phonological processes. The analyses that they suggest include (a) feature and position plus feature analysis of substitutions, (b) analysis of context-sensitive patterns, (c) syllable structure analysis, (d) analysis of idiosyncratic structures, and (e) analysis of possible phonological strategies.

Lund and Duchan advocate narrow phonetic transcription of single words from an articulation test and spontaneous sample. They analyze feature changes according to manner, place, and voicing, and then describe patterns in terms that other authors call phonological processes: stopping, frication, nasalization, and others for manner errors; fronting, backing, and others for place errors; and voicing and devoicing for voicing errors.

Under context-sensitive patterns, they examine assimilation, coalescense (the collapsing of two

TABLE 4.10
Classification of Phonological Processes According to Grunwell (1985)

Structural simplifications		Example	
Developmental			
Weak syllable deletion	/metə/		for *tomato*
Final consonant deletion (including clusters)	/bæ/		for *bad*
	/des/		for *desk*
Vocalization	/wɑdo/		for *water*
Reduplication	/bɑbɑ/		for *bottle*
Consonant harmony	/gɔg/		for *dog*
Syllable initial cluster reduction	/nek/		for *snake*
Unusual			
Vocalic support of final consonants	/bædə/		for *bad*
Initial consonant adjunction	/wæbu/		for *apple*
Vowel insertion	/pəliz/		for *please*
Dissimilation	/baɪt/		for *pipe*
Perseveration	/lɪptɪp/		for *lipstick*
Metathesis	/æks/		for *ask*
Systemic simplifications			
Developmental			
Fronting	/ti/		for *key*
Stopping	/ti/		for *see*
Gliding	/wo/		for *row*
Context-sensitive voicing	/do/		for *toe*
Glottal replacement	/bæʔ/		for *back*
Glottal insertion	/beʔbiʔ/		for *baby*
Unusual			
Backing	/ko/		for *toe*
Backing in terminations	/mæk/		for *mat*
Tetism	/to/		for *foe*
Labial realizations of fricatives	/fi/		for *see*
Lateral realizations of sibilants	/ɬi/		for *see*
Weakening of plosives	/si/		for *tea*
Affrication of plosives	/tsi/		for *tea*
Denasalization	/do/		for *no*

Source: Phonological Assessment of Child Speech by Pamela Grunwell, 1985, San Diego: College Hill Press. Used by permission.

syllables into one, e.g., *spaghetti*—[skɛti]), and transposition of sounds (e.g., *asked*—[ækst]).

Possible problems with the syllable structure of words include weak-syllable deletion (*pajamas* —[dʒɑməs]), reduplication of syllables (*baby* —[bibi]), addition of syllables (*book*—[bʊki]), and restricted syllable structure, including cluster reduction (*drum*—[dʌm]) and final consonant deletion (*cat*—[kæ]).

Finally, Lund and Duchan consider it important to look for patterns that are not common among children with normally developing or delayed speech and therefore not listed. In addition, some children may use strategies that are the result of the application of a number of rules. For example, cluster reduction, final consonant omission, and weak-syllable deletion may result in the child producing only CV structures for words. Other possible strategies include avoidance or selection of certain words based on their phonological structure.

The authors advocate completing the analysis in the following order:

1. Recognize and ignore productions that are typical of everyday speech patterns of normal speakers.
2. Transcribe a formal articulation test using narrow transcription.
3. Obtain a narrow transcription of a sample of spontaneous speech.
4. Make a listing transcript for each sound in error, including correct as well as error productions. Examine for context effects.
5. Identify syllable structure patterns and idiosyncratic forms.
6. Complete a substitution analysis.
7. Make an inventory of the sounds that the child produces, both those that match and those that do not match the target.
8. Complete deep testing to confirm suspected patterns and elicit sounds that were not included in the sample.
9. Complete an intelligibility analysis using both familiar and unfamiliar listeners in context-bound and context-free situations.
10. Complete a phonological repair analysis to determine sounds that the child repairs spontaneously and when asked to repeat.

Like the procedures to be described at the end of this chapter, this analysis offers the possibility of obtaining thorough information regarding the child's phonological system without the need to purchase specific testing and charting materials. Some will see this as an advantage for cost and flexibility; others may prefer the structure that specific materials provide.

Natural Process Analysis. Shriberg and Kwiatkowski (1980) use only the following eight natural processes in their analysis: (a) final consonant deletion, (b) velar fronting, (c) stopping, (d) palatal fronting, (e) liquid simplification, (f) cluster reduction, (g) assimilation, and (h) unstressed-syllable deletion. They base their choice of these natural processes on three factors:

1. The process must have phonological reality based on the fact that (a) it changes a more complex articulatory structure to a less complex one and (b) it occurs across languages.
2. It must frequently occur in children with delayed speech.
3. It must be able to be scored reliably by clinicians.

This last criterion caused Shriberg and Kwiatkowski to omit one process that is well established in the phonological literature: voicing-devoicing. Further, distortions and omissions are considered to be phonetic errors and are not included in the Natural Process Analysis. The final difference between this method and most process analyses is that only one process is allowed to account for a given sound change. Rule ordering is not included. This means that if the child substituted t/ʃ, only stopping would be coded. Palatal fronting would not be noted for this substitution.

Shriberg and Kwiatkowski advocate obtaining a sample of approximately 200 to 225 words and using the first 90 different words for analysis. The analysis is to be completed in a specific order, scanning the sample for each of the eight processes in the order listed. This procedure is based on the assumption that this order best demonstrates the most likely processes to occur. For example, if a child produces the word *dog* as /dɔd/, the substitution of d/g would automatically be counted as velar fronting rather than progressive assimilation because all instances of velar fronting are to be coded before assimilation is assessed for remaining uncoded forms. The authors recommend that, following the process analysis, the clinician reexamine the data for phonetic errors (distortions and omissions) and for uncoded deletions and substitutions. The clinician should also determine the variables associated with inconsistent process use.

The Shriberg-Kwiatkowski analysis is more streamlined and less time-consuming than the Ingram analysis. However, one criticism is that some useful data may be lost due to the analysis of only 90 different words and to the prescribed order for conducting the analysis.

Unless careful attention is given to the suggested reexamination of the data, less common or idiosyncratic processes may be missed.

Shriberg has also designed a series of computer programs called Programs to Examine Phonetic and Phonologic Evaluation Records (PEPPER). The programs provide information about the pho-

netic inventory, features, and phonological processes.

The Assessment of Phonological Processes— Revised. Hodson's revised version (1986a) of the Assessment of Phonological Processes (1980) uses 50 single-word responses to objects and pictures. All English consonants and common consonant clusters are included in the words. Following transcription of the sample words, the data are transferred to a phonological process assessment sheet where applicable processes are checked off across the row. Hodson uses the classification of processes shown in Table 4.11.

TABLE 4.11
Classification of Phonological Processes According to Hodson (1986)

Process	Example	
Segment omissions		
Syllable reduction	/teto/	for *potato*
Consonant sequence reduction	/pun/	for *spoon*
Prevocalic singleton		
consonant omission	/u/	for *shoe*
Postvocalic singleton		
consonant omission	/bʌ/	for *bus*
Class deficiences		
Stridents	/i/	for *see*
	/ti/	for *see*
Velar obstruents	/ʌn/	for *gun*
	/dʌn/	for *gun*
Liquid (l)	/aɪt/	for *light*
	/waɪt/	for *light*
	/wiə/	for *wheel*
	/bo/	for *blow*
Liquid (r)	/aɪt/	for *right*
	/waɪt/	for *right*
	/beə/	for *bear*
	/bwɪŋ/	for *bring*
Nasals	/do/	for *no*
	/bĩ/	for *bean*
Glides	/ɛs/	for *yes*
	/beɪt/	for *wait*
Miscellaneous error patterns		
Glottal replacement	/kæʔ/	for *cat*
Epenthesis	/təres/	for *trace*

The number of occurrences for each of the processes and the percentage of occurrence for the 10 most common are recorded on a summary sheet. A list of phonemes produced by the child is also included on this sheet.

Hodson also provides two screening instruments, which include 12 words each. One is primarily for preschool children, but can also be used for elementary-school-aged children. The other is for elementary school-aged children who evidence difficulty producing complex multisyllabic words. There is also a Spanish version (1986b) of the complete test.

The number of processes to be examined in the complete analysis may be somewhat unwieldy; however, the analysis procedure is simple and clear enough that the large number of processes can be checked in a reasonable amount of time. Only single-word stimuli are used for the analysis. Hodson justifies this decision on the basis of the difficulty of understanding spontaneous speech produced by children with severe articulation disorders. This is an important consideration in work-

TABLE 4.11 *(continued)*

Process	Example	
Stopping	/dʌm/	for *thumb*
Fronting	/do/	for *go*
Backing	/kʌg/	for *tub*
Gliding	/weɪ/	for *ray*
Vowelization	/kɑə/	for *car*
Vowel deviations	/it/	for *it*
Metathesis	/æks/	for *ask*
Migration	/moʊks/	for *smoke*
Reduplication	/mumub/	for *music box*
Coalescence	/fok/	for *smoke*
Affrication	/tsi/	for *see*
Deaffrication	/ʃiz/	for *cheese*
Palatalization	/ʃu/	for *sue*
Depalatalization	/su/	for *shoe*
Assimilations		
Nasal	/nʌn/	for *sun*
Labial	/fwɛtɚ/	for *sweater*
Velar	/gɔg/	for *dog*
Alveolar	/tɝtɪ/	for *turkey*
Voicing alterations		
Prevocalic voicing	/do/	for *toe*
Prevocalic devoicing	/piz/	for *bees*
Postvocalic devoicing	/bæt/	for *bad*
Minimal place of articulation shifts		
Sibilant distortions	/θʌn/	for *sun*
Substitution of /f, v, s, z/ for /θ, ð/	/fʌm/	for *thumb*

ing with highly unintelligible children. Hodson's analysis, as well as the next two to be described, may be particularly useful for assessing children with low intelligibility. The use of toys and allowing the child to select and name them in the order that she chooses are advantages for use with young children. This strategy is also likely to elicit some connected speech.

Hodson's analysis is also available as a computer program. The clinician types in the client's production of the 50 words, and the program reports the child's processes in order of frequency of occurrence with percentages for each. It also provides a severity rating for the child. This analysis takes only minutes to complete. Clinicians with large caseloads can therefore complete phonological analysis on many of their children in a reasonable amount of time. However, two cautions are in order. First, some data may be lost due to the confines of the data entry process. For example, there must be a one-to-one relationship between target consonants and substitutions so that added sounds cannot be included. Second, there is always a danger in determining severity, and thus priority for therapy, based on purely objective data. When subjecting research data to computer analysis, students are always taught to "eyeball" the data to determine if the answer seems logical based on the data. Similarly, the clinician should always examine the child as well as the computer results.

The Phonological Process Analysis. Weiner's procedure (1979) includes a protocol for obtaining the sample to be analyzed as well as a system for analysis. Action pictures are used to elicit phonemes in single words and in sentences through delayed imitation. For example, the response "back" is elicited by saying:

> Here is Uncle Fred's back. An elephant is standing on Uncle Fred's _____ [back]. What is the elephant doing? [Standing on Uncle Fred's back.]

Forms are provided for identifying 16 processes in the sample obtained from the pictures. The processes are grouped under the general headings of (a) syllable structure processes, which simplify the structure of syllables, (b) harmony processes, which are based on assimilation, and (c) feature contrast processes, which account for substitutions that are not related to neighboring sounds. The syllable structure processes are deletion of final consonants, cluster reduction, weak-syllable deletion, and glottal replacement. The harmony processes are labial assimilation, alveolar assimilation, velar assimilation, prevocalic voicing, final consonant devoicing, manner harmony, and syllabic harmony (reduplication). Feature contrast processes include stopping, affrication, fronting, gliding of fricatives, gliding of liquids, vocalization, denasalization, and neutralization.

The data are summarized by profiling the child's phonetic inventory, determining the proportion of occurrence of the 16 processes in the test words and in nontest words, and deciding whether or not the process operates in the child's speech. Weiner sets the criterion for inclusion in the phonetic inventory at four or more examples of the phoneme, but gives no clear-cut criteria for determining the presence of a process.

One advantage of Weiner's model is that it includes a strategy for eliciting the sample. However, despite the fact that it is time-consuming to administer, this strategy may not produce a sample that is fully representative of the child's speech due to the fact that the speech is imitated. A second advantage is that the process analysis is simple and straightforward. Excessive paperwork is avoided. This analysis is also available as a computer program.

Bankson and Bernthal (1982b) examined the phonological processes that were identified through the delayed word imitation task and the delayed sentence imitation task on this test, and found that the two procedures did not differ significantly. They concluded that the clinician may obtain the same results by using only one of the two procedures. They suggest that completing both provides a more in-depth sample, but supplement-

The Khan-Lewis Phonological Analysis. The Khan-Lewis analysis (1986) uses the data from the Sounds-in-Words Subtest of the Goldman-Fristoe Test of Articulation. The words are completely transcribed phonetically, and the data are transferred to a form that analyzes 12 developmental phonological processes, which are divided into "suppression groups" according to whether they are suppressed first, intermediate, or last in normal development. These 12 processes are as follows:

suppressed first
    deletion of final consonants
    initial voicing
    syllable reduction
    palatal fronting
    deaffrication
intermediate suppression
    velar fronting
    consonant harmony
    stridency deletion
suppressed last
    stopping of fricatives and affricates
    cluster simplification
    final devoicing
    liquid simplification

Each of these is given a developmental phonological process rating from 0 (no occurrence) to 4 (highest occurrence) according to the number of times that they occur in the sample.

Three other nondevelopmental processes may also be noted: deletion of initial consonants, glottal replacement, and backing to velars. In addition, there is a chart for defining the client's phonetic inventory in the initial, medial, and final positions.

This procedure is convenient because it uses data from the Goldman-Fristoe Test of Articulation, which is popular and quick and easy to administer. The worksheet is clear, and the analysis is not time-consuming in comparison to some other procedures. Additional data over those obtained from the Goldman-Fristoe test itself are included because the whole word, not just the target phoneme, is analyzed; however, only single word pro-

ductions are available. Information that might be obtained from connected speech is not included.

Assessing Productive Phonological Knowledge. In their handbook, Elbert and Gierut (1986) present a brief description of the current strategies for evaluating phonologically disordered speech and one different viewpoint. Information about the child's phonological knowledge is gleaned from her performance in a spontaneous, continuous speech sample supplemented with spontaneous single words. They suggest that the sample include target minimal pairs such as *cat-bat* and morphophonemic alterations such as *dog-dogs* or *run-running*. There are three components of the analysis:

1. The Breadth of the Distribution of Sounds includes a phonetic inventory (all sounds that the child produces), a phonemic inventory (those sounds that the child uses contrastively), and the distribution of the phonemes by word position and in morphemes. The elicited minimal pairs and morphophonemic alterations are useful in determining this information.

2. The Use of Phonological Rules encompasses two types of rules: (a) static or phonotactic rules, which include constraints on the inventory of sounds, the word positions in which they can occur, and the allowable sequences and (b) dynamic rules, which include allophonic rules and neutralization rules. When a child has knowledge of one phoneme, but produces it differently in different contexts, the child is using an allophonic rule. When the child has knowledge of two phonemes, but collapses them into one in certain contexts, she is applying a neutralization rule. These rules act on sounds that exist in the child's phonemic inventory.

3. The Nature of the Child's Lexical Representations is determined by the correspon-

dence of the child's production to the adult target. To the extent that the child's production of words is like the adult model, she demonstrates knowledge of the rules that associate sound with meaning.

Following analysis of these three components, the child's phonological knowledge of a given phoneme or sound class can be classified as follows:

Type 1 knowledge: Adult-like lexical representations for all morphemes in all word positions; no phonological rules apply. If the child demonstrates this type of knowledge for all phonemes, she has an adult-like system; however, the child may display this type of knowledge for only some sound classes.

Type 2 knowledge: Adult-like representations for all target morphemes in all word positions; dynamic phonological rules apply. This child will include the phoneme in her repertoire, but production errors will occur.

Type 3 knowledge: Adult-like lexical representations in all word positions, but only for some target morphemes. This child uses "fossilized" forms defined as incorrect words that persist beyond when the child has acquired a phonological rule that should correct the sound production.

Type 4 knowledge: Adult-like lexical representations in some word positions for all target morphemes. The child can produce the sound, but only in certain word positions.

Type 5 knowledge: Adult-like lexical representations in some word positions for some target morphemes. This child would have fossilized forms and positional constraints. Elbert and Gierut note that they have not actually seen children who display this type of knowledge.

Type 6 knowledge: Non-adult-like lexical representations in all word positions for all target morphemes. The child does not have the sound in her inventory.

By ranking productive phonological knowledge along this continuum, the clinician can determine the ease with which the child may learn a target sound. Type 1 knowledge represents the most knowledge of the sound, whereas type 6 represents the least. The child will have most difficulty learning those sounds for which she has type 6 knowledge.

Although this is a different method of classifying the child's phonological system and although the terminology is somewhat different, it is based on the same principles as other methods, i.e., the child's phonetic inventory, the rules or processes that exist, and the variability in the system.

The classification system is based on a traditional examination of consistency of production.

A Procedure for Completing Phonological Analysis. It is not necessary to use a published procedure for analysis. The following method for doing a phonological process analysis incorporates elements from the systems already discussed. The data in Table 4.2 are used to illustrate this analysis.

1. Transcribe the sample phonetically as a list of words as described earlier (Table 4.2). The beginning clinician may then find it useful to group the words according to their initial and final consonants. However, this step may seem wasteful to the experienced clinician, who may prefer to scan the original transcript for phonemes, word structures, and substitutions.

2. Analyze the syllable structures. A list of the different word structures found in the sample should be made. Prior to tabulation, the beginning clinician may want to list the word structure beside each word as in Table 4.2. With experience comes the ability to list the different patterns while scanning the sample. The word structures for this example are V (5), CV (19), CVV (9), CVCV (13), VVCV (1), and CVCVCV (1). From the analysis, two things become obvious: (a) There is a limited repertoire of word structures and (b) syllable-final consonants are omitted. One other detail should be examined. There is a relatively large number of CVV word structures in the sample considering the rarity of this form in English. This should alert the clinician to examine the origin of the CVV structures. It can be seen that they come from two sources: (a) two omis-

sions of intersyllable consonants and (b) three vocalizations (substitution of a vowel for a consonant) of final consonants. The second issue will appear later in the analysis.

3. Analyze substitutions and omissions. They can be recorded on the transcription sheet. Omissions should be recorded as syllable-initiating or syllable-terminating. An attempt should be made to code errors as substitutions rather than distortions whenever possible because substitution data provide greater opportunity for examining consistencies. For example, a narrow phonetic transcription might reveal the following substitutions: ʃ/s, ʒ/z, c/ʃ, j/ʒ, c/t, ɟ/d (see Table 4.3). Inspection of these substitutions reveals that all of the phonemes are produced further back in the mouth than normal. If a broad transcription had been used, most of these phonemes would have been coded as distorted. Marking them as such gives no information about the pattern of error.

Once all substitutions and omissions have been recorded, a summary list can be made. In this case, substitutions are: p/f, d/θ, d/ð, d/s, d/z, w/l, t/tʃ, d/dʒ, d/ʃ, w/r, w/j, t/k, d/g, p/pl, d/tr, d/dr, d/st, t/kl, d/kr, ə/l, ə/r, ə/ɚ, ʌˀ/ɜ·. All final consonants in the sample are deleted. Semivowels become vowels.

4. Following the listing of substitutions, omissions, and distortions, examine the data for phonemes in the child's repertoire. The distortion column is ignored for this analysis. The following lists of sounds should be made: (a) phonemes always used correctly, (b) phonemes used correctly anywhere in the sample (note word position), (c) phonemes appearing in the sample as substitutions, but never used correctly, and (d) phonemes that were not represented in the sample words.

5. Examine the substitution and omission columns for phonological processes. The distortion column continues to be ignored at

this point. The following order of analysis is suggested: (a) Scan the omission column for final consonant deletion, number of times it does and does not occur, and phonemes for which it applies and (b) scan the substitutions for stopping, fronting of palatals and/or velars, gliding or liquid simplification, cluster reduction, assimilation, voicing or devoicing, and other processes. Notation should be made of which phonemes are affected.

Examination of the number and kinds of processes will enable the clinician to predict the degree of homonymy in the child's speech and the level of speech intelligibility (already known from listening). A greater number of processes will produce more homonymy and therefore less intelligibility. However, the specific types of processes also contribute differentially to intelligibility. For example, the child who exhibits deletion processes and stopping will have more homonymous forms than children who exhibit other processes. The clinician who desires a more precise measure of homonymy can use the procedure outlined by Ingram (1981).

The relative importance of determining the phonemic repertoire and analyzing the phonological processes may vary from child to child. The phonemic repertoire determination may include the most important information for a child with a very severe articulation problem. For children who exhibit articulation characteristic of the first 50 words described by Ingram (1976), the process analysis would reveal many processes, but the more meaningful information might be that the child uses only four consonants. For example, examine the sample below:

ball	bɔ	candy	dænɪ
cat	dæ	light	aɪ

down	daʊ	drum	dʌ
no	no	broke	bo
there	dɛˀ	go	do
tummy	dʌmɪ	put	bʊ
Mama	mɑmɑ	that	dæ
rabbit	æbɪ	cheese	di
show	do	Daddy	dædɪ
zipper	dɪbˀ	sit	dɪ
pretty	bɪdɪ	shoe	du

Assuming this to represent the child's complete repertoire, her consonant inventory includes /b/, /d/, /m/, and /n/.

Process analysis would reveal the following processes operating in the child's speech: stopping, velar fronting, palatal fronting, final consonant deletion, cluster reduction, voicing, and deletion of initial liquids. This analysis tells us that the child uses most major processes and needs work on eliminating all of them. It may fail to account for the absence of liquids because initial consonant omission is not a commonly discussed process.

Although the information can be expressed either way, it may be equally useful in this case to describe the features of the phonemes that the child uses rather than the changes made. The full repertoire includes only the following classes of sounds:

Manner	*Place*
stop	bilabial
nasal	alveolar
voiced	

Only voiced bilabial and alveolar stops and nasals are used, and only in syllable-initiating positions. The feature analysis indicates that the child needs help in developing fricatives, glides and liquids, palatals, velars, and unvoiced sounds.

Neither analysis may represent the information as clearly as simply saying that the child uses only four consonants (/b, m, d, n/) in only syllable-initiation position. Obviously, this repertoire needs expansion in many directions. The real decision is the ordering of features to be learned or processes to be eliminated. The phonemic repertoire data have given the clearest picture of the child's current status. The process or feature analysis will help to direct the therapeutic procedures.

6. Analyze the child's phoneme preferences. Weiner (1981) suggests that some children may demonstrate a preference for the use of certain phonemes not necessarily consistent with the child's phonological processes. Such preferences may look like processes at first glance, but closer analysis shows that the preference is more widespread than the process would predict. For example, Weiner mentions a child who substituted /θ/ for all initial fricatives, affricates, liquids, and glides. Weiner points out that initially this child's sample might be interpreted as exhibiting a fronting process, but the substitution of /θ/ for /f/ and /w/ does not reflect fronting. In addition /g/ is produced correctly. Based on the children he observed, Weiner gives four characteristics of sound preferences: (a) One or a few phonemes were substituted for a manner class, (b) sound preference was more common in the initial position, (c) sound preference was more likely to affect nonlabial and voiceless sounds, and (d) fricatives were more often affected than other manner classes. This does not mean that a given substitution must meet all of these characteristics to reveal a sound preference. When a particular sound is especially prevalent as a substitution and it does not fit with the child's phonological patterns, sound preference is a possibility.

For children with severe articulation disorders, what may initially look like exceptions to a phonological process may be better explained by sound preference. It is important to examine the possibility of sound preference because different therapeutic techniques are indicated for remediation of processes and sound preferences (Weiner, 1981).

Choosing an Analysis Procedure

The clinician may be confused about which of the phonological analysis procedures to choose. Several studies have investigated whether different analysis procedures suggest the same or different remediation targets.

Benjamin and Greenwood (1983) compared the results obtained from three assessment procedures, the Assessment of Phonological Processes (Hodson, 1980), Procedures for the Phonological Analysis of Children's Language (Ingram, 1981), and the Phonological Process Protocol (Khan & Lewis, 1982). They used these procedures to measure the percentage of occurrence of five processes in 18 children. The processes were final consonant deletion, cluster reduction, stopping, fronting, and gliding. They found good agreement among the three procedures despite the fact that different samples were used for each. Gliding was the least consistent across analyses.

Dyson and Robinson (1987) used the Assessment of Phonological Processes (Hodson, 1980), Natural Process Analysis (Shriberg and Kwiatkowski, 1980), and a modified form of the Procedures for the Phonological Analysis of Children's Language (Ingram, 1981) to analyze the speech of five children. Paden and Moss (1985) analyzed three children's speech using the same procedures. Both studies found that similar therapy targets were selected using all three procedures despite the fact that the procedures varied according to whether single words or conversational speech was analyzed. Any differences in target processes were due largely to definition of terms. Findings from the three studies suggest that (1) use of both single words and conversational speech may be useful, (2) no one procedure may provide all of the information needed to select targets, and (3) reliability need not be a major factor in choosing a test to evaluate the major processes. The clinician may

therefore consider issues such as time needed for completion, number of processes to be evaluated, type of sample available or obtainable, and intelligibility and interest level of the child.

Looking Beyond Standard Assessment Procedures

Idiosyncratic patterns have been noted frequently enough in phonologically disordered children (Dunn & Davis, 1983; Grunwell, 1981; Ingram, 1976; Leonard & Brown, 1984; Leonard & Leonard, 1985; Weiner, 1981) to warrant close examination of speech samples for unusual patterns, sound preferences, and the contexts in which these phonomena occur. Camarata and Gandour (1984) argue that phonological process analysis may not be sufficient for describing idiosyncratic phonological systems. These authors found that the process analysis did not adequately describe the system of a child whose use of stops was conditioned by vowel height. The child used [d] before high vowels and [g] before nonhigh vowels. This pattern was captured by writing context-sensitive rules that specify the sound change and the phonetic environment in which it occurs.

Further support for going beyond the phonological process analysis is provided by Klein and Spector (1985), who found that children's process use was related to syllable stress. Increased process use, as well as a larger number of atypical productions, occurred in syllables of reduced stress.

Similarly, Pollock and Schwartz (1988) observed a relationship between syllable structure and position and the development of segments in a phonologically disordered child whom they studied over 4 years. Some assessment programs (especially Grunwell, 1985) suggest procedures for analyzing such interrelationships; however, in at least some cases, a really thorough analysis will require the clinician to be creative in developing a strategy for examining the child's unique system.

It has been suggested here that clinicians can design their own analysis procedures rather than use a published test. Lowe (1986) further suggested that clinicians can design formats for analyzing phonological processes using single-word articulation tests. He presented a form for use with the Goldman-Fristoe Test of Articulation (Goldman & Fristoe, 1986) and the Templin-Darley Tests of Articulation (Templin & Darley, 1969). While major processes were identified by using these forms, more thorough analysis would be required to describe less obvious patterns.

The conclusion that should be drawn is that the best decisions will be made by clinicians who select assessment strategies based on thorough understanding of the principles and procedures and the needs of individual clients, and who interpret their own findings using sound clinical judgment.

Using the Assessment Results

The value of any assessment procedure lies in its usefulness in planning remediation and making predictions about success. One problem in using diagnostic results to plan therapy is the difficulty of determining exactly where an observed breakdown actually occurs in the phonological-articulatory system. Winitz makes this point in chapter 9 and provides the following example. Consider the difficulty that exists in trying to establish whether a child's difficulty has resulted from a breakdown in the phonological system or whether it is a motor planning or production problem. Often a phonological rule can be used to describe the consistency of an articulation error, but it does not necessarily follow that the primary cause of difficulty lies in a defective phonological system. For example, a rule stating that a target sound is omitted in consonant blends may define a generalization that exists because a breakdown has occurred at any of a number of points in the sound production process. A radiologic or spectrographic examination may reveal unusual articulatory relationships that suggest errors in timing or overall coordination of the component sounds of blends. In this particular case, the phonological rule describes the consistency of the patterned error on blends; it does not adequately explain it, and furthermore, this interpretation might mislead one to believe that the primary reason for the error is at the underlying phonological level and not elsewhere. For this reason, it is important to examine all aspects of the phonological-articulatory system and to be open to all possible explanations for a given problem.

Making predictions is the second important outcome of assessment. In early sections of this chapter, research regarding the predictive value of tests of stimulability and discrimination was discussed. A third factor in making predictions involves the severity of the articulation problem itself. Van Riper and Erickson (1969) used this as a basis for the Predictive Screening Test of Articulation, which was designed to predict which first-grade children would correct their articulation errors by third grade without clinical intervention. This prediction was based on the number of errors on the screening test.

In addition to the number of errors the child exhibits, the types of errors may also be related to the severity of the problem. Renfrew (1966) discusses the great difficulty encountered in therapy with clients who use consonants correctly in initial position of words but omit medial and nearly all final consonants. She refers to these omissions as a persistent ''open-syllable'' pattern and describes intelligent children who become aware of their disability to the extent of adding a consonant, which is usually incorrect, after giving a one-word response. This added consonant is produced as a separate syllable, and Renfrew reports that such children seem to find it impossible to make the transition from vowel to consonant in the same syllable.

Panagos (1974) explained the open-syllable problem identified by Renfrew as but one symptom of a more generalized language disorder in which children with delayed language development systematically reduce syllable complexity. He relates the problem to deeper levels of cognitive and linguistic development and discusses it in terms of simplified rule systems by which the child operates. A number of studies have suggested this relationship between language and articulation disorders (Gross, St. Louis, Ruscello, Hull, 1985; Leonard, Miller, & Brown, 1980; Matheny & Panagos, 1978; Menyuk & Looney, 1972; Schwartz, Leonard, Folger, & Wilcox, 1980; Shriner, Holloway, & Daniloff, 1969; Whitacre, Luper, & Pollio, 1970). In general, it has been found that children with articulation errors score more poorly on formal tests of syntax (Marquardt & Saxman, 1972; Saxman & Miller, 1973; Smit & Bernthal, 1983). There is also a relationship between phonological errors and other syntactic measures, such as morphological omissions (Menyuk, 1964; Paul & Shriberg, 1982; Smit & Bernthal, 1983b) and sentence structure complexity (Menyuk, 1964; Paul & Shriberg, 1982). It has been shown that linguistic complexity may promote articulation errors (Dunn & Barron, 1982; Panagos, Quine, & Klich, 1979) and that phonological complexity and syntactic complexity may interact in producing errors in both domains (Paul & Shriberg, 1982).

Campbell and Shriberg (1982) also found an interaction between phonological errors and pragmatics. The children in their study demonstrated more phonological processes on unstressed words than on stressed and on those stressed words that were topics rather than those that were comments. The comment is the new information in the sentence, and may be considered to be more necessary to communicate early. Likewise, stressed words usually carry important information.

This suggested relationship between phonological errors and other linguistic deficits indicates need for evaluating the language of children with

articulation problems. Description of language evaluation procedures is not within the realm of this text, but it is important to note here that the clinician should be aware of the potential language problems of articulation-disordered children and be prepared for such assessment.

Shriberg (1982) and Shriberg and Kwiatkowski (1982a, 1982b) have attempted to develop procedures for assessing severity of articulatory involvement and deriving a classification system. They examined the contributions of four factors in determining severity: (a) percentage of consonants correct, (b) severity ratings of judges, (c) percentage of intelligible words, and (d) suprasegmental ratings (loudness, quality, phrasing, stress, rate, pitch). They found that percentage of consonants correct was the major predictor of the judges' severity ratings, but they were also influenced by age and suprasegmentals. The authors suggested the following procedures for classifying clients as mild, moderate or severe:

1. Tape a continuous speech sample. Repeat the client's utterances for subsequent analysis.
2. Calculate percentage of consonants correct from the tape.
3. Score the six suprasegmentals on a 3-point rating scale.
4. Use percentage of consonants correct as the major weighting factor, but also account for age and suprasegmentals.

SUMMARY

Thorough and accurate assessment is a necessary prerequisite for any remediation program, but assessment is not an activity that is complete before therapy begins. Continual evaluation and reevaluation is important throughout the remediation process in order to determine the appropriateness of

ongoing procedures, to suggest needed changes, and to make decisions regarding termination.

This chapter has presented a variety of procedures to be used for assessment. Any evaluation of articulation includes obtaining an adequate sample of speech, which generally includes both single-word productions and spontaneous conversation. Traditional methods have usually analyzed substitutions, omissions, and distortions in single-word samples. Tests that evaluate sounds in a variety of phonetic contexts are also available.

More recent linguistic approaches to analyzing articulation have been developed in response to the notion that treating patterns of error rather than individual phonemes can lead to more effective and efficient remediation. These assessment methods are based on examination of the child's rule system. Distinctive-feature analysis and phonological-process analysis are two methods of describing the child's rules and determining how they differ from the standard system.

In addition to the articulation test or phonological analysis, a thorough evaluation should include any or all of the following, depending on the child's symptoms and needs: orofacial examination, stimulability testing, and perhaps auditory discrimination testing. Other aspects of any communication assessment such as case history, hearing evaluation, language assessment, etc., have not been discussed here.

Each clinician must select those evaluation strategies that are appropriate for a particular situation. The best assessment protocol is one that is based on the kind of careful attention to detail that goes into developing formal tests, but is designed by the clinician to fit the needs of the client and the therapeutic program.

REFERENCES

Aungst, L. F., & Frick, J. V. (1964). Auditory discrimination ability and consistency of articulation of /r/. *Journal of Speech and Hearing Disorders, 29*, 76–85.

Bankson, N. W., & Bernthal, J. E. (1982a). Articulation assessment. In N. J. Lass, J. L. Northern, D. E. Yoder, & L. V. Reynolds (Eds.), *Speech, language and hearing* (Vol II). Philadelphia: W. B. Saunders.

Bankson, N. W., & Bernthal, J. E. (1982b). A comparison of phonological processes identified through word and sentence imitation tasks of the PPA. *Language, Speech and Hearing Services in Schools, 13*, 96–99.

Bankson, N. W., & Bernthal, J. E. (1983). In the defense of the traditional articulation test battery. In J. L. Locke (Ed.), *Assessing and treating phonological disorders: Current approaches. Seminars in speech and language, 4*. New York: Thieme-Stratton.

Benjamin, B. J., & Greenwood, J. L. (1983). A comparison of three phonological assessment procedures. *Journal of Childhood Communication Disorders, 7*, 19–27.

Bernstein, D. K. (1978, November). *More of the same about different*. Paper presented at the American Speech-Language-Hearing Association Annual Convention, San Francisco.

Bernthal, J. E., & Bankson, N. W. (1981). *Articulation disorders*. Englewood Cliffs, NJ: Prentice-Hall.

Camarata, S., & Gandour, J. (1984). On describing idiosyncratic phonologic systems. *Journal of Speech and Hearing Disorders, 49*, 262–266.

Campbell, T., & Shriberg, L. (1982). Associations among pragmatic functions, linguistic stress, and natural phonological processes in speech-delayed children. *Journal of Speech and Hearing Research, 25*, 547–553.

Carter, E. T., & Buck, M. W. (1958). Prognostic testing for functional articulation disorders among children in the first grade. *Journal of Speech and Hearing Disorders, 23*, 124–133.

Chomsky, N. (1968). *Language and mind*. New York: Harcourt, Brace & World.

Chomsky, N., & Halle, M. (1968). *The sound pattern of English*. New York: Harper & Row.

Compton, A. J., & Hutton, J. S. (1978). *Compton-Hutton phonological assessment*. San Francisco: Carousel House.

Costello, J. (1975). Articulation instruction based on distinctive features theory. *Language, Speech and Hearing Services in Schools, 6,* 61–71.

Curtis, J. F. (1956). Disorders of articulation. In W. J. Johnson, S. Brown, J. Curtis, C. Edney, & J. Keaster (Eds.), *Speech handicapped school children* (Rev. ed., pp. 92–153). New York: Harper & Row.

Curtis, J. F., & Hardy, J. C. (1959). A phonetic study of misarticulation of /r/. *Journal of Speech and Hearing Research, 2,* 244–257.

Diedrich, W. M. (1983). Stimulability and articulation disorders. *Seminars in Speech and Language, 4*(4), 297–311.

Dubois, E. M., & Bernthal, J. E. (1978). A comparison of three methods of obtaining articulatory responses. *Journal of Speech and Hearing Disorders, 43,* 295–305.

Dunn, C., & Barron, C. (1982). A treatment program for disordered phonology: Phonetic and linguistic considerations. *Language, Speech, and Hearing Services in Schools, 13,* 100–109.

Dunn, C., & Davis, B. (1983). Phonological process occurrence in phonologically disordered children. *Applied Psycholinguistics, 4,* 187–207.

Dworkin, J. (1978). Differential diagnosis of motor speech disorders: The clinical examination of the speech mechanism. *Journal of the National Student Speech and Hearing Association, 8,* 37–62.

Dworkin, J., & Culatta, R. (1980). *D-COME: Dworkin Culatta oral mechanism examination.* Nicholasville, KY: Edgewood Press.

Dyson, A. T., & Robinson, T. W. (1987). The effect of phonological analysis procedure on the selection of potential remediation targets. *Language, Speech and Hearing Services in Schools, 18,* 364–377.

Elbert, M., & Gierut, J. (1986). *Handbook of clinical phonology: Approaches to assessment and treatment.* San Diego: College Hill Press.

Elbert, M., & McReynolds, L. (1978). An experimental analysis of misarticulating children's generalization. *Journal of Speech and Hearing Research, 21*(1), 136–150.

Elbert, M., Shelton, R., & Arndt, W. (1967). A task for evaluation of articulation change: 1. Development of methodology. *Journal of Speech and Hearing Research, 10,* 281–288.

Faircloth, M. A., and Faircloth, S. R. (1970). An analysis of the articulatory behavior of a speech-defective child in connected speech. *Journal of Speech and Hearing Disorders, 35,* 51–61.

Farquhar, M. S. (1961). Prognostic value of imitative and auditory discrimination tests. *Journal of Speech and Hearing Disorders, 26,* 342–347.

Fisher, H., & Logemann, J. (1971). *The Fisher-Logemann test of articulation competence.* Boston: Houghton Mifflin.

Fluharty, N. B. (1976). Fluharty preschool speech and language screening test. Hingham, MA: Teaching Resources.

Fudala, J. (1974). *Arizona articulation proficiency scale.* Los Angeles: Western Psychological Services.

Gallagher, T. M., & Shriner, T. H. (1975a). Articulatory inconsistencies in the speech of normal children. *Journal of Speech and Hearing Research, 18,* 168–175.

Gallagher, T. M., & Shriner, T. H. (1975b). Contextual variables related to inconsistent /s/ and /z/ production in the spontaneous speech of children. *Journal of Speech and Hearing Research, 18,* 623–633.

Goldman, R., & Fristoe, M. (1969, 1986). *Test of articulation.* Circle Pines, MN: American Guidance Service.

Goldman, R., Fristoe, M., & Woodcock, R. (1970). *The Goldman-Fristoe-Woodcock test of auditory discrimination.* Circle Pines, MN: American Guidance Service.

Gross, G. H., St. Louis, K. O., Ruscello, D. M., & Hull, F. M. (1985). Language abilities of articulatory-disordered school children with multiple or residual errors. *Language, Speech and Hearing Services in Schools, 16,* 171–186.

Grunwell, P. (1981). The nature of phonological disability in children. New York: Academic Press.

Grunwell, P. (1982). *Clinical phonology.* Rockville, MD: Aspen Systems.

Grunwell, P. (1985). *Phonological assessment of child speech.* San Diego: College Hill Press.

Ham, R. E. (1958). Relationship between misspelling and misarticulation. *Journal of Speech and Hearing Disorders, 23,* 294–297.

Hodson, B. W. (1980). The assessment of phonological processes. Danville, IL: Interstate.

Hodson, B. W. (1986a). *The assessment of phonological processes—revised.* Danville, IL: Interstate Press.

Hodson, B. W. (1986b). *Assessment of phonological processes—Spanish.* San Diego: Los Amigos.

Hoffman, P. R., Schuckers, G. H., & Ratusnik, D. L. (1977). Contextual-coarticulatory inconsistency of /r/ misarticulation. *Journal of Speech and Hearing Research, 20,* 631–643.

Hoffman, P. R., Stager, S., & Daniloff, R. G. (1983). Perception and production of misarticulated /r/. *Journal of Speech and Hearing Disorders, 48,* 210–215.

Ingram, D. (1976). *Phonological disability in children.* New York: Elsevier.

Ingram, D. (1981). *Procedures for the phonological analysis of children's language.* Baltimore: University Park Press.

Jakobson, R., Fant, C. G. M., & Halle, M. (1963). *Preliminaries to speech analysis.* Cambridge: MIT Press.

Johnson, J. P., Winney, B. L., & Pederson, O. T. (1980). Single word versus connected speech articulation testing. *Language, Speech, and Hearing Services in the Schools, 11*(3), 175–179.

Jordan, E. P. (1960). Articulation test measures and listener ratings of articulation defectiveness. *Journal of Speech and Hearing Research, 3*(4), 303–319.

Kent, R. D., Kent, J. F., & Rosenbek, J. C. (1987). Maximum performance tests of speech production. *Journal of Speech and Hearing Disorders, 52,* 367–387.

Khan, L., & Lewis, N. (1982). *Phonological process protocol.* Field Test Edition.

Khan, L., & Lewis, N. (1986). *Phonological analysis.* Circle Pines, MN: American Guidance Service.

Kisatsky, T. J. (1967). The prognostic value of Carter-Buck tests in measuring articulation skills of selected kindergarten children. *Exceptional Children, 34*(2), 81–85.

Klein, H. B., & Spector, C. C. (1985). Effect of syllable stress and serial position on error variability in polysyllabic productions of speech-delayed children. *Journal of Speech and Hearing Disorders, 50,* 391–402.

Kresheck, J. D., & Socolofsky, G. (1972). Imitative and spontaneous articulatory assessment of four-year-old children. *Journal of Speech and Hearing Research, 15,* 729–733.

Ladefoged, P. (1975). *A course in phonetics.* New York: Harcourt Brace Jovanovich.

Leonard, L. B., & Brown, B. L. (1984). Nature and boundaries of phonologic categories: A case study of an unusual phonologic pattern in a language-impaired child. *Journal of Speech and Hearing Disorders, 49,* 419–428.

Leonard, L. B., & Leonard, J. S. (1985). The contribution of phonetic context to an unusual phonological pattern: A case study. *Language, Speech and Hearing Services in Schools, 16,* 110–118.

Leonard, L., Miller, J., & Brown, H. (1980). Consonant and syllable harmony in the speech of language disordered children. *Journal of Speech and Hearing Disorders, 45,* 336–345.

Locke, J. L. (1980a). The inference of speech perception in the phonologically disordered child. Part I: A rationale, some criteria, the conventional tests. *Journal of Speech and Hearing Disorders, 45,* 431–444.

Locke, J. L. (1980b). The inference of speech perception in the phonologically disordered child. Part II: Some clinically novel procedures, their use, some findings. *Journal of Speech and Hearing Disorders, 45,* 445–468.

Lowe, R. J. (1986). Phonological process analysis using three position tests. *Language, Speech and Hearing Services in Schools, 17,* 72–79.

Lund, N. J., & Duchan, J. F. (1978). Phonological analysis: A multifaceted approach. *British Journal of Disorders of Communication, 13,* 119–126.

Lund, N. J., & Duchan, J. F. (1983). *Assessing children's language in naturalistic contexts.* Englewood Cliffs, NJ: Prentice-Hall.

Madison, C. L. (1979). Articulatory stimulability reviewed. *Language, Speech and Hearing Services in Schools, 10*(3), 185–190.

Marquardt, T., & Saxman, J. (1972). Language comprehension and auditory discrimination in articulation deficient kindergarten children. *Journal of Speech and Hearing Research, 15,* 382–389.

Mason, R., & Simon, C. (1977). An orofacial examination checklist. *Language, Speech and Hearing Services in Schools, 8,* 155–163.

Matheny, N., & Panagos, J. M. (1978). Comparing the effects of articulation and syntax programs on syntax and articulation improvements. *Language, Speech and Hearing Services in Schools, 9,* 57–61.

McDonald, E. T. (1964). *A deep test of articulation –picture form.* Pittsburgh: Stanwix House.

Menyuk, P. (1964). Comparison of grammar of children with functionally deviant and normal speech.

Journal of Speech and Hearing Research, 7, 109–121.

Menyuk, P., & Looney, P. (1972). Relationships among components of the grammar in language disorder. *Journal of Speech and Hearing Research, 15,* 395–406.

Milisen, R. (1954). A rationale for articulation disorders. In R. Milisen & Associates (Eds.), The disorder of articulation: A systematic and clinical and experimental approach. *Journal of Speech and Hearing Disorders,* Monograph Suppl. 4, 5–18.

Monnin, L. M., & Huntington, D. A. (1974). Relationship of articulatory defects to speech-sound identification. *Journal of Speech and Hearing Research, 17,* 352–366.

Moore, W. H., Burke, J., & Adams, C. (1976). The effects of stimulability on the articulation of /s/ relative to cluster and word frequency of occurrence. *Journal of Speech and Hearing Research, 19,* 458–466.

Olmsted, D. L. (1971). *Out of the mouths of babes: Earliest stages in language learning.* The Hague: Mouton.

Paden, E. P., & Moss, S. A. (1985). Comparison of three phonological analysis procedures. *Language, Speech and Hearing Services in Schools, 16,* 103–109.

Panagos, J. M. (1974). Persistence of the open syllable reinterpreted as a symptom of language disorder. *Journal of Speech and Hearing Disorders, 39,* 23–31.

Panagos, J. M., Quine, M. E., & Klich, R. J. (1979). Syntactic and phonological influences on children's articulation. *Journal of Speech and Hearing Research, 22,* 841–848.

Parker, F. (1976). Distinctive features in speech pathology: Phonology or phonemics? *Journal of Speech and Hearing Disorders, 41,* 23–29.

Paul, R., & Shriberg, L. (1982). Associations between phonology and syntax in speech delayed children. *Journal of Speech and Hearing Research, 25,* 536–547.

Paynter, E. T., & Bumpas, T. C. (1977). Imitative and spontaneous articulatory assessment of three-year-old children. *Journal of Speech and Hearing Disorders, 42,* 119–125.

Pendergast, K., Dickey, S., Selmar, J., & Soder, A. (1969). *Photo articulation test.* Danville, IL: Interstate.

Pollock, K. E., & Schwartz, R. G. (1988). Structural aspects of phonological development: Case study of a disordered child. *Language, Speech and Hearing Services in Schools, 19,* 5–16.

Powers, M. J. (1957). Functional disorders of articulation: Symptomatology and etiology. In L. E. Travis (Ed.), *Handbook of speech pathology.* New York: Appleton-Century-Crofts.

Renfrew, C. E. (1966). Persistence of the open syllable in defective articulation. *Journal of Speech and Hearing Disorders, 31,* 370–373.

Ritterman, S. I., Zook-Herman, S. L., Carlson, R. L., & Kinde, S. W. (1982). The pass/fail disparity among three commonly employed articulatory screening tests. *Journal of Speech and Hearing Disorders, 47,* 429–433.

St. Louis, K. & Ruscello, D. (1981). *The oral speech screening examination.* Baltimore: University Park Press.

Sander, E. K. (1972). When are speech sounds learned? *Journal of Speech and Hearing Disorders, 37,* 55–63.

Saxman, J., & Miller, J. (1973). Short term memory and language skills in articulation deficient children. *Journal of Speech and Hearing Research, 16,* 721—730.

Schwartz, R., Leonard, L., Folger, M., & Wilcox, M. (1980). Early phonological behavior in normal-speaking and language-disordered children: Evidence for a synergistic view of linguistic disorders. *Journal of Speech and Hearing Disorders, 45,* 357–377.

Secord, W. (1981a). *C-PAC: Clinical probes of articulation consistency.* Columbus, OH: Merrill.

Secord, W. (1981b). *T-MAC: Test of minimal articulation competence.* Columbus, OH: Merrill.

Shelton, R. L. (1978). Speech sound discrimination in the correction of disordered articulation. *Allied Health and Behavioral Sciences, 1,* 176–194.

Shriberg, L. D. (1982). Diagnostic assessment of developmental phonological disorders. In M. A. Crary (Ed.), *Phonological intervention: Concepts and procedures.* San Diego: College-Hill Press.

Shriberg, L. D., & Kwiatkowski, J. (1980). *Natural process analysis.* New York: Wiley.

Shriberg, L. D., & Kwiatkowski, J. (1982a). Phonological disorders. I: A diagnostic classification system. *Journal of Speech and Hearing Disorders, 47,* 226–241.

Shriberg, L. D., & Kwiatkowski, J. (1982b). Phonological disorders. III: A procedure for assessing severity of involvement. *Journal of Speech and Hearing Disorders, 47,* 422–456.

Shriberg, L. D., & Kwiatkowski, J. (1985). Continuous speech sampling for phonologic analysis of speech-delayed children. *Journal of Speech and Hearing Disorders, 50,* 323–334.

Shriner, T. H., Holloway, M. D., & Daniloff, R. G. (1969). The relationship between articulatory deficits and syntax in speech defective children. *Journal of Speech and Hearing Research, 12,* 319–325.

Siegel, G. M., Winitz, H., & Conkey, H. (1963). The influence of testing instruments on articulatory responses of children. *Journal of Speech and Hearing Disorders, 28,* 67–76.

Singh, S., & Frank, D. C. (1979). A distinctive feature analysis of the consonantal substitution pattern. In H. H. Walsh (Ed.), *Phonology and speech remediation: A book of readings.* Houston: College Hill Press.

Singh, S., & Polen, S. (1972). Use of a distinctive feature model in speech pathology. *Acta Symbolica, 3,* 17–25.

Smit, A. B., & Bernthal, J. E. (1983a). Voicing contrasts and their phonological implications in the speech of articulation-disordered children. *Journal of Speech and Hearing Research, 26,* 486–499.

Smit, A., & Bernthal, J. (1983b). Performance of articulation-disordered children on language and perception measures. *Journal of Speech and Hearing Research, 26,* 124–136.

Smith, M. W., & Ainsworth, S. (1967). The effects of three types of stimulation on articulatory responses of speech defective children. *Journal of Speech and Hearing Research, 10,* 333–338.

Snow, K., & Milisen, R. (1954). The influence of oral versus pictorial presentation upon articulation testing results. *Journal of Speech and Hearing Disorders,* Monograph Supplement 4, 29–36.

Sommers, R. K., Leiss, R. H., Delp, M. A., Gerber, D. F., Smith, R. M., Revucky, M. V., Ellis, D., & Haley, V. A. (1967). Factors related to the effectiveness of articulation therapy for kindergarten, first, and second grade children. *Journal of Speech and Hearing Research, 10,* 428–437.

Spriestersbach, D. C., & Curtis, J. F. (1951). Misarticulation and discrimination of speech sounds. *Quarterly Journal of Speech, 37,* 483–491.

Templin, M. C. (1947). Spontaneous versus imitated verbalization in testing articulation in preschool children. *Journal of Speech and Hearing Disorders, 12,* 293–300.

Templin, M. C. (1957). Templin speech sound discrimination test. In M. C. Moore (Ed.), *Certain language skills in children.* Minneapolis: University of Minnesota Press.

Templin, M. C., & Darley, F. L. (1969). The Templin-Darley Tests of Articulation. Iowa City, IA: Bureau of Educational Research and Service, University of Iowa.

Travis, L. E. (1931). *Speech pathology.* New York: Appleton-Century.

Travis, L. E., & Rasmus, B. (1931). The speech-sound discrimination ability of cases with functional disorders of articulation. *Quarterly Journal of Speech, 17,* 217–226.

Turton, L. J. (1980). Developmental bases of articulation assessment. In W. D. Wolfe & D. J. Goulding (Eds.), *Articulation and learning* (2nd ed.). Springfield, IL: Charles C. Thomas.

Van Riper, C., (1947). *Speech correction principles and methods* (2nd ed.). New York: Prentice-Hall.

Van Riper, C. (1972). *Speech correction principles and methods* (5th ed.). Englewood Cliffs, NJ: Prentice-Hall.

Van Riper, C., & Erickson, R. (1969). A predictive screening test of articulation. *Journal of Speech and Hearing Disorders, 34,* 214–219.

Van Riper, C., & Irwin, J. (1958). *Voice and articulation.* Englewood Cliffs, NJ: Prentice-Hall.

Walsh, H. (1974). On certain practical inadequacies of distinctive feature systems. *Journal of Speech and Hearing Disorders, 39,* 32–43.

Weiner, F. F. (1979). *Phonological process analysis.* Baltimore: University Park Press.

Weiner, F. (1981). Systematic sound preference as a characteristic of phonological disability. *Journal of Speech and Hearing Research, 46,* 281–285.

Weiner, P. S. (1967). Auditory discrimination and articulation. *Journal of Speech and Hearing Disorders, 32,* 19–28.

Weismer, G., Dinnsen, D., & Elbert, M. (1981). A study of the voicing distinction associated with omitted, word-final stops. *Journal of Speech and Hearing Disorders, 46,* 320–327.

Wepman, J. (1973). *Auditory discrimination test* (rev. ed.). Palm Springs: Language Research Association.

Whitacre, J. D., Luper, H. L., & Pollio, H. R. (1970). General language deficits in children with articulation problems. *Language and Speech, 13,* 231–239.

Winitz, H. (1975). *From syllable to conversation.* Baltimore: University Park Press.

Wise, C. (1957). *Applied phonetics.* Englewood Cliffs, NJ: Prentice-Hall.

Woolf, G., & Pilberg, R. (1971). A comparison of three tests of auditory discrimination and their relationship to performance on a deep test of articulation. *Journal of Communication Disorders, 3,* 239–249.

Zehel, Z., Shelton, R. L., Arndt, W. B., Wright, V., & Elbert, M. (1972). Item context and /s/ phone articulation test results. *Journal of Speech and Hearing Research, 15,* 852–860.

APPENDIX 4.1 Assessment Instruments Available Commercially

Articulation Tests

Arizona Articulation Proficiency Scale (ASPS). Janet Barker Fudala and William M. Reynolds. Los Angeles: Western Psychological Services, 1963, 1970, 1974, 1986. Cost: $64.00; picture test cards, protocol booklet, 10 survey forms, manual; additional forms (pad of 100), $13.50. Time: 20 minutes.

Articulation Testing and Treatment: A Sensory-Motor Approach, Eugene T. McDonald. Pittsburgh, PA: Stanwix House, 1964. Cost: $18.00; individual record sheet, screening (50 sheets per pad), $.75; teacher report form, screening (50 sheets per pad), $1.25.

Austin Spanish Articulation Test (ASAT), Elizabeth Carrow. Allen, TX: Teaching Resources Corporation, 1974. Cost: $19.00; examiner's manual and test stimuli, 130 pages; test booklet, 4 pages. Time: 25 minutes.

Clinical Probes of Articulation Consistency (C-PAC), Wayne Secord. San Antonio: The Psychological Corporation, 1981. Cost: $79.00; manual, storytelling manual, spirit master articulation probes. Time: 5 minutes per consonant probe, 10 minutes per vowel probe.

A Deep Test of Articulation, Picture Form, Eugene T. McDonald. Pittsburgh, PA: Stanwix House, 1964. Cost: $18.00; individual record sheet, screening (50 sheets per pad), $.75; teacher report form, screening (50 sheets per pad), $1.25.

A Deep Test of Articulation, Sentence Form, Eugene T. McDonald. Pittsburgh, PA: Stanwix House, 1964. Cost: $13.50; individual record sheet, screening (50 sheets per pad), $.75; teacher report form, screening (50 sheets per pad), $1.25.

The Denver Articulation Screening Examination (DASE), Amelia F. Drumwright. Denver: Ladoca Project and Publishing Foundation, Inc., 1971. Cost: $6.50, Denver Articulation Manual Workbook; picture cards (per set), $1.25; test forms (per 25), $1.75; 1-hour training and proficiency film, $400.00; 1-hour training and proficiency video cassette, $150.00; rental of training and proficiency film (per week), $50.00; rental of training and proficiency video cassette (per week), $40.00. Time: Picture form, 20–45 minutes; sentence form, 8–10 minutes, administration; 10–20 minutes, scoring.

Goldman-Fristoe Test of Articulation (GFTA), Ronald Goldman and Macalyne Fristoe. Circle Pines, MN: American Guidance Service, 1969, 1972, 1986. Cost: $62.00; test plates in easel, 25 response forms, manual; additional response forms (package of 25), $6.50. Time: 15 minutes for Sounds in Words Subtest.

Integrated Articulation Test, Orvis C. Irwin. Published in Orvis C. Irwin, *Communication variables of cerebral palsied and mentally retarded children*. Springfield, IL.: Charles C. Thomas, 1972. Two equivalent forms, Part Tests A through E and Alternate Part Tests A through E. Cost: $29.75. Manual and test forms are not available except as a part of the book.

Photo Articulation Test (PAT), Kathleen Pendergast, Stanley E. Dickey, John W. Selmar, and Anton L. Soder. Danville, IL: Interstate Printers and Publishers, Inc., 1969. Short and long forms available. Cost:

Predictive Screening Test of Articulation (PSTA) (3rd ed.), Charles Van Riper and Robert L. Erickson. Kalamazoo, MI: Western Michigan University, Continuing Education Office, 1973. Cost: $1.50. Manual, 18 pages; score sheet, 5 pages. Time: 7–8 minutes.

Screening Deep Test of Articulation, Eugene T. McDonald. Pittsburgh, PA: Stanwix House, 1968. Cost: $18.00; individual record sheet, screening (50 sheets per pad), $.75; teacher report form, screening (50 sheets per pad), $1.25.

Screening Speech Articulation Test (SSAT), Merlin J. Mecham, J. Lorin Jex, and J. Dean Jones, Salt Lake City, UT: Communication Research Associates, Inc., 1970. Cost: manual, 30 pages, $4.50; score sheets, $2.50 for pad of 25; test booklet, 30 pages. Time: Picture portion: 5–8 minutes; consonants in sentences: 3–5 minutes; vowels in sentences: 2 minutes; blends in words: 1 minute.

The Templin-Darley Tests of Articulation (2nd ed.), Mildred C. Templin and Frederic L. Darley. Iowa City: University of Iowa Bureau of Educational Research and Service, 1969. Cost: $6.00, manual, 38 pages, Appendix A (test words), Appendix B (test sentences); reusable overlays for scoring, $1.00 set of nine; test response forms, 4 pages, $.10 each; specimen set, $6.00 postpaid. Time: variable.

Test of Minimal Articulation Competence (T-MAC), Wayne Secord. San Antonio: The Psychological Corporation, 1981. Cost: $45.00: manual, 25 record forms; additional forms (pack of 25) $17.00. Time: 10–20 minutes, 3–5 minutes for screening.

Weiss Comprehensive Articulation Test (W-CAT), Curtis Weiss. Hingham, MA: Teaching Resources, 1978. Cost $54.00; picture cards in easel, sentence card, 50 response forms, manual; additional forms (pad of 50) $12.50. Time: 20 minutes.

Phonological Assessment Procedures

The Assessment of Phonological Processes—Revised, Barbara W. Hodson. Danville, IL: The Interstate Publishers and Printers, Inc., 1986. Cost: $39.95. Extra recording forms (pad of 48), $5.00; extra phonological analysis summaries (pad of 48), $5.00; extra screening forms (pad of 96), $5.00.

Compton-Hutton Phonological Assessment, Arthur J. Compton and Stanley Hutton. San Francisco: Carou-

sel House, 1978. Cost: $35.00. Additional forms (set of 25), $4.25.

The Khan-Lewis Phonological Analysis (KLPA), Linda M. L. Khan and Nancy P. Lewis. Circle Pines, MN: American Guidance Service, 1986. Cost: $33.50. Scoring forms (package of 25), $25.00. Time: 15–40 minutes for analysis.

Natural Process Analysis, Lawrence Shriberg and Janet Kwiatkowski. New York: John Wiley and Sons, 1980. Cost: $29.95.

Phonological Analysis: a Multifaceted Approach, described in Nancy J. Lund and Judith F. Duchan, *Assessing children's language in naturalistic contexts*. Englewood Cliffs, NJ: Prentice-Hall Inc., 1987. Cost: $19.95.

Phonological Assessment of Child Speech, Pamela Grunwell. San Diego: College-Hill Press, 1985. Cost: $42.00.

Phonological Process Analysis, Frederick Weiner. Baltimore: University Park Press, 1979. Cost: $19.95.

Phonological Processes: Assessment and Intervention Program, Allan K. Bird and Anne P. Higgins. Allen, TX: DLM Teaching Resources. Cost: $150.00.

Procedures for the Phonological Analysis of Children's Language, David Ingram. Baltimore: University Park Press, 1981. Cost: $17.00. Scoring forms, $9.50.

Computer Programs for Phonological Assessment

Comprehensive Phonemic Inventory for School Age Children, Stephen Blache. Waltham, MA: College-Hill Press, 1986. Cost: $68.00.

Computer Analysis of Phonological Processes, Barbara W. Hodson. Stonington, IL: PhonoComp, 1985. Cost: $85.00.

Lingquest 2, Phonology Analysis, copyright 1982, Michael W. Palin and Dennis R. Mordecia, distributed exclusively by Merrill Publishing Co., Columbus, Ohio. Cost: $495.00.

Process Analysis Version 2.0, Frederick Weiner. State College, PA: Parrot Software. Cost: $79.95.

Programs to Examine Phonetic and Phonological Evaluation Records, Lawrence D. Shriberg. Madison, WI: University of Wisconsin Software Development Distribution Center. Cost: $495.

APPENDIX 4.2 Orofacial Examination Checklist

Client name: _____ Age: _____ Date: _____
Examiner: _____

I. Facial Characteristics
  A. General appearance: normal color ____; normal symmetry ____; adenoid facies ____; other _____
  B. Frontal view
    1. eye spacing: normal (one eye apart) ____; hypertelorism ____; other _____
    2. zygomatic bones: normal ____; hypoplasia ____; other _____
    3. nasal area: septum (straight) ____; or deviated ____; nares ____; columella ____; septum/turbinate relationship ____; turbinate color ____; other notations _____
    4. vertical facial dimensions:
      a. upper (40% of face) ____; other notations _____
      b. lower (60% of face) ____; other notations _____
    5. lips: cupid's bow present ____; muscular union ____; neuromotor functioning—/i/ ____; /u/ ____; /p-p-p/ ____; other notations _____
  C. Profile
    1. normal (straight or convex) linear relationship between bridge of nose, to base of nose, to chin ____;
      retrusion $\begin{cases} \text{maxilla ____;} \\ \text{mandible ____;} \end{cases}$ protrusion $\begin{cases} \text{maxilla ____;} \\ \text{mandible ____;} \end{cases}$
    2. mandibular plane: normal ____; steep ____; flat ____
  D. General notations:

II. Intraoral Characteristics
  A. Dentition
    1. general hygiene: good ____; needs improvement ____; caries ____; gingival hyperplasia or recession ____
    2. occlusal relationships ("bite on your back teeth" and separate cheek from teeth with tongue depressor)
      a. first molar contacts:
        Class I—normal molar occlusion (mandibular molar is one-half tooth ahead of maxillary molar) ____
        Class I malocclusion (normal molar relationship with variations in other areas of dentition) ____
        Class II malocclusion (maxillary ahead of mandibular first molar) ____
        Class III malocclusion (mandibular molar more than one-half tooth ahead of maxillary molar) ____
      b. biting surfaces: normal vertical overlap (overbite) ____; excessive vertical overlap A____/ P____; normal horizontal overlap (overjet) ____; excessive horizontal overlap A____/ P____; crossbite (mandibular tooth or teeth outside or wider than maxillary counterpart, or maxillary tooth or teeth inside

mandibular counterpart) ____; notation of teeth involved ____; open bite (gap between biting surfaces) A____/ P____

    c. sibilant production with teeth in occlusion: normal /s/ ____; /z/ ____; /f/ ____; /v/ ____

B. Hard palate ("extend your head backward")
    1. midline coloration: normal (pink and white) ____; abnormal (blue tint) ____
    2. lateral coloration: normal ____; torus palatinus (blue tint surrounding a raised midline bony growth) ____
    3. posterior border and nasal spine: normal ____; short ____
    4. general bony framework: normal ____; submucous cleft ____; cleft ____; repaired cleft ____; other _____
    5. palatal vault: normal relationship between maxillary arch/vault ____; narrow maxillary arch/high vault ____; wide maxillary arch/flat vault ____; other _____
    6. general notations _____

C. Soft palate or velum (Examiner's eye level should be client's mouth level. Client's head erect, mouth three-fourths open, and tongue not extended out of mouth.)
    1. midline muscle union (say "ah"): normal (whitish-pink tissue line) ____; submucous cleft (blue tint with A-type configuration during phonation) ____; cleft ____; repaired cleft ____
    2. length: effective (closure of nasopharyngeal port possible during phonation) ____; ineffective (hypernasality noted) ____
    3. velar dimple (where elevated soft palate buckles during phonation): normal 80% of total velar length (or 3–5 mm above tip of uvula) ____; other notations _____
    4. velar elevation: normal (up to plane of hard palate) ____; reduced ____; other _____
    5. range of velar excursion (up and back stretching during phonation): excellent ____; moderate ____; minimal ____
    6. presence of hypernasality during counting: 60s ____; 70s ____; 80s ____; 90s ____
    7. general notations: regarding air loss of unphonated sounds (nasal emission) and nasal resonance on phonated sounds _____

D. Uvula
    1. shape: normal ____; bifid ____; other _____
    2. position: midline ____; lateral ____

E. Fauces
    1. open isthmus ____; tonsillar obstruction of isthmus ____
    2. tonsil coloration: normal (pinkish) ____; inflamed ____

F. Pharynx
    1. depth between velar dimple and pharyngeal wall on "ah": normal ____; deep ____; other _____
    2. Passavant's pad: present during physiologic activity? _____
    3. adenoidal surgery (ask client); intact ____; removed ____; date of tonsil/adenoid removal _____
    4. gag response: positive ____; negative ____; weak ____
    5. general notations: _____

G. Tongue
    1. size: normal ____; macroglossia (rare) ____; microglossia ____
    2. diadochokinetic rate—an estimate of neuromotor maturation for speech (observe consistency and pattern of rapid movements during the 15-repetition sequence)
        a. normal movement patterns: tuh ____; luh ____; kuh ____; puh-tuh-kuh ____; describe variations _____
        b. mandibular assist: normal (until age 7½) ____; possible neuromotor delay for speech (after 7½) ____
    3. lingual frenum: normal (tongue tip to alveolar ridge when mouth is one-half open) ____; short ____
    4. general notations: _____

III. General Observations and Other Findings

Source: "Orofacial Examination Checklist" by R. M. Mason and C. Simon, 1977, *Language Speech & Hearing Services in the Schools, 8,* pp. 161–163. Copyright 1977 by the American Speech-Language-Hearing Association, Rockville, Maryland. Reprinted by permission.

APPENDIX 4.3 Time-by-Count Measurement of Diadochokinetic Syllable Rate

Norms for syllable production in seconds/criterion count taken from oscillographic analyses of responses of 384 children, 24 boys and 24 girls at each age shown. Scores represent time, in seconds, required for 20 repetitions of single syllables (that is, pʌ), 15 repetitions of bisyllables (that is, pʌtə), and 10 repetitions of pʌtəkə.

Age	pʌ	tʌ	kʌ	fʌ	lʌ	pʌtə	pʌkə	tʌkə	pʌtəkə
6 Mean	4.8	4.9	5.5	5.5	5.2	7.3	7.9	7.8	10.3
SD	0.8	1.0	0.9	1.0	0.9	2.0	2.1	1.8	3.1
7 Mean	4.8	4.9	5.3	5.4	5.3	7.6	8.0	8.0	10.0
SD	1.0	0.9	1.0	1.0	0.8	2.6	1.9	1.8	2.6
8 Mean	4.2	4.4	4.8	4.9	4.6	6.2	7.1	7.2	8.3
SD	0.7	0.7	0.7	1.0	0.6	1.8	1.5	1.4	2.1
9 Mean	4.0	4.1	4.6	4.6	4.5	5.9	6.6	6.6	7.7
SD	0.6	0.6	0.7	0.7	0.5	1.6	1.5	1.7	1.9
10 Mean	3.7	3.8	4.3	4.2	4.2	5.5	6.4	6.4	7.1
SD	0.4	0.4	0.5	0.5	0.5	1.5	1.4	1.2	1.5
11 Mean	3.6	3.6	4.0	4.0	3.8	4.8	5.8	5.8	6.5
SD	0.6	0.7	0.6	0.6	0.6	1.1	1.2	1.3	1.4
12 Mean	3.4	3.5	3.9	3.7	3.7	4.7	5.7	5.5	6.4
SD	0.4	0.5	0.6	0.4	0.5	1.2	1.5	1.1	1.6
13 Mean	3.3	3.3	3.7	3.6	3.5	4.2	5.1	5.1	5.7
SD	0.6	0.5	0.6	0.5	0.5	0.8	1.5	1.3	1.4

Source: "Time-by-Count Measurement of Diadochokinetic Syllable Rate" by S. G. Fletcher, 1972, *Journal of Speech and Hearing Research, 15,* p. 765. Copyright 1972 by the American Speech-Language-Hearing Association, Rockville, Maryland. Reprinted by permission. (The Fletcher Time By Count Test of Diadochokinetic Syllable Rate is available from Pro-Ed Inc., 5341 Industrial Oaks Blvd., Austin, TX 48735.)

PART TWO

General Considerations in Treatment

As noted in the introduction, the treatment of articulatory and phonological disorders has a considerable history. During that history a number of different approaches have been used, each of them bringing some new contribution to what we know about helping children talk better. This section presents an overview of remediation methods. The discussion deals with underlying principles, general procedures, and research directed toward identifying effective methods and verifying the value of specific procedures. In this section, four general approaches to therapy will be described: the traditional approach (chapter 5), the behavioral approach (chapter 6), linguistic approaches (chapter 7), and communication-centered therapy (chapter 8). These approaches are not discrete; each of them shares some aspects with the others. It may be that the best approach is one that combines elements of all of them.

This section also considers two areas of special concern. One is the role of auditory factors in articulatory and phonological learning (chapter 9), and the other is the need for special methods in working with individuals whose articulation problems are caused by organic pathologies (chapter 10).

CHAPTER 5 The Traditional Approach to Treatment

During the first 4 decades of this century, early "speech correctionists" laid the foundations for what we now know as the *traditional approach to articulation therapy*. Pioneers such as Mosher (1929), Scripture and Jackson (1927), Borden and Busse (1929), Ward (1923), Peppard (1925), and Travis (1931) were among the first to set forth their ideas about how to treat clients with articulation problems. They were followed by such experts as West, Kennedy, and Carr (1937), Nemoy and Davis (1937), and Stinchfield and Young (1938).

As this chapter shows, these clinicians emphasized the proper positioning of the articulators, that is, correct phonetic placement and a variety of drill activities for the different speech sounds. They also stressed and taught their clients the importance of good listening skills.

In 1939, Charles Van Riper published the now classic work *Speech Correction: Principles and Methods*. In this book, Van Riper was the first to set forth the *stimulus approach,* a general set of guidelines to be used in articulation therapy, rather than a series of exercises and drills. As he stated, "[although] most texts in speech correction give a host of drill material for the various speech sounds, this text will ignore such drill and will concentrate

upon techniques and policies" (Van Riper, 1939, p. 208). His text was the first to describe an organized scheme for articulation treatment.

Traditional articulation therapy today is no doubt more closely tied to Van Riper and his stimulus approach than to anyone else, even though the practice of articulation therapy has evolved throughout the years since Van Riper first wrote about it. Since 1939, Van Riper's text has been revised six times (1947, 1954, 1963, 1972, 1978, and most recently in 1984 with Lon Emerick). Clearly, his approach has stood the test of time. It has changed in certain ways over the years because other therapy methods have influenced Van Riper's thinking as well as clinicians' use of his approach. On the other hand, at least some aspects of the traditional approach are incorporated in most if not all other approaches to articulation treatment. One of them, the *discrimination approach,* emerged from the writings of Van Riper.

Van Riper's approach will be discussed in depth later in this chapter. First, other traditional treatment methodologies will be surveyed. Some of these methods were predecessors of Van Riper's approach and served to influence its development. Others were developed afterward and could be considered spin-offs. For example, one approach focuses primarily on discrimination, whereas another emphasizes stimulation. Both of these are

This chapter was written by **Wayne A. Secord.**

stressed heavily by Van Riper. Some of these later methods, as well as behavioral and linguistic approaches (discussed in chapters 6 and 7), have had an impact on Van Riper's writings and on clinical practices derived from them.

AN OVERVIEW OF TRADITIONAL METHODS

Phonetic Placement

The *phonetic placement approach,* aspects of which are still being used by speech pathologists today, was first described by Scripture and Jackson (1927). This approach stresses the correct positioning of the articulators and the correct use of the breath stream. It does not rely on listening skills or discrimination training. Assuming that each speech sound is always produced in only one way, the clinician teaches the client how to place the lips, tongue, and jaw and how to breathe for each misarticulated sound. Tongue depressors, the clinician's fingers, mirrors, other devices, and diagrams may be used. The approach relies heavily upon drill to stabilize the production of each learned sound. Because the approach requires the client to form each target sound consciously, it may be difficult to transfer the skills learned to conversational speech. The phonetic placement approach can be used with individuals or with groups. According to Van Riper (1978), it may be particularly useful with people with hearing impairments.

The Moto-Kinesthetic Approach

The *moto-kinesthetic approach* of Edna Young and Sara Stinchfield-Hawk (Stinchfield & Young, 1938) is related to the phonetic placement approach. However, each sound is taught as part of a specified stimulus syllable, word, phrase, or sentence. The client lies down, to encourage relaxation, while the clinician manipulates the client's articulators to stimulate correct production of the target sound. At the same time, the clinician says the sound while the client watches. Thus the client simultaneously receives tactile, kinesthetic, auditory, and visual feedback. Because of the one-to-one nature of the therapy techniques, the kinesthetic approach can only be used on an individual basis. Today this approach is largely used with clients with neurogenic impairments, including cerebral palsy. Aspects of the moto-kinesthetic approach, particularly the stimulations used to elicit new sounds, are often used in traditional therapy, as will be seen later in this chapter.

The Stimulus Approach

The *stimulus approach,* first advocated by Charles Van Riper in 1939, focuses on the single misarticulated target sound. The approach begins with intensive ear training and proceeds to production of the sound in isolation, in syllables, in words, in phrases, in sentences, and in conversation. It includes work to stabilize correct sound production in therapy and in settings outside of therapy. This method provides the very core for the traditional approach to treatment and is discussed in depth later in this chapter.

The Group Method

The *group method* proposed by Ollie Backus and Jane Beasley (1951) emphasizes the client as a whole person with many behaviors, of which speech is only one. Backus and Beasley treated groups of clients with a variety of speech disorders rather than one type of disorder (such as articulation problems). The focus is on using speech in a meaningful context, to communicate with the clinician and other members of the group. In addition to improvement in speech skills, goals include personal adjustment and social-skills growth. The group activities involve conversational practice of the target sound and feedback on misarticulations. The approach is, in part, based on the idea of learning as a process that moves from the whole to the parts and back to the whole. The group communication situation provides the whole, or the starting point, while individual work on speech sounds is the part. An important aspect is the warm, accepting atmosphere of the group and the group's dynamics.

Integral Stimulation

The *integral stimulation approach* advocated by Robert Milisen (1954), like the moto-kinesthetic approach, involves use of as many sources of feedback as possible, particularly auditory and visual feedback. In contrast to the traditional approach of Van Riper, however, it begins with production rather than auditory discrimination. Stress is put on successful production of the first target sounds, which are therefore very carefully chosen for stimulability and frequency in speech (to provide motivation for learning).

Servotheory Approach

Edward Mysak (1959) described the *servotheory approach* to articulation treatment, stressing the need for the client to discriminate the error sound and the correct target. Mysak emphasized *error-sound sensitivity* and *error-sound measuring processes* and the related processes of *correct-sound seeking and approximating* and *correct-sound tracking*. In the first stage of therapy, the client learns to discriminate quickly and accurately correct and incorrect articulations in a variety of linguistic contexts. In the second stage, the client produces the sound in different words until correct production is more and more consistent. Next, the clinician provides direct instruction until the sound is mastered.

Sensory-Motor Approach

According to Eugene McDonald (1964a), the functional unit of speech production is the syllable. It is the unit on which the *sensory-motor approach* is structured. Based upon his and others' work in the

area of motor phonetics, McDonald has outlined a systematic program that utilizes the coarticulatory effects of context in both assessment and treatment. That program has had a profound influence on our thinking with respect to how articulation disorders should be managed. It is presented in detail in chapter 13 by Richard Shine, a proponent of the sensory-motor approach and a former doctoral student of Dr. McDonald.

Discrimination Approach

According to Harris Winitz (1969, 1975; Winitz & Bellerose, 1962, 1963), the key to articulation treatment of children is speech sound discrimination. After identifying the contexts in which a client misarticulates a target sound, the clinician teaches the child to discriminate the error sound. When the child can discriminate between the error and the target sounds in sentences, speech production begins. The clinician uses common toys or other objects whose names contain the error and target sounds and gets the child to play with them. The child must use the correct name to obtain the toy. Thus correct articulation is naturally rewarded. In more difficult cases, progressively more difficult sound contrasts might be used. Winitz begins training with the error sound rather than the target sound, and continues to focus on the error sound except when teaching the child to discriminate between his own error and the target. For a more complete discussion of the importance of discrimination training in articulation therapy, see chapter 9 of this text.

Nonsense Approach

The goal of the *nonsense approach* developed by Adele Gerber (1973) is to facilitate carryover of learned target sounds from deliberate use (as in the therapy setting) to spontaneous conversational speech. Thus Gerber does not present techniques for acquiring sounds, except for /r/. Once the client (usually a school-aged child or adolescent) has mastered deliberate production of the target sound, the clinician systematically trains the child to use the target in nonsense materials. The materials start with simple CV, VCV, and VC syllables and proceed gradually to entire conversations in nonsense words and then use of nonsense words in meaningful contexts. At each level, the nonsense material is produced with conversational juncture, speed, stress, and so forth. Once the nonsense words can be produced spontaneously in meaningful sentences, real target words from the child's vocabulary are introduced. Eventually those words are used in sentences and conversational speech. The child is also taught techniques for monitoring his own speech. All procedures emphasize conversational speed and prosody.

THE TRADITIONAL APPROACH

This section presents an in-depth look at the traditional approach as it is practiced by speech pathologists today. Before beginning therapy, the clinician performs all necessary assessments, both for diagnosis and intervention planning (see chapter 4 on assessment). A tentative treatment plan and tentative therapy targets are selected, though changes are often made during the course of therapy.

Most clinicians who use the traditional approach direct therapy toward one sound, or at most two sounds, at a time. For example, if /s/ is the target, it is likely that the client also misarticulates its cognate, /z/, at least occasionally. Thus both /s/ and /z/ may be chosen as initial therapy targets. Some clinicians do use a "bombardment" approach; that is, they direct treatment toward many error sounds simultaneously. This, however, is the exception rather than the rule. Typically, clinicians have treated only a small number of sounds at once.

Several factors are involved in deciding which sounds to treat first. Perhaps the most important consideration is the chronological age of the client;

the target sound should be developmentally appropriate for the child. A second important factor is the frequency of the sound in English phonology. Sounds that occur frequently make good therapy targets because their remediation may result in noticeable improvements in the intelligibility of the client's speech. Another consideration is stimulability; that is, the clinician looks for sounds that the client can produce correctly by imitating the clinician's exaggerated model. Stimulable sounds usually respond more favorably to treatment than other sounds. Another factor is the extent to which the client produces errors. Sounds that the client can sometimes produce correctly are good targets for therapy because the correct productions provide a point of departure for treatment. Finally, the clinician might consider sounds that the client produces with relatively minor errors. If the client produces the sound with only a very mild distortion of the target, for instance, only a slight "fine tuning" may be needed.

In choosing the initial therapy targets, the clinician takes all these factors, and perhaps others, into consideration. He weighs all the possibilities and may trade one advantage for another. For example, a clinician may choose to treat a more severe, unstimulable error over a less severe, stimulable sound because the target sound occurs frequently in English and is also the first sound in the client's name ("Wudy" for "Rudy"). Although it sounds complicated, speech pathologists go through this process frequently. With experience, the decision-making process becomes easier.

Once assessment is complete and the initial therapy targets have been chosen, it is time to begin the actual course of therapy. As mentioned previously, early practitioners stressed procedures for placement of the articulators and use of the breath stream. Therapy was implemented through a series of drills and exercises. Before Van Riper, texts on articulation treatment were filled with diagrams and lists of tongue and speech exercises, as well as exercises for listening for certain acoustic properties of sounds and discriminating between error sounds and the target.

In 1939, Van Riper outlined the first general guidelines, seven steps to use in treating articulation disorders.

(1) The speech defective[1] must be convinced that he has errors which he must eradicate. (2) The causes of the disorder, if still existent, must be eliminated. If those causes are no longer present, their influence must be counteracted. (3) Through intensive ear training, the old word configurations are broken down so that the correct sound and the error may be isolated, recognized, identified, and discriminated. (4) Through various methods, the speech defective must be taught to produce the correct sound in isolation and at will. (5) The new and correct sound must be strengthened. (6) The new sound must be incorporated within familiar words, and the transition to normal speech must be accomplished. (7) The use of the sound must be made habitual, and the error must be eliminated. (p. 209)

Although the traditional approach has evolved through the years, Van Riper's contributions of emphasis on ear training and on stabilizing the new sound and transferring its use to conversational speech are still crucial to the approach. In the seven editions of his book (as well as a text written with John Irwin in 1958), he has assembled a cohesive approach to articulation treatment.

That approach, as practiced today, has four major stages: (a) sensory–perceptual training (ear training), (b) production training (establishment), (c) stabilization, and (d) transfer and carryover. An important fifth stage is *maintenance*. These stages are summarized in Table 5.1. In the words of Van Riper and Emerick,

The hallmark of traditional articulation therapy lies in its sequencing of activities for (1) sensory-perceptual training, which concentrates on identifying the standard sound and discriminating it from its error through scanning and comparing; (2) varying and correcting the various productions of the sound until it is produced correctly; (3) strengthening and stabilizing the correct production; and finally, (4) transferring the new speech skill to everyday communication situations. This process is usually carried out first for the standard sound in isolation, then in the syllable, then in a word, and finally in sentences. (p. 193)

Thus, this approach has four operational levels— the sound in isolation, the syllable, the word, and

TABLE 5.1
Course of Therapy

1. Sensory-perceptual training (ear training)
   Identification
   Isolation
   Stimulation
   Discrimination
2. Production training
   Sound establishment/sound acquisition
3. Production training—Sound stabilization
   Isolation
   Nonsense syllables
   Words
   Phrases
   Sentences
   Conversation
4. Transfer and carryover
5. Maintenance

the sentence. It can be depicted as a staircase (Figure 5.1), a program of clear-cut levels through which a client must pass on the way to correct production of an error sound. It is useful because it gives both the clinician and the client a clear direction; they know at any time what has been accomplished and what is still to be done. It is not necessary to enter the ''Van Riper staircase'' at the bottom. If, for instance, a client can say an error sound correctly in isolation and in syllables but not at the word level and beyond, therapy might well begin by training in words.

Sensory-Perceptual Training (Ear Training)

The goal of this stage of therapy is to define a standard for the target sound. The client is not required to actually produce the sound. Rather, the emphasis is on developing an auditory model that will serve as an internal standard against which comparisons can be made. This helps the client become aware that he is indeed making errors. When therapy moves to production training, the client will use this image as a basis to vary productions and evaluate them.

[1]The term *speech defective* is dated and no longer used.

133

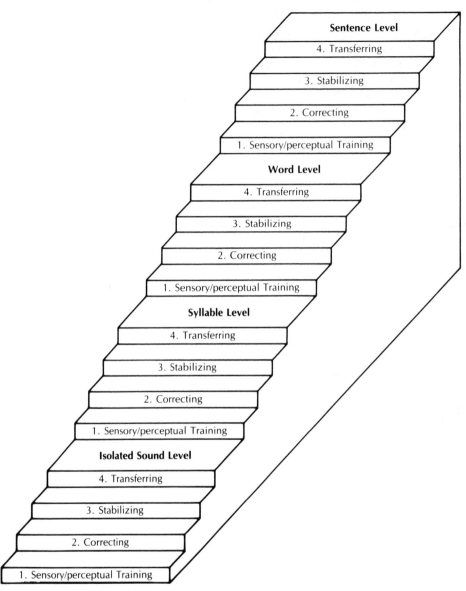

Sentence Level

4. Transferring

3. Stabilizing

2. Correcting

1. Sensory/perceptual Training

Word Level

4. Transferring

3. Stabilizing

2. Correcting

1. Sensory/perceptual Training

Syllable Level

4. Transferring

3. Stabilizing

2. Correcting

1. Sensory/perceptual Training

Isolated Sound Level

4. Transferring

3. Stabilizing

2. Correcting

1. Sensory/perceptual Training

FIGURE 5.1

Design of articulation therapy. (*Source:* Charles Van Riper, Lon Emerick, SPEECH CORRECTION: An Introduction to Speech Pathology and Audiology, 7th Edition, ©1984, p. 194. Reprinted by permission of Prentice-Hall, Inc., Englewood Cliffs, NJ.)

Sensory-perceptual training is composed of four phases. They are:

1. identification
2. isolation
3. stimulation
4. discrimination

Identification. The goal of this phase of sensory-perceptual training is to teach the client the auditory, visual, and tactile-kinesthetic properties of the target sound. The client learns to identify the target sound in isolation against a background of several possibilities composed of similar and dissimilar properties. Once the client identifies the sound, the clinician describes its inherent acoustic, visual, and movement features. With a young child, the sound /t/ becomes the "ticking sound," the /s/ becomes the "snake sound," and the /k/ becomes the "coughing sound." With older children and adults, much more sophisticated acoustic and anatomical descriptions may be more appropriate and useful. The clinician describes and demonstrates the sight, sound, and feel of the sound. When this phase of sensory-perceptual training is complete, the client should be able to recognize the sound in isolation and perceive, if not describe, a number of its important characteristics.

Isolation. In this phase of sensory-perceptual training, the client is expected to use the new recognition skills to isolate the target sound when it is produced against a backdrop of other speech sounds. That is, he must be able to locate the target when the clinician produces a word, phrase, or sentence using it. The clinician might, for example, give a child two cards, one with a happy (smiling) face and one with a sad (frowning) face. The clinician would say, "When I say a word, I want you to show me the happy face if it has your sound in it. If it doesn't, show me the sad face." The clinician then utters words one at a time, and the child responds by displaying the appropriate card after each stimulus word. The clinician can increase the difficulty of the task by presenting a series of words or even a sentence and asking the child to signal each word that contains the target sound. The child can next be asked to identify the position of the target in the stimulus word—initial (beginning), medial (middle), or final (end). This task is quite common in sensory-perceptual training. Again, the focus of this phase is on the location of the target sound in various phonetic contexts.

Stimulation. In this third phase of sensory-perceptual training, the clinician presents the target

sound in a variety of ways. The sound may be presented at different intensities (loudnesses), perhaps with the use of a tape recorder. In a group therapy setting, other clients may be asked to produce the target sound. The client is, in effect, bombarded with instances of the target. In addition to varying loudness, the clinician may present samples quickly or slowly, of long or short duration. The client may be asked to listen to sentences or even paragraphs containing several uses of the sound. Even tongue twisters can be used. In each case, the client is asked to identify the target sound as it occurs. The goal of this phase is to elevate the client's sensitivity to the phonetic properties of the sound and further develop a complete, internalized auditory model of the target.

Discrimination. Discrimination, the final phase of sensory-perceptual training, may be the most important because it is the basis for developing the client's learning, detecting, and correcting skills. Therapy is still focused on listening, rather than producing sounds. The task at this point is to make external comparisons; that is, the client listens to the productions of the clinician and compares them to the internal auditory image of the sound that he has developed. This is known as an *interauditory* comparison (where the client compares someone else's production with the image), as opposed to an *intra-auditory* comparison (in which the client would compare his own production with the image). This discrimination is the last interauditory skill learned before training shifts to enhancing the client's skill in listening to his own speech.

The ability to make external comparisons does not necessarily mean that the client can make accurate internal (intra-auditory) comparisons (Aungst & Frick, 1964). Thus the efficacy of sound discrimination training is a matter of some controversy today (see, for example, Dickson, 1962; Sonderman, 1971; Williams & McReynolds, 1975). The ability to produce a target sound at least inconsistently, that is, to have some internal production model, may be important (Lapko & Bankson, 1975).

Van Riper presents sensory-perceptual training as a stage that precedes production training, but some clinicians feel that sensory-perceptual training and early establishment of production of new sounds should go hand in hand. They feel that the more a client knows about his own production, the better will be the auditory image for the target sound.

Van Riper and Emerick (1984) describe two tasks in discrimination training, error detection and error correction. In error detection the client is to uncover errors produced on purpose by the clinician. He may be required, for instance, to stop the clinician whenever the target sound is produced incorrectly. The clinician usually produces a series of target sounds with an intentional mistake, probably of the type most often made by the client. The "mistake" can occur within the context of a series of words, a passage, or even a tongue twister, to make it more difficult if appropriate. These tasks could be called "ear twisters"; they are useful in developing discrimination skills.[2]

Error correction is an extension of error discrimination. At this point the client is asked to explain why the sound was in error and perhaps what needs to be done to correct it. For example, for /s/ the client might say, "You forgot to close your teeth" or "You stuck your tongue out; you have to keep it in your mouth." The clinician might reply, "Okay, how's this?" and then produce the target in the way the client described.

This last phase is often the bridge to the client's first analyses of his own productions, the first time the client really begins to take a critical look at

how he is making errors. The client now has available at least some rudiments of the perceptual equipment needed to begin making internal comparisons, has learned about many aspects of the sound to be learned, and is thus more apt to make good judgments about his own productions and to make better judgments more quickly.

In the last phase of sensory-perceptual training, the focus shifts to intra-auditory discrimination. Van Riper and Emerick (1984) contend that this process involves learning how to recall, perceive, and predict errors. As experienced clinicians know, there is a natural time sequence involved in error recognition. At first, most clients will recognize their errors only some time after they have occurred. Clearly, to be able to make the important self-corrections necessary for more automatic accurate production, one needs to be able to detect one's own errors immediately as they occur. What's more, it is necessary to be able to predict the sounds and sound combinations that are likely to lead to errors. Thus this last phase of sensory-perceptual training, though often not heavily emphasized, is crucial to the ongoing process of automatic self-monitoring of speech. These skills will also be needed throughout the remainder of therapy, but at this point the emphasis on discrimination is primary rather than secondary.

Teaching intra-auditory discrimination is not easy. Moment-to-moment appraisals of one's own speech are often difficult to learn. Some clinicians use signals to help their clients immediately recognize their errors. Any signal—a light, a tone, slapping the table—that alerts the client that he has made an error can be used. Clinicians also use shadowing techniques, such as simultaneous talking with the client. Here the clinician may either speak more loudly at exactly the moment the client makes the error or stop talking altogether. Amplification techniques, especially those where the client can hear his own voice but more loudly, are also effective (Van Riper, 1963).

One final aspect of discrimination training is learning how to predict sounds and sound combinations where errors are likely to occur. The clinician may provide activities, such as circling letters in an oral reading passage where an error

---

[2]Consider carefully the appropriateness of tasks such as these for very young children. This task, in particular, requires a child to be able to use language to comment on the correctness or appropriateness of the language itself (metalinguistic awareness). Although this ability is observed in normally developing children as early as age 4, it is important to consider carefully the age and linguistic abilities of each client.

might occur or speaking more loudly on likely targets in sample words or sentences. In each case, the client must identify the places where errors are most likely to occur. Again, almost any activity that provides practice in predicting errors will help the client develop self-discrimination and correction skills. (For several exercises for all phases of sensory-perceptual training, see Van Riper, 1963.)

Conclusion. Sensory-perceptual training (ear training) consists of four phases: identification, isolation, stimulation, and discrimination. It is the first phase of articulation therapy, but it does not end when therapy moves to production training. In reality, training in listening and self-correction often continues throughout the course of therapy. As a new, more difficult production level is undertaken, the problem of intra-auditory discrimination may arise again. The ultimate goal of sensory-perceptual training is to provide the client with the skills necessary to correct his or her own errors throughout the process of therapy. This ability is essential if the client is to learn automatic, correct, and fluent speech.

One final caution: The effectiveness of sound discrimination training is a matter of some dispute today. It is undoubtedly an outgrowth of concern that clinicians and researchers have with regard to the overall efficacy of auditory discrimination testing. For more information on this dispute, refer to the section on assessment of auditory discrimination in chapter 4.

Production Training (Sound Establishment)

The second major stage of treatment usually begins after the client has learned to identify the acoustic features of the new sound to be learned; that is, when the client can recognize the characteristics of the new sound and make some correct judgments about whether a given production is correct or incorrect. (Again, some clinicians who use traditional methods begin with eliciting at least some instances of the sound before training sound awareness.) The focus of production training is to

evoke and establish a new sound pattern that will replace the client's error pattern.

It is not necessarily easy to evoke the correct sound. Van Riper and Emerick (1984), as in previous editions of Van Riper's work, stress the notions of *varying* and *correcting* the attempts at the sound. The client must learn to change the way he produces the sound. As Van Riper and Emerick say,

> Long-practiced habits are very resistant to change. . . . Variation must precede approximation. By this we mean something similar to what happens when a person learns to shoot an arrow at a target. When he shoots and misses, he must first know that his second shot will have some chance of hitting a different part of the target, preferably a spot closer to the bull's-eye. But he must vary and he must try to correct. This same procedure occurs in articulation therapy. (p. 199)

Thus, no matter what approach the clinician uses to elicit the new sound, the client will most probably have to vary and correct productions of that sound before he can produce the sound consistently and accurately.

Secord (1981a) has described in depth several commonly used approaches to eliciting new sounds. They include (a) auditory stimulation/imitation, (b) use of context, (c) phonetic placement, (d) the moto-kinesthetic method, and (e) sound approximation.

Auditory Stimulation/Imitation. The very first method used to elicit new sounds is auditory stimulation (Bernthal & Bankson, 1981; Irwin, 1965; Milisen, 1954; Powers, 1971; Van Riper, 1978; Weiss, Gordon & Lillywhite, 1987). The clinician provides one or several examples of the target sound and requires the client to repeat it. This widely used technique is probably the best-known method (if not the easiest to implement) of eliciting new sounds.

Auditory stimulation can be handled in several different ways. If the sound can be produced in isolation, the clinician might present two or three instances of the correct sound. If the sound can only be produced in a syllable, the clinician would present the target syllable two or three ways. (Some authorities feel that only certain sounds, such as continuants /s, z, f, v, θ/, to name a few, can be produced in isolation, and that others, such as stops and affricates, must be produced in syllables. Others feel that no sound can actually be produced in isolation.) The client then attempts to produce the sound correctly. The clinician may ask the client to say the sound loudly and softly, to prolong it, or produce short bursts of the sound. Next the client might be asked to describe how the sound feels. He will definitely be asked to vary productions on the road to producing the correct form.

Auditory stimulation is often combined with other methods for establishing new sounds. For example, the clinician might use phonetic placement (described later) to help the client produce the sound the first few times and then revert to auditory stimulation for practice. It is common clinical practice to use a combination of methods to elicit new sounds.

Again, the clinician must stress varying and correcting. At this point in therapy, the client is trying to learn accurate and deliberate production. Many attempts will fall short of this goal, so the client may need to be encouraged to continue trying. These varying and correcting responses improve the client's internalized model of the correct production. Just as early sensory-perceptual training responses are unsure and unstable, early production responses will vary. That is, the establishment of an internalized model of the correct sound, whether auditory or motor, requires a great deal of trial-and-error learning.

Use of Context. Often a client will be able to produce a target sound in some contexts but not in others because of the coarticulatory effects of adjacent sounds. That is, adjacent sounds make it easier for the client to produce a sound in some contexts. Those contexts are called *facilitating*

contexts (McDonald, 1964a). They are specific phonetic environments—syllables or words, singularly or in combination—where a sound that is usually produced incorrectly is produced correctly. The clinician may use those contexts in therapy. Two methods of identifying facilitating contexts are deep testing (McDonald, 1964b) and using probes of articulation consistency (Secord, 1981b). (See chapter 4 for a discussion of these two methods and chapter 13 for a thorough account of McDonald's approach in the development of facilitating contexts.)

The facilitating contexts will often be familiar words or word combinations. Correct production in these contexts is used as a point of departure for establishing the sound. For instance, assume that Josh, who lisps, can say /s/ correctly in the word *outside*. A clinician might break *outside* into its components *out* and *side* and use the second part *(side)* as a place to begin training for /s/. Because Josh can already say the sound correctly, the clinician needs to expand on this correct use. (McDonald, 1964a, has described the sensory-motor approach, a complete approach to treatment based on early use of facilitating phonetic contexts.)

Using contexts in words, such as in *outside* for Josh, is important because these words, which Van Riper calls *key words,* become a standard for production. Josh will learn to compare his other attempts to produce the /s/ sound with the /s/ in *outside* and will develop other words from this base. As another example, assume that Sara could correctly say *hats*. The clinician might have her hold the ending sound so long that she, in effect, begins to produce the /s/ by itself (in isolation). Thus, the key word can be, and often is, a starting block for producing the target in isolation.

If the client can produce the sound correctly in several contexts, production training might begin at the word level. However, this would only be the case if the client has relatively accurate and consistent production at the important isolation and syllable levels. Key words can also be used in the paired stimuli method of articulation therapy. This specific, behavioral approach is discussed in detail in chapter 6.

Some clients will not present any facilitating contexts and will not be able to produce the target sound in response to auditory stimulation. In that case, the clinician will need to teach the client directly how to say the target sound. The remaining techniques to be discussed are suited to that purpose.

Phonetic Placement. As we have seen, for years speech clinicians have been using diagrams, instruments, and exercises to show their clients where and how to position their speech organs to pronounce specific sounds correctly. Scripture and Jackson (1927) are probably most responsible for what is today known as the *phonetic placement method*. Clinicians still frequently use this method to help teach clients how to place the articulators correctly, to modify the breath stream, and to voice sounds appropriately. It is designed to give the client as many clues as possible to use in producing a difficult sound. The clinician may use a variety of diagrams, applicators, or instruments to explain the correct production. One very commonly used tool is a mirror, either large or hand-held, to enable the client to see his own production of the sound. Weiss and his colleagues (1987, p. 186) have summarized several of the many techniques and devices used in the phonetic placement method.

1. manipulating or holding articulators in place with tongue depressors or sticks
2. manipulating articulators with clinician's fingers
3. giving verbal description and instruction
4. applying breath indicator to mouth and nose
5. making graphic records; for example, spectrogram
6. feeling breath stream with hand or seeing effects of breath stream on a tissue
7. observing clinician and self in mirror while producing sounds
8. feeling laryngeal vibration
9. observing diagrams, pictures, or drawings of articulators while producing certain sounds

10. observing palatograms of articulators while producing certain sounds

The variety of techniques available in the phonetic placement method is limited only by the clinician's imagination.

As mentioned, this method is often used in combination with other methods discussed in this section. For example, a clinician might extract a target sound from a key word and present it several times via auditory stimulation. As the client responds, the clinician could give moment-to-moment phonetic placement instructions to help the client vary and correct the response. For an exhaustive list of phonetic placement techniques, see Secord (1981a). Here are some examples for eliciting /s/. Techniques marked with an *M* are especially effective if a mirror is used; those followed by an asterisk are especially good for lateral /s/.

M   Demonstrate the feature characteristics of /s/:
Tongue tip-blade nearly touching the alveolar ridge
Slow release of air over the tongue toward the cutting edges of upper central incisors
Vocal cords silent

M   1.   Demonstrate this procedure in a mirror step-by-step first and then allow the client to demonstrate the same. Tell the client to:
     a. Raise the back of the tongue so he can feel his upper back teeth.
     b. Place the tip of the tongue behind his upper front teeth and then pull it away from them just a bit.
     c. Close his teeth so that they are barely touching. The clinician should then hold the tip of his finger in front of the center of the client's mouth and say: "Blow air slowly over your tongue toward my finger."

M   2.   For /s/ with the tongue tip down:
     a. Raise back of the tongue to upper back teeth.
     b. Place tongue tip behind lower central incisors. (You may need a tongue depressor for this.)

    c. Close the teeth.

    d. Initiate /s/.

3. To develop a central air flow, a variety of techniques are available:

    a. Draw a small target and hold it in front of mouth. Tell the client to make a bull's-eye with the /s/.

    b. Hold your fingertip about three inches from the client's nose. Ask him to force the /s/ outward and upward toward your finger, or have the client use his own finger.

    c. Have the client close his teeth and direct the air flow for /s/ through a straw.

    d. Use a tongue depressor and trace a line through the center of his tongue to give the client the idea of a trough before attempting /s/.

    e. Have the client brush the lower gums with his tongue while attempting to say /s/.

    f. Tell the client to pucker his lips and then fully retract them. Push the tongue forward and say /s/.

    g. Place the client's finger at the very center of the teeth and have him attempt /s/.

M 4. Use a tongue depressor to explain precise points of contact in the mouth. Then place the tongue depressor just behind the teeth. Ask the client to hold it there with his tongue tip. The small opening created when you remove the tongue depressor is almost the distance necessary for air to pass in order to secure /s/.

5. Instruct the client to close the teeth and rapidly bring the back of the tongue up against the lower teeth while attempting /s/.

6. Tell the client to groove the tongue and then attempt /s/.

7. Tell the client to brush the upper gums with his tongue tip while he attempts /s/.

8. Instruct him to close his teeth and bring his lips together tightly. Then slowly open the lips to allow the /s/ to escape. (Secord, 1981a, pp. 21–22)

The Moto-Kinesthetic Method. Developed by Edna Young and Sara Stinchfield-Hawk in the late 1930s, the moto-kinesthetic method is similar to phonetic placement. In fact, according to Sommers (1983), it is perhaps the ultimate extension of the general phonetic placement concept. It differs from other phonetic placement techniques, however, in its stress on patterns of movement in articulation and an increasing awareness of kinesthetic movements to guide articulation.

In this method, the clinician uses his own hands to manipulate the client's articulators. In this way the clinician forces the client to notice where the movement begins, how much tension or pressure is needed, the overall shape and direction of the movement, and the timing of the movements. The clinician thus helps the client use the tactile and kinesthetic senses to feel the way the sound is produced. The clinician may also provide visual and auditory stimulation to improve the client's sensory image of the correct production. Here is an example of the correct moto-kinesthetic stimulation for /s/, based on Young and Hawk (1955): Place the thumb and forefinger of your left hand at the corners of the upper lip. Place the thumb and forefinger of your right hand on the corners of the lower lip. If the occlusion is normal, push the lower jaw into the position of a normal bite; then pull the lower jaw down to create an ever so slight opening between the teeth. Ask the client to blow air through the teeth.

More detail on the moto-kinesthetic method can be found in Young and Hawk's 1955 book. A brief summary of each moto-kinesthetic stimulation for all consonants, vowels, and diphthongs can be found in Secord (1981a).

Today the moto-kinesthetic method is primarily used as an adjunct to phonetic placement. In fact, many of the stimulations are no doubt perceived as phonetic placement techniques. The moto-kinesthetic method is used for the most part to evoke correct speech sounds for the first time.

Sound Approximation. *Sound approximation* refers to two similar approaches, progressive approximation and modification of other sounds (Van Riper, 1978). Both involve the behavioral learning principle known as *shaping*. In progressive approximation, the clinician evokes a series of sounds or sound segments that gradually approximate the target response, until the actual target-sound is produced. Van Riper described progressive approximation as follows:

> The clinician joins the client and makes the same error the client makes. She then shows the client a series of transitional sounds, each of which comes a little closer to the standard sound until finally the standard sound is produced. Each little modification the client makes that comes a bit closer to the goal is rewarded. Those variations that move away from the target sound are ignored. (1978, p. 188)

Thus the clinician begins with the client's error and gradually modifies it, using his own finely tuned discrimination skills to guide the client's productions. Many clinicians know and use this method—for instance, with a client who has a distorted /ɝ/ that resembles the /ʊ/ in *put*. The client initially produces the error /ʊ/ in isolation and is then guided by the clinician's instructions to produce sounds that come closer and closer to the target /ɝ/.

The second type of sound approximation method is modification of other sounds. Here the clinician uses another sound or sounds already in the client's repertoire as a point of departure for the target sound. The clinician instructs the client to produce a known sound and then to adjust the articulators in certain ways while continuing to produce the known sound. Each articulatory adjustment is a movement that comes closer to the position necessary for the target sound. This method is often used with nonspeech sounds such as coughing to elicit a /k/ or growling to elicit /ɝ/. Once the client produces a sound that is close to the target, the clinician can use a variety of other techniques, such as auditory stimulation and further phonetic placement instruction, to bring the production precisely on target. Here are several clinical examples for /s/.

1. Instruct the client to bring his or her teeth together and "slurp" inhaled air, then exhale this air as /s/.

2. Shape /s/ from /θ/. Instruct the client to prolong /θ/ as in *think*. Tell him or her to gradually bring the tongue into the mouth over the back of the top teeth and along the alveolar ridge to the vicinity for /s/ while saying /θ/.
   a. Same procedure but use a tongue depressor to guide the movement.
   b. Tell the client to do the same but use the tongue tip to "point" to the back of the teeth and the gum ridge.
   c. Tell the client to say a list of initial-position /θ/ words slowly, pushing the tongue inward and upward to the alveolar ridge as the /θ/ sound is uttered.
3. Shape /s/ from /t/. Instruct the client to make rapid productions of /t/ and prolong the last one into /s/.
4. Shape /s/ from [tʰ]. Tell the client to say /t/ with a great amount of plosion. This considerably aspirated [tʰ] will result in the German affricate /ts/. Ask the client to prolong the second sound in /ts/, resulting in tsssssss. Then the /t/ is dropped.
5. Shape /s/ from /i/. Instruct the client to say /i/, then gradually close the teeth and say /s/.
6. Shape /s/ from /ʃ/. Tell the client to say /ʃ/, smile and push the tongue a little forward.
7. Shape /s/ from /z/. Tell the client to whisper a /z/ or hold a hand on his throat while producing /z/, then turn off the voicing.
8. Shape /s/ from /n/. Tell the client to place the tongue at the position for /n/ and then to release the tongue a little bit and force air over the tongue.
9. Shape /s/ from /l/. Tell the client to put the tongue up for /l/, close the teeth and remove the tongue a little bit, and then blow air over the tongue.
10. Shape /s/ from /h/. Instruct the client to

close the teeth first, then prolong /h/ while gradually raising the tongue tip.

11. Shape /s/ from /f/. Instruct the client to lift the tongue tip slowly while prolonging /f/ and gradually bringing the front teeth together.

Conclusion. This section has described five ways to establish correct production of an error sound. Most of these eliciting methods have been used for years. For a complete discussion of eliciting techniques, see Nemoy and Davis (1954), Secord (1981a), and Bosley (1981).

Production Training (Stabilization)

When a client has learned to make the target sound accurately though deliberately, the next task is to stabilize that correct response at the simplest level of production—isolation. As shown in Figure 5.1, isolation is the first in a series of stabilization levels that are each assumed to be of increasing complexity and difficulty. The client must master the target sound at each of these levels. The task is *stabilization,* that is, developing the ability to say the target sound relatively easily and quickly.

Not all clinicians begin at the isolation level. Some insist that the syllable level is the appropriate entry point. They point out that evidence suggests that the syllable is the basic element of speech and that, while not all phonemes can be produced in isolation, all can be produced in syllables. Still other clinicians begin stabilization training at the word level because words are more meaningful. After all, phonemes are units used to signal changes in meaning. Advocates of beginning with isolated sounds or syllables, however, believe that there is often too much interference between the client's habitual error sound and the new sound if it is used in a meaningful context (a word). They feel that this interference is reduced by early stabilization work in isolation and/or syllables.

No matter what stabilization level is chosen as the beginning point, as the client enters each level,

ability to produce the sound is weak and generally unstable. As the client leaves the level, however, production should be consistently accurate and fluent. Stabilization at one level is considered a prerequisite for entry to the next level, and increases the client's chances for success at that next level.

Isolation. Beginning with isolation, then, the goal is to develop a stronger, more consistently correct response. This response will serve as a foundation for later, more complicated phonetic alterations. Often the clinician will use a mirror in isolation work. The mirror further extends the visual cues learned in the establishment stage.

The following list presents some common tasks used in isolation training:

1. practicing prolonging the target
2. varying the number of productions emitted at any one time
3. varying the intensity with which the sound is produced
4. whispering the new sound
5. starting and stopping production in response to the clinician's signal
6. simultaneously talking and writing the new sound (This technique has been highly recommended by Van Riper, 1963.)
7. responding to large and small letters that represent the target by using loud or soft sounds depending on the size of the letter cues
8. playing ''speech games'' in which the child responds by producing the target sound a certain number of times when it is his turn
9. playing with a deck of cards with different numbers used to indicate to the child the number of times to produce the sound
10. switching from one sound to another and then back to the target so that the target is said immediately after the client has repositioned the articulators (This technique is used later in training.)

Throughout treatment at this level, the client is instructed to concentrate on how the sound ''feels''; that is, on such characteristics as where the tongue is during production, where the airstream is going, what the productions look like in the mirror, and what happens when an error is produced.

Many clients, even young children, become quite adept at analyzing their own productions. They may come to know as much about their error responses as they do about what they need to do to say the sound correctly. Again, the clinician may continue using sensory-perceptual training during stabilization work in isolation. The client who continues to practice varying and correcting isolated productions and to develop auditory self-monitoring skills is likely to progress nicely in this stage.

Toward the end of the isolation phase, most clinicians begin to give tasks that facilitate movement from simple isolated productions to production in syllables. The client whose productions are stable at one level will typically have little trouble moving to the next level, but the smart clinician will prepare the client for this step. For example, the client may occasionally be able to produce a few simple syllables without much trouble. Before the clinician moves on to the syllable level, the training sessions should incorporate a few of the simple syllables to help smooth the transition. One very useful principle here is the behavioral "itsy bitsy" principle—"think small." The steps from one level to the next should be small enough to ensure success for the client.

Nonsense Syllables. During this phase, the goal is to develop more consistently correct productions in a variety of nonsense-syllable contexts. At this point, training in nonsense syllables offers certain advantages over practice in meaningful words. First, the clinician can use nonsense syllables for any target sound to practice the sound in a wide variety of phonetic contexts. For example, for /s/, contexts could include:

/si/	(CV)	prevocalic
/is/	(VC)	postvocalic
/isi/	(VCV)	intervocalic
/sib/	(CVC)	initial
/bis/	(CVC)	final

Any of the stressed vowels could then be substi-

tuted for /i/, creating more nonsense syllables to be used in practice. By producing a wide variety of nonsense syllables, the client practices the target sound in all different syllable positions. This practice helps prepare for connected speech, which requires accuracy in sequentially initiating and terminating syllables, as well as in producing the sound between syllables.

The clinician might also use the target sound in nonsense clusters, such as /**spi**/ and /**tips**/. This practice helps ready the client to produce complex cluster words. The clinician can develop nonsense clusters that foreshadow real words. If the client is going to have to master the cluster /ts/, as in the word *outside,* for instance, the clinician might provide practice in the nonsense clusters /itsi/, /ætsi/, and /etsi/. This practice builds a stable base of motor readiness for learning cluster contexts (see Secord, 1981b; Winitz, 1975).

A second advantage of using nonsense syllables is reducing the interference of the client's habitual error sound. Just as correct phonemes signal changes in meaning, so can error phonemes signal changes in meaning for the client. Consider a rapid drill activity for Cindy, a 7-year-old who substitutes /θ/ for /s/.

Clinician: Say /saɪ/ five times.
Cindy: saɪ
      saɪ
      saɪ
      saɪ
      saɪ
Clinician: Good! Now say /si/.
Cindy: si
    si
    si
    si
    si
Clinician: Great! What do you do with your eyes?
Cindy: /θi/ (thee)

It is easier for Cindy to produce the /s/ as a nonsense syllable because there is very little competition from her articulatory programming for /θ/.

However, she still uses /θ/ as the meaningful insertion to signify what you do with your eyes; you "thee." Thus, using nonsense syllables allows Cindy to learn to produce /s/ more easily.

To summarize, most clinicians who use traditional methods use nonsense syllables to provide practice in a variety of phonetic contexts and syllabic positions and to reduce interference from the old error. With Cindy, the clinician might use a nonsense-syllable diagram such as the one shown in Figure 5.2. Cindy would be told to say /s/ and combine it with the vowels in the diagram. Thus she might produce:

sa	/se/
se	/si/
si	/saɪ/
so	/so/
soo	/su/

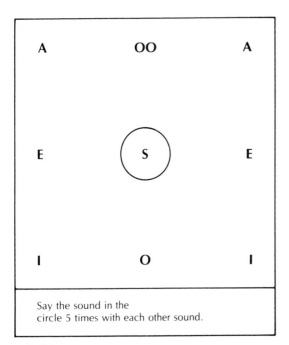

A   OO   A

E   S   E

I   O   I

Say the sound in the circle 5 times with each other sound.

FIGURE 5.2
Nonsense syllable diagram used with a second-grade student.

She can also combine the vowels and a following /s/:

as	/es/
es	/is/
is	/aɪs/
os	/os/
oos	/us/

Intervocalic combinations can be created with /s/ between two instances of each vowel or two different vowels.

asa	/ese/
ese	/isi/
oso	/oso/
ase	/esi/
esa	/ise/

The clinician can simply sequentially point to the sounds Cindy is to produce.

The focus of training might next shift to nonsense words. For example, a clinician might first present an activity where familiar objects are given funny or silly nonsense names that contain the child's target sound. Then the clinician might have the child play a "fill-in," or cloze, game in which the clinician describes the object and the child tells its nonsense name. The purpose here is to get the child accustomed to using the target sound as part of a nonsense word that has a referent, the object described.

Next, Cindy might use the nonsense words in simple phrases or sentences to increase the length of utterance that she can say containing her target sound. From there the focus of training might shift to nonsense words used in a conversational or even storytelling frame. A clinician might conduct a session using silly names created for characters in a child's story or for puppets. For example, the clinician might say,

"Tell me about /sæbo/ and /sæbi/, the two pirates who searched for buried treature," or

"This is /sibɑ/, a little lost puppy. Tell me how /sibɑ/ got home."

Thus the child continues to use nonsense words, but the activity resembles tasks that will later be accomplished with real words.

Some clinicians carry nonsense training quite far. They may have the client tell a story using a wide variety of nonsense words or use nonsense words in conversational responses. The only difference between these activities and those used later for sentence and conversation stabilization training is the set of target words. Again, using nonsense words helps make the transition to the word level easier and increases the chances of success.

Words. When the client is able to produce the target sound in nonsense syllables relatively easily and quickly, therapy moves to stabilization training in words. Table 5.2 outlines a series of substages commonly used in this phase, though some clinicians use even smaller steps. The treatment plan moves from simple, one-syllable words to complex, multisyllable examples. While this scheme may be varied in practice, it is typical of the progression most frequently used. The goal is to teach the client to produce the target sound in the almost endless variety of phonetic contexts in which it can occur in words. He must be able to say the sound when it abuts a number of other consonants and vowels, as well as in the simplest CV, VC, or CVC words.

Clearly, the task is a challenging one. The client needs to learn not only simple words like *so, say,* and *us,* but also complex words such as *successful* or even *necessary.* It is equally challenging for the clinician, who must assure that the client can *fluently* produce these numerous contexts in order

eventually to stabilize all those complex productions in even longer and more complex connected speech utterances.

Again, some clinicians will skip early stabilization training in isolation and/or syllables and begin with words. They may attempt to elicit correct productions first in simple VC or CV one-syllable words or may begin with words or word contexts produced correctly during the initial assessments. Those words may be used as a beginning point for treatment, the first training words from which other, similar words are developed. As mentioned before, these clinicians may feel that words are a more useful, natural beginning point because they are everyday communication tools.

Once an initial core of correctly produced words is established, the clinician may return to the scheme shown in Table 5.2. Sensory-perceptual training procedures may be used before or concurrently with further work on production. The clinician may also continue to stress self-monitoring throughout the remaining course of treatment.

The clinician's first task in word stabilization training is to choose the set of target words. Some clinicians prefer to use a small group of highly familiar, meaningful words, adding a few words at a time as the client masters the first ones. Others begin with a few words and then add a great many more when the client can consistently produce the

TABLE 5.2
Substages of Word-Level Stabilization Training

Substage	Syllables	Examples for /s/
1. Initial prevocalic words	1	sun, sign, say
2. Final postvocalic words	1	glass, miss, pass
3. Medial intervocalic words	2	kissing, lassie, racer
4. Initial blends/clusters	1	star, spoon, skate
5. Final blends/clusters	1	lost, lips, rocks
6. Medial blends/clusters	2	whisper, outside, ice-skate
7. All word positions	1–2	[any of above]
8. All word positions	any	signaling, eraser, therapist
9. All word positions; multiple targets	any	necessary, successful

first targets accurately. The first practice group often will consist of names of familiar people, objects, or pets, or familiar slang words. Because the client will use these frequently occurring words relatively often, the new, correct production can be reinforced by parents, friends, and other people. These words will also be of greater interest to the client and no doubt will be more meaningful than a group of randomly chosen words.

Throughout this stage, sensory-perceptual training activities should be used at least occasionally so that the client continues to develop the ability to monitor his own productions of the target words and correct errors where necessary. With both adults and children who cannot monitor their own productions well, it is best to use a very small group of words at the outset, perhaps 10 to 15 words at each substage (prevocalic, postvocalic, and intervocalic). The client should practice only those words and the clinician should reinforce only those words when produced correctly, ignoring errors in all words other than the 30 to 45 targets. This procedure helps clients to remember the specific words they can say and are responsible to monitor. It also lets parents and other family members be more aware of the specific words to reinforce or remind the client to correct. When a small group of words is used, it is easier to develop "speech awareness" in the client. Frequently the correct production of this small target group will easily generalize to other words; the client's ability to self-monitor also often improves.

One commercially available program (discussed in chapter 6) using this approach of a very small group of initial training words is the S-PACK (Mowrer, Baker, & Schutz, 1968). This behavioral instructional program uses only about 30 words, which have been programmed for use up to and including conversational tasks. Mowrer has demonstrated considerable improvement using only this small group of training words.

Some clients simply do not have any beginning words in which they can produce their targets correctly, even though they can produce them cor-

rectly in nonsense syllables. They find the competition from the error response too great. In this case, the clinician must again "think small," using techniques that gradually step over the gap from nonsense syllables to teach the client how to produce the target sound in words. Van Riper and Emerick (1984) list three types of techniques used for this purpose:

1. reconfiguration
2. simultaneous talking and writing
3. signaling

to which we can add:

4. creating simple words from complex contexts

The idea behind *reconfiguration* is to teach the client "that words are made up of sound sequences and that these sound sequences can be modified without losing the unity of the word" (Van Riper & Emerick, 1984, p. 208). Again, with Cindy (who lisps, substituting /θ/ for /s/ at the beginning of words), the clinician might use a sentence involving initial /s/: *Cindy has a dog named Sir*. First, Cindy is told to substitute another sound, perhaps /p/, for one of her nonerror sounds: *Cindy has a pog named Sir*. Next, she uses her new, target sound for other sounds, but not in the error words: *Cindy has a ssssog named Sir*. She then substitutes /p/ for the initial /s/ in the sentence: *Pindy has a dog named Pir*. The next step is to speak the sentence but omit all instances of initial /s/: *___indy has a dog named ___ir*. Finally, Cindy is instructed to use her new sound in the blank spaces: *SSSS(C)indy has a dog named SSSSir*.

In *simultaneous talking and writing,* the clinician again chooses words using the target sound. The client says and writes the sound, first by itself, then in one-syllable words, then in the first syllable of multisyllable words, then in whole words. Next the client may alternate the letter and the whole word, and finally may write only the letter as he pronounces the whole word.

Signaling techniques use "preparatory sets" to allow the client to combine the target sound with the rest of the word. The client might draw out the target sound until the clinician gives a prearranged signal; then a vowel or the rest of a word is added. For instance, Cindy may sit with her eyes closed saying *sssss*. When the clinician rings a bell, Cindy immediately and automatically says *ir*. Van Riper and Emerick (1984, p. 208) recommend requiring the child to say the word twice, *sssss* [bell] *irsir*.

If Cindy says the target correctly but then produces the error before the rest of the word *(sthir),* the clinician may ask her to begin by forming her mouth for the vowel that begins the rest of the word *(ir)*. This simple task of preforming the mouth often solves the problem, as may the use of pairs of words in which the first ends with the vowel of the second. (For more on these three techniques, see Van Riper & Emerick, 1984, pp. 208–209.)

Creating simple words from complex contexts is another form of using context. The clinician uses the results of deep testing (McDonald, 1964b) or a test of articulation consistency (e.g., Secord, 1981b) to identify those contexts in which the target can be produced correctly. To use the example of the child who can correctly say *outside,* the clinician may be able to break that word in half, retaining the second syllable, *side*. Using this word as a key word, as in the paired stimuli method (see chapter 6), the clinician can pair *side* with other words such as *out, sign, sight,* and *sigh*. Once the client can use his sound in a few words, development of other words becomes much easier.

Activities used in word-level stabilization training have several goals. One important goal is eliciting a large number of responses to give the client practice in production and evaluation. A second purpose is to provide a wide variety of exercises to keep the therapy sessions from becoming meaningless drill (though, unfortunately, considerable drill work is often needed). Some emphasis is usually placed on self-correction skills, with continued reminders and special practice on judging correct and incorrect productions. Clinicians usually reward self-correction skills at this point because treatment will soon move to much longer and phonetically more complex utterances. It is then much more difficult to give immediate reinforcement for correct responses.

The therapy tasks may include speech games, making things, drill work, speech dittoes, and so forth. For examples of some commonly used activities, see the list of activities in Appendix 5.1.

To summarize, there are three main purposes of stabilization training at the word level:

1. to provide numerous opportunities for practice in a variety of increasingly more complex word contexts
2. to stabilize correct sound productions at each substage (initial, final, medial, etc.)
3. to develop further the ability to self-monitor correct and incorrect sound productions

As in other levels, the ultimate goal of training is consistent, correct production of the target sound with ease and speed.

Phrases. At this point some clinicians choose to work on stabilization training using the target sound in short (two- to four-word) phrases. This practice is in keeping with the "think small" philosophy. It may help ensure that the jump from words to sentences is not so great that the client encounters difficulty. Again, it is important for the client to be successful (to some degree) at each stage. Thus, many clinicians insert one or more sessions of phrase work between work on words and sentences, while others consider phrases to be a level equal in stature (and possibly in time devoted) to words and sentences. Usually, however, the client who has mastered stabilization at the word level is ready to proceed to sentence practice, and most clinicians will begin the sentence level with short sentences in any case.

Sentences. Once the client is able to produce the target sound consistently in words, the likelihood of breakdown at the sentence level is reduced. In a few cases, stabilization training may begin at the sentence level. This is likely only when the client cannot produce the target sound at any simpler level but can produce it in certain contexts in running speech. For example, Don may be able to produce /r/ correctly only when it occurs after the word *are*, as in *The boys are running*. In that case, the clinician might build on that base.

Just as practice at the word level is carefully sequenced to ensure success, practice at the sentence level is also structured by level of difficulty and complexity. Table 5.3 outlines a simple scheme for structuring sentence practice. Following such a scheme will enable the client to make steady progress in producing sentences and to become more skilled at monitoring his or her own productions as the utterances become more complex. In other words, the difficulty of the exercises must be carefully sequenced to develop both production and perception skills.

In addition to controlling the level of complexity of the practice sentences, the clinician should control the phonetic environment. Early sentence practice might use simple one-syllable words and then move to examples of more complex clusters.

Some clients may have difficulty making the transition to sentences. In that case the clinician may choose to have the client practice only a limited number of words that he knows well in the various word positions (initial, medial, and final). Van Riper (1978) listed several techniques the clinician can use to help establish production in sentences: slow-motion speech, echo speech or shadowing, unison speaking, the corrective set, and role playing.

In *slow-motion speech,* the clinician and the client say the target sentence together, but very

TABLE 5.3
Substages of Sentence-Level Stabilization Training

Sentence Description	Instances of Target Sound
1. Simple short sentence	1
2. Sentences of various lengths	1
3. Simple short sentence	2 or more
4. Sentences of various lengths	2 or more

slowly. This oral drill may be preceded by performing simple motor tasks, such as walking, in slow motion. For the speech exercise, the clinician may sit behind and slightly above the client so that the client can hear the difficult words clearly.

Shadowing is one form of echo speech. In this activity, the client repeats the clinician's speech as quickly and automatically as possible, one word at a time. Interestingly, children can learn to do this more easily than adults can. A second form of *echo speech* has the client repeat a series of words, a phrase, or a sentence, after the clinician has given a signal. The signal should include a gesture or prompt that the client also repeats.

Unison speech employs sentences or phrases that have already been identified. Often using hand tapping or other signals of rhythm, the clinician and client speak in unison. Again the client follows the clinician's physical movements and the prosody of the clinician's speech. Each phrase or sentence is spoken several times.

An activity that most children enjoy is correcting the clinician. The *corrective set* uses this practice. The clinician will do or say something obviously wrong and ask the child to correct it. When the child is beginning to enjoy correcting the clinician's mistakes, the clinician produces some utterances that contain the child's common error. Often the child will be able to say the sentence accurately in order to correct the clinician.

Some children are able to speak correctly when they are acting or *role playing,* though they cannot produce their target sounds in sentences when they are "being themselves." Thus dramatics, theater, and storytelling may all be vehicles for getting a child to become involved in another role and therefore to speak correctly.

When the client can fluently produce the target sound in sentences and can skillfully monitor his own speech, it is time to tackle even longer connected speech utterances. It is time for conversation.

Conversation. Most clinicians today do at least some work on stabilizing production in conversation in the therapy setting before moving on to settings outside the treatment room. This conversational therapy usually moves from very structured tasks, where the responses are planned or known, to unstructured tasks, as in everyday speech.

In structured tasks, the clinician controls the task so that only specific words using the target sounds are practiced. One such task is telling silly stories. The clinician might create a deck of cards picturing objects whose names contain /s/ in different positions. The child turns five cards face up and then must tell a story using all five of the objects. He is responsible for saying the target sound correctly in all of the object names but not in any other words. If the client makes errors in other words, the clinician pays little, if any, attention to those mistakes.

Another structured activity involves using a simple map where all of the locations and street names contain the client's target sound. Figure 5.3 shows a map highlighting the sound /s/. The clini-

cian asks the client questions that require the sound in the answer.

Clinician: Now you're on Ca*ss* *S*treet at the Bu*s* *S*tation. How do you get to the ca*s*tle?
Child: You go up *S*ea*s*ide Drive and turn left on Ra*ce S*treet till you get to the Big *S*ea. The ca*s*tle is on top of *S*ailboat Point looking out on the Big *S*ea.

Here again the clinician has structured the task so that the client uses the target in known contexts within a ''conversation.'' The client is aware of when the sound will be used, which helps with both production and self-monitoring.

There are myriad structured tasks like these and the ones described in Appendix 5.1. The point is to

FIGURE 5.3
Map incorporating /s/ for structured conversation training.

structure the task so that the specific response opportunities are known to both clinician and client.

Once the client can perform the structured tasks without trouble, it is time to attempt use of the target sound in conversation, where no constraints are placed on the client. That is, the client's responses will consist of connected speech on any topic. The client is now asked to monitor his own speech and to correctly produce all occurrences of the target sound.

For some clients, however, the jump from structured conversational tasks to unstructured ones may be too large. In keeping then with our "think small" philosophy, it might be appropriate to provide some intermediate steps that consist of a combination of structured and unstructured activities. This will help to sequence the difficulty level gradually. If the client's productions at the unstructured conversational level are consistently poorer than at the level before, then some of this bridging work should be provided.

Typical unstructured therapy tasks include answering open-ended questions. "Tell me the things you would do if you won a million dollars in the state lottery." "What movies have you seen lately? Tell me about them." "What did your family discuss at dinner last night?"

If the client can read fairly well, reading can be used for conversational training (both unstructured and structured). It elicits continuous, flowing speech, and the extent of structure can easily be controlled. For example, the clinician could choose a reading passage and have the client go through it and circle all instances of the target. Then the client reads the passage out loud. This task is highly structured because all instances are known ahead of time. Later the client can perform the unstructured task of reading the passage out loud without looking it over first. Finally, the client can tell the clinician what the passage was about—a completely unstructured task.

The clinician can also prepare preset reading passages incorporating several instances of the cli-

ent's sound. Those instances can be marked in boldface, in a different color, or with a capital letter. Again, this task is very structured. The same passages can later be given to the client with the signals removed.

When the client has acquired the ability to converse in unstructured conversation easily and rapidly, most of the treatment within the therapy setting is finished.

The focus of therapy now shifts to enlarging the therapy setting.

Transfer and Carryover

Consider the child who has just carried on a completely unstructured conversation in therapy and made no errors. As he leaves the room at the end of the session, he turns to the clinician and says, "Thee you Friday, Mither Thecord"—100% correct in conversation during therapy, 100% *incorrect* at the door! Unfortunately, this is not an uncommon experience. It almost seems as if an aura of correct speech surrounds the client during therapy and disappears at the door.

The clinician's challenge, then, is to enlarge the therapy situation to include all important settings in the client's life; to expand the learning environment so that the client recognizes cues to correct speech outside the therapy room. This process is called *transferring* the newly learned skills. The term *transfer,* first used in the traditional approach in the late 1960s and early 1970s, was borrowed from the behavioral approach. It refers to the extension of learned behaviors from the original setting to other settings. (Chapter 6 has a more complete discussion of transfer. See also Mowrer, 1982.)

Carryover refers to the ability to use the new sound in conversation. It is not unusual to hear a clinician complain that "the sound just doesn't carry over" or "there is little carryover." What the clinician means is that the client performs well in therapy but cannot remember to say the sound correctly at home or with friends. The cues that help control the almost automatic correct production in therapy either do not exist outside the therapy setting or are not strong enough to help maintain the learned skill in other situations.

Many clinicians use the terms *transfer* and *carryover* interchangeably. However, some use *carryover* to refer to only the conversation stage of therapy. To still others, *carryover* signifies retention of the skill after therapy work on the sound is complete.

Again drawing on Van Riper and Emerick (1984, pp. 213–216), there are several techniques the therapist can use to develop the client's transfer and carryover skills. One simple activity is giving *speech assignments*. The clinician designs very specific assignments for the client to carry out at home, in school, in the office. The assignments should be individually designed for the client's ability levels and environments. The clinician should also ask for a report on how the client fared during the next therapy session. This simple tactic often provides the motivation necessary for the client to succeed.

A second useful practice is to have the client or someone else, perhaps a classmate, *check* the client's speech and record errors.[3] The client could simply mark an index card every time an error is produced during dinner conversation. Another possibility is to assign a simple *penalty* for each error. However, "painful and highly emotional penalties should not be used" (p. 214). Instead, the penalties could be game-like. One variation is to give rewards (points, stars on a card) for correct production and take those rewards away (one at a time) for errors. (Behaviorists call this *response cost*; see chapter 6).

The clinician can also, with the help of the client's family, set up *nucleus situations* in which correct speech is required. Everyone makes speech errors. Requiring the client to have perfect speech at all times can have the effect of making him nervous and too self-conscious, possibly causing

the errors to increase. Therefore, certain situations can be chosen to be targets for correct speech. The reading group for a second grader or all coffee breaks for an adult might be good choices. When the client makes a mistake in the nucleus situation, it should be penalized "good-naturedly but emphatically" (p. 214). Most clients will be able to transfer correct speech to this limited number of situations, and the correct speech often generalizes to other situations.

Yet another approach is *negative practice*, requiring the client occasionally to say the word incorrectly. Research shows that the occasional deliberate production of a habitual response a person is trying to eradicate helps make him more conscious of the habit and helps make it more vivid. It also has the same effect as providing a penalty for the error, even though no penalty is given. This approach should not be taken until the client can consistently produce the correct sound when asked.

It is very important to *use the new sound in various types of speaking*. The client must be able to use the new sound in sending messages, in interacting socially, in thinking, in expressing emotions. The clinician may need to set up a nucleus situation for each of these types of expression to ensure the client's facility in each of them.

Finally, the client must learn to use the proprioceptive sense to monitor his own speech. That is, it is not enough to be able to hear whether a production is correct; the client must also be able to feel it. Exercises to increase proprioceptive awareness of the correct positions and movements of speech include speaking with earplugs, speaking while wearing earphones that supply a masking noise, whispering, and speaking in pantomime. In schools, contrived tasks, such as talking with teachers, meeting with the janitor to give a specific message, or talking in reading groups while self-monitoring, can be used. Some clinicians use parents or other paraprofessional speech aids to work with students outside the clinical setting. In addi-

---

[3]A word of caution is given here concerning the use of peers as speech monitors. This can sometimes be a socially touchy situation and should therefore be handled carefully.

tion, there are some commercially available programs that can be used in transfer work.

Maintenance. A last part of therapy that is often neglected is *maintenance* (another concept drawn from behaviorists). Maintenance refers to retention of the newly learned skill after the course of therapy is complete. Some clinicians do not dismiss their clients after all transfer work has been completed. Instead, they see the client on a decreasing basis, perhaps once a week for a month, and then once a month for a few months, then once every 3 months, every 6 months, and so on, for periodic checks. Some clinicians who practice in schools make periodic checks in the child's classroom for some months and then check back once a year. These checks serve as a clinical reminder to the client to continue to use the new skills.

SUMMARY

This chapter has presented an in-depth look at the traditional approach to articulation therapy. One hallmark of this approach is its flexibility. As we have seen, over the years it has been influenced by a variety of other approaches—the sensory-motor approach, the moto-kinesthetic approach, the behavioral approach, and others. Clinicians who advocate these and other approaches often use many aspects of the traditional approach with their individual clients. And in practice today, they continue to pick and choose from the best techniques available to tailor a therapy plan.

To summarize, the path of traditional therapy involves the stages of sensory-perceptual training, over which there is considerable dispute today; sound establishment; stabilization; transfer; carryover; and maintenance. These processes are implemented through a wide variety of specific techniques, which may involve listening, imitating, physical modeling, and lots of drill and practice. Training almost always focuses on one sound at a time. When one sound is corrected, another, if necessary, is treated and so forth until all error sounds have been corrected. As you will see later, more contemporary approaches often treat several sounds at one time. Even though the stages of traditional therapy are clearly structured, the practice of therapy itself is often highly creative. Combining techniques and activities and responding to the individual needs of each client provides a highly stimulating and satisfying challenge.

REFERENCES

Aungst, L., & Frick, J. (1964). Auditory discrimination ability and consistency of articulation of /r/. *Journal of Speech and Hearing Disorders, 28,* 76–85.

Backus, O., & Beasley, J. (1951). *Speech therapy with children.* Boston: Houghton Mifflin.

Bernthal, J., & Bankson, N. (1988). *Articulation and phonological disorders* (2nd ed.). Englewood Cliffs, NJ: Prentice-Hall.

Borden, R., & Busse, A. (1929). *Speech correction.* New York: F. S. Crofts.

Bosley, E. (1981). *Techniques for articulatory disorders.* Springfield, IL: Charles C. Thomas.

Dickson, S. (1962). Difference between children who spontaneously outgrow and children who retain functional articulation disorders. *Journal of Speech and Hearing Research, 5,* 263–271.

Gerber, A. (1973). *Goal: Carryover.* Philadelphia: Temple University Press.

Irwin, R. (1965). *Speech and hearing therapy.* Pittsburgh: Stanwix House.

Lapko, L., & Bankson, N. (1975). Relationship between auditory discrimination, articulation stimulability and consistency of misarticulation. *Perceptual and Motor Skills, 40,* 171–177.

McDonald, E. (1964a). *Articulation testing and treatment: A sensory-motor approach.* Pittsburgh: Stanwix House.

McDonald, E. (1964b). *A deep test of articulation.* Pittsburgh: Stanwix House.

Milisen, R. (1954). The disorder of articulation: A systematic clinical and experimental approach. *Journal of Speech and Hearing Disorders,* Monograph Suppl. 4.

Mosher, J. (1929). *The production of correct speech sounds.* Boston: Expression.

Mowrer, D. (1982). *Methods of modifying speech behaviors.* Columbus, OH: Merrill.

Mowrer, D., Baker, R., & Schutz, R. (1968). *S-programmed articulation control kit.* Tempe, AZ: Educational Psychological Research Associates.

Mysak, E. D. (1959). A servomodel for speech therapy. *Journal of Speech and Hearing Disorders, 24,* 144–149.

Nemoy, E., & Davis, S. (1937). *The correction of defective consonant sounds.* Boston: Expression.

Nemoy, E., & Davis, S. (1954). *The correction of defective consonant sounds* (rev. ed.). Boston: Expression.

Peppard, H. (1925). *The correction of speech defects.* New York: Macmillan.

Powers, M. (1971). Clinical and educational procedures in functional disorders of articulation. In L. Travis (Ed.), *Handbook of speech pathology and audiology.* Englewood Cliffs, NJ: Prentice-Hall.

Scripture, M., & Jackson, E. (1927). *A manual of exercises for the correction of speech disorders.* Philadelphia: F. A. Davis.

Secord, W. (1981a). *Eliciting sounds: Techniques for clinicians.* San Antonio, TX: Psychological Corporation.

Secord, W. (1981b). *C-PAC: Clinical probes of articulation consistency.* San Antonio, TX: Psychological Corporation.

Sommers, R. (1983). *Articulation disorders.* Englewood Cliffs, NJ: Prentice-Hall.

Sonderman, J. (1971, November). *An experimental study of clinical relationships between auditory discrimination and articulation skills.* Paper presented at the convention of the American Speech and Hearing Association, San Francisco.

Stinchfield, S., & Young, E. (1938). *Children with delayed or defective speech: Motor-kinesthetic factors in their training.* Stanford, CA: Stanford University Press.

Travis, L. (1931). *Speech pathology.* New York: Appleton-Century.

Van Riper, C. (1939). *Speech correction: Principles and methods.* Englewood Cliffs, NJ: Prentice-Hall.

Van Riper, C. (1947). *Speech correction: Principles and methods* (2nd ed.). Englewood Cliffs, NJ: Prentice-Hall.

Van Riper, C. (1954). *Speech correction: Principles and methods* (3rd ed.). Englewood Cliffs, NJ: Prentice-Hall.

Van Riper, C. (1963). *Speech correction: Principles and methods* (4th ed.). Englewood Cliffs, NJ: Prentice-Hall.

Van Riper, C. (1972). *Speech correction: Principles and methods* (5th ed.). Englewood Cliffs, NJ: Prentice-Hall.

Van Riper, C. (1978). *Speech correction: Principles and methods* (6th ed.). Englewood Cliffs, NJ: Prentice-Hall.

Van Riper, C., & Emerick, L. (1984). *Speech correction: An introduction to speech pathology and audiology.* Englewood Cliffs, NJ: Prentice-Hall.

Van Riper, C., & Irwin, J. (1958). *Voice and articulation.* Englewood Cliffs, NJ: Prentice-Hall.

Ward, I. (1923). *Defects of speech.* New York: E. P. Dutton.

Weiss, C., Gordon, M. E., & Lillywhite, H. (1987). *Clinical management of articulatory and phonological disorders.* St. Louis: Mosby.

West, R., Kennedy, L., & Carr, A. (1937). *The rehabilitation of speech.* New York: Harpers.

Williams, G., & McReynolds, L. (1975). The relationship between discrimination and articulation training in children with misarticulations. *Journal of Speech and Hearing Research, 18,* 401–412.

Winitz, H. (1969). *Articulatory acquisition and behavior.* Englewood Cliffs, NJ: Prentice-Hall.

Winitz, H. (1975). *From syllable to conversation.* Baltimore: University Park Press.

Winitz, H., & Bellerose, B. (1962). Sound discrimination as a function of pretraining conditions. *Journal of Speech and Hearing Research, 5,* 340–348.

Winitz, H., & Bellerose, B. (1963). Effects of pretraining on sound discrimination learning. *Journal of Speech and Hearing Research, 6,* 171–180.

Young, E., & Hawk, S. (1955). *Moto-kinesthetic speech training.* Stanford, CA: Stanford University Press.

APPENDIX 5.1   Activities to Use with Children

Sound Discrimination

Pick and Poke (individual). Randomly glue pictures of objects whose names contain target cognate sounds on a piece of poster board. Under each picture, punch three holes to represent the initial, medial, and final positions. (You may wish to paste reinforcers around the holes.) Mark the target sounds on one side edge of the board. Next to one (e.g., /k/), place a long piece of red yarn; next to the other (e.g., /g/), a piece of green yarn. The ends of the yarn should be wrapped with masking tape to make it easier to poke with them and to keep them from unraveling. Poke the pieces of yarn through the edge of the board and glue them to the back.

To play, name the pictures one at a time. The child decides which sound was heard and pokes the appropriate piece of yarn through a hole under the picture.

Variation. Require the child to indicate which position the sound was heard in by selecting the appropriate hole.

Polly's Apron Pocket (individual/group). Make an apron from construction paper or cloth. It should have at least one pocket. Give the child a group of flashcards with objects or words on them. The child places those cards containing the target sound in the apron pocket.

Variation. The apron will need three pockets. Instruct the child to place the flashcards in the pockets according to whether the target sound appears in the initial, medial, or final position.

Stabilization

Coffee Can (individual). Decorate a coffee can and its plastic lid with contact paper. Punch holes in the lid. Thread pieces of yarn of different colors and different lengths through the holes, tying a knot at each end of each string. As the child pulls each string, he must sustain the target sound until the string stops at the other end.

Variation. Have the child repeat a syllable rather than prolong an isolated sound.

The Bubble Blower (individual). Draw a chart with a little girl in the corner blowing bubbles of three different sizes. In each bubble write the target sound or syllable. Give the child an ice-cream-stick pointer. As the child points to each bubble, he says the sound, changing intensity with the size of each bubble.

Syllable Dice (individual). Construct two large blank cardboard dice and laminate them. Mark the dice with syllables made up of the target sound combined with various vowels. Use two different consonants for the two dice. The child rolls the dice and reads off the two-syllable combination shown.

Syllable Cups (individual). Decorate styrofoam cups and write a target sound on the bottom (used as the top) of each one. Write vowels on ice-cream sticks. Have the child tap each cup with a vowel, repeating the syllable five times.

Duration Lines (individual). Make a deck of cards with lines of various lengths on them. The child picks a card and repeats the target syllable for the "length" of the line on the card. If the child can do it, he gets to keep the card; if not, it goes back on the pile.

Froggy Jump (individual). Draw a bunch of lily pads on one piece of poster board and a frog on another. Cut the frog out. On each lily pad, write a syllable using the target sound and a vowel. The child moves the frog from lily pad to lily pad, saying the repeating or alternating syllables.

Syllable Spin (individual). Make a cardboard spinner divided into sections. Label each section with a syllable using the target and a vowel. Have the child spin and quickly say the syllable the spinner lands on.

Duration Cards (individual). Construct index cards with patterns of long and short lines. For instance, one row would have a line all the way across the card, the second would have a line halfway across, the next would have two short lines and a long line, and so forth. The child repeats the sound in a pattern matching each line on the card. Begin with a simple one-pattern sequence and build up to three- and four-pattern sequences.

Automobile Strips (individual). Cut strips of construction paper into long and short strips to represent long and short variations. Give the child a small model car to "drive" along the strips, making the appropriate vocalizations. Strips can be rearranged to make different patterns.

Hotdog (individual). Draw an exaggeratedly long dog. Give the child an ice-cream stick to represent a bone. The child moves the bone out of the "hotdog" and sustains the target sound as the bone is moved from the dog's tail to its mouth.

Snoopy (individual). Draw a picture of Snoopy and a chart showing a series of dishes of dog food. Cut out Snoopy and attach him to an ice-cream stick. The child moves Snoopy to each dog dish full of food. Targets can be written on Snoopy and on the dishes.
Variations. Use a series of doghouses and a different dog. Have the child move the dog from house to house. Or use Woodstock and a series of trees or a fish and a series of bowls.

Wiggly Worm (individual). Draw a chart with a worm that goes up and down. Divide the worm into sections. The child moves his finger up and down the worm. He increases the sound in loudness as he moves up and decreases it as he moves down.

Mountain Road (individual). Draw a scene with a series of mountains on it. The child moves a model car along the top of the mountains, changing the intensity of his vocalizations as he goes.

Uncover the Picture (individual). Put a picture of an object such as a drum, a butterfly, or a pair of glasses on a piece of poster board covered with contact paper. Cut up pieces of construction paper and tape them over the picture to conceal it. Have the child say his sound or word a given number of times. If it is said correctly, the child can take a piece of construction paper off in order to reveal the picture.

Dominoes (individual). Make a set of dominoes with the target sound rather than dots. Have the child make the sound the number of times that it appears on the domino.
Variation. Use two different sounds on the domino set. This activity can be used with words as well.

Sound Tic-Tac-Toe (2 children). Create a tic-tac-toe board with each section marked with a vowel. Each child has a series of markers with his target sound. As the child places a marker, he must say the syllable it makes. When a child wins, he must repeat all the syllables in the winning row.

Fishing for Sounds (individual/group). Cut fish out of poster board and attach a safety pin through each one. Write target syllables on each fish. Create a "pole" from a string and a magnet. Have the children go fishing and say the targets they catch.

S-M-I-L-E (individual/group). On a ditto draw round faces with eyes and nose. Do not put on the mouth. Have the child say five (or any preferred number) good sounds. After saying five good sounds, he can draw a smile on the face.
Variation. Follow each single sound with a smile for a correct sound or a frown for an error. These activities can also be used with words.

The Kitty Cat (individual/group). Cut a cat out of construction paper and place it on a flannel board. As the child says his sound a required number of times, he can place a construction paper spot on the cat. The cat's name should include the target sound.

Egg Carton Toss (individual/group). Number the spaces in an egg carton. Have the child toss a paper clip into the carton. He must say the sound, word, or sentence the number of times indicated. Picture cards can be used to show the target word or sentence.

Paste an Apple on the Tree (individual/group). Draw a ditto of a tree. Every time the child says five correct syllables or words, he may paste an apple on the tree. (Apples can be made from punches out of red construction paper.)

Variations. Paste spots on a cow, petals on a flower, and so forth.

Animal Homes (individual/group). Create a chart with pictures of a tree, a zoo cage, a pond, and a barn. Cut out pictures of animals that would live in one of these four places. Have each child choose an animal and place it in its home, while saying the animal's name. (Note: Many animal names have /s/ and /r/ sounds.)

Find the Target (individual/group). Create 12 flashcards or pictures of objects whose names contain the target sound. First, the child is asked to name the object shown. Then the clinician displays the cards. If the target were /s/, the clinician might say, "I'm going to pretend that this piece of paper [a blank card] is soap. You close your eyes. I'll hide the soap under one of the other cards. You must guess which card the soap is under. Say, Is the soap under the pencil?" The child must ask the carrier question until he finds the soap. He looks under the cards himself.

Variation. With a group, have the children each take one turn looking for the target. The one who finds it gets to hide it next, though the clinician supplies the carrier phrase.

Animal Cards (group). Create a deck of cards with pictures of animals on them. The deck should include four matching pictures of each animal. Place the pack face down and have each child pick a card in turn. The object of the game is to get as many matches as possible.

Variations. The child must say a syllable or word a given number of times, or say it and use it in a sentence, before he is allowed to pick a card. Or the child can be required to describe the card drawn, using at least one word with his sound.

Ladderboard (group). Draw a ladder with each rung numbered. The numbers indicate the number of times the player is required to say his target sound or word. If it is said correctly, the child can move to the next rung. The object is to get to the top rung of the ladder.

Racetrack (group). Create a racetrack divided into spaces on a piece of poster board. Each child is given a colored marker that represents his horse. In addition, each child has a stack of cards with pictures of names of objects using that child's sound (or word). In turn, each one rolls a die, moves the number of spaces shown on the die, draws that same number of cards, and says the sounds on the cards. If all the sounds are said correctly, the child's marker stays where it is. For each sound said incorrectly, the marker is moved back two spaces. Either the clinician or the other children judge the productions.

Variation. Children at the sentence level can be required to put the target words into a sentence.

Spin the Arrow (group). Construct a cardboard spinner divided into wedges. Write words around the edge of the circle and give each word a number between 1 and 10. Each child spins and says the word on which the spinner stopped the number of times indicated. If the child says it correctly, he receives that many points. The first child to reach a designated number of points wins. (The point value of the words should be based on their difficulty.)

Word Bingo (group). On a ditto, draw enough nine-section bingo boards with pictures of objects in the sections so that each child can have a different board. Each object name should use the target sound. Cut the pictures out of one copy and place them face down in a box. The clinician draws a picture from the box and the children look to see if they have that picture on their cards. If a child finds the picture, he says the word a required number of times or uses it in a sentence, and can then place a chip on the picture. The first child to fill a row going across, down, or diagonally wins.

Variation. The first child to cover all nine sections wins.

Good Speech Land (group of 3 to 5). Create a ditto with 30 blanks and a color key showing the colors red, green, black, orange, blue, and yellow. Copies should be given to the children the day before the game is to be played. The children are to fill in the blanks with words using their target sounds. Cut out small squares, triangles, and diamonds of construction paper in the six game colors. These should be pasted on a piece of poster board in 5 rows of 12 shapes each, with colors and shapes arranged at random. Label the top of the chart "Good Speech Land."

To play the game, give each child a marker. Each child places his marker at the end of one of the rows. One child is the caller. The caller sits facing away from the group with his word list and color key. The caller reads three words from the word list and the players move their markers one space for each word called. The caller then says a color from the color key. Any player whose marker is on that color must move the marker back to the beginning to start again. The others can keep moving ahead. The game proceeds this way until one player wins by reaching the top of the row—"Good Speech Land." That player becomes the new caller.

The Shopping Game (group). Use poster board to create a spinner and a game board depicting four colored groups (red, blue, yellow, and green) of six stores each (florist, groceries, gifts, cards, pets, and so forth). Draw houses at the corners of the board to be starting points. The spinner should have 24 sections, representing the numbers 1 through 6 combined with each color. The first player spins and moves to the block of stores with the color indicated. He chooses one store to enter, then names an item that could be bought at that store. The name of the item must contain that player's target sound. He must say the name the number of times indicated on the spinner. Poker chips can be used as a reward, with the child receiving one chip for each time the word is said correctly. The winner is the child with the most chips at the end of the session.

Carryover

Around the Town (individual/group). Create a board showing streets of your community with familiar stores and other buildings labeled. The child must tell a story about a trip to the bank, to the zoo, and so forth—what he would do or buy at each place.

Road Map (group). Draw a map with made-up street and place names using the target sound. Make pairs of cards with place names from the map. Each child draws a card and moves a token to that place on the map. While moving on the roads, the child must say each street name correctly. If not, he does not keep the card and does not move. At the end of the session, the child with the greatest number of cards wins.

Variation. Require the children to describe their paths or to answer questions about the destinations.

Password (group). Make a set of cards picturing objects whose names contain the target sound. Each player is given a few cards. The first player says a carrier phrase that is a clue to the "password"—"I'm thinking of something hot." Other players guess the password, using full sentences such as "Are you thinking of the sun?" If the guess is wrong, the first player gives another clue. The player who guesses correctly gets the card and says a sentence using the password. The second player then gives a clue to his password. At the end of the session, the player with the most new cards wins.

CHAPTER 6 The Behavioral Approach to Treatment

One of the most important and obvious roles performed by the speech-language pathologist (SLP) is to assist individuals to modify some aspect of their communicative behavior. Treatment programs that SLPs design for this purpose can be evaluated primarily in terms of how efficient they are and the resulting permanency of the behavioral changes sought. The purpose of this chapter is to describe effective procedures that have been used to modify communicative behaviors. It is hoped that, through the use of these procedures, SLPs can improve their therapy techniques and thus bring about more effective and permanent changes in the communication skills of their clients.

The procedures described in this chapter have evolved from research conducted by such noted learning theorists as J. Watson, E. L. Thorndike, C. Hull, and, more recently, B. F. Skinner. One of the primary interests of these psychologists was to identify laws of learning that apply to all living organisms, specifically those laws that govern human learning. Their research techniques were modeled after those used in the natural sciences, including physics, biology, chemistry, and medicine.

Donald E. Mowrer, Ph.D., is a professor of speech pathology in the Department of Speech and Hearing Disorders, Arizona State University, Tempe, Arizona.

Several learning theorists were seeking a construct that would explain how organisms learn. They wanted an explanation analogous to Graham's (1951) mathematical equation,

$$Y = f(x) \text{ under } c.$$

The elements in this equation are as follows: y is an event or response, like the bursting of a rubber balloon. The equal sign (=) stands for the word "is." f means "a function of" or "is directly related to." (x) refers to a stimulus, such as a specific amount of air pressure sufficient to rupture a balloon. c represents a set of conditions, such as the strength of the rubber of the balloon as well as the atmospheric pressure. What Graham's law says when applied to inflating a balloon is that, as the balloon is inflated, a point will be reached when the balloon can no longer contain any increase in air pressure. It will rupture. The amount of air pressure needed to rupture the balloon can be specified in advance when the physical properties of the rubber are known. Given this knowledge, we can both control and predict the occurrence of the balloon's rupture.

Laws of this type are common in physics. These laws allow us to predict the occurrence of many events in our daily lives. For example, a specified amount of foot pressure applied to the brakes of a car will bring the car to a halt within a specified number of feet given certain conditions such as temperature, moisture on the surface, type of road surface, weight of the car, and so on. In another instance, water becomes gaseous when it is heated past 212° F. at sea level. A ball will attain a prescribed speed as it rolls down a 12-inch, 45° inclined plane. Thus, following Graham's equation, it is possible to predict and to control certain events.

Assuming that lawful relationships observed in the natural sciences may also occur in human learning, Skinner (1956) sought to discover similar lawful relationships in the behavior of animals. He conducted a series of experiments designed to identify the variables responsible for behavioral change. After he and his colleagues accumulated and analyzed massive amounts of animal responses resulting from a series of experiments, the conclusions were published in an impressive text entitled *Cumulative Record* (Skinner, 1959). From these observations, Skinner formulated a number of laws that seemed to govern behavior. One of the laws Skinner identified dealt with the effects that consequences of a behavior have on the rate of behavior. Simply stated, when a desired event (such as food) follows a specific behavior (such as a bar press), that behavior is more likely to occur in the future under similar conditions. Conversely, when a behavior (bar press, for example) is followed by an aversive event such as shock, that behavior is less likely to occur in the future when the conditions are similar. This latter condition was described as *punishment*.

What Skinner and others were seeking could be expressed as a modification of Graham's equation used to describe observed relationships in the natural sciences. The functional relationship of stimuli and responses in a learning situation might be expressed as $R = f(S)$ under c. To clarify this concept, consider the often cited hungry pigeon pacing about a small cage in search of food. The pigeon approaches a red disk mounted on the wall of the cage and pecks it. Actually, the pigeon could be taught to peck it through a series of trials called *successive approximation* but, to make a long story short, let's just assume the pigeon happens to peck the disk within a few minutes after being placed in the cage. Immediately after pecking, a food pellet plunks into his food dish! After eating, again he happens to peck the disk, and again, food drops into the dish. The pecking behavior continues until we conclude the pigeon has been "taught" to peck the disk.

We can apply each part of Graham's equation to the pigeon pecking experiment. First, R would consist of the pigeon's pecking response, and S would be the food stimulus dispensed in the dish. The conditions (c) would be the red disk. We could now say that pecking, the response, is controlled by its consequences, the presentation of food when the conditions of a red disk are present. We could also make predictions about pecking behavior. We could say that, given the hungry bird, he will peck at a red disk when given the opportunity in the future. Finally, we could say that the pigeon has "learned" to peck at the red disk as a result of the consequences of pecking.

Now suppose the color of the disk is changed to green, and suppose the pigeon pecks the green disk but, as a consequence, no food is delivered. Soon, the rate of the pigeon's pecking behavior diminishes, perhaps to zero pecking. But when the color of the disk is changed from green to red, the pigeon resumes a high rate of pecking, which is followed by food pellets. Thus, as a result of the differential consequences (food versus no food) of pecking at two different stimuli (green and red), the pigeon is said to have learned a discrimination task; that is, peck when red is presented, don't peck when green is presented. If all pigeons learn this discrimination task when the consequences are controlled in this manner, we can make a general statement about the nature of pigeon learning. Furthermore, if rats, pigs, goats, and cockroaches as well as humans also learn this red–green discrimination task under similar conditions, then we can formulate a law of learning for discrimination tasks.

Once stimulus–response relationships are identified, we can predict and control behavior by manipulating the consequences of the behavior. This was one of Skinner's major findings, and it is the framework upon which the treatment of articulation, as described in this chapter, is founded. Put simply, those who control the consequences of a behavior control the frequency of the behavior. Thus, we can increase the number of correct speech responses an individual produces and decrease the number of incorrect responses simply by controlling the consequences we administer following the production of correct and incorrect responses. In this way, we can bring about prescribed changes in articulation. As stated earlier, modifying articulation is one of our chief goals. The client who comes to us substituting /t/ for /k/, distorting /r/, or lisping should leave our treatment program articulating these sounds correctly in most or all speaking situations. Knowing how to change behavior is an important key to effective articulation treatment. In this chapter we will draw heavily from the research findings of the learning theorists in an attempt to apply a scientific rationale to the treatment of articulation errors.

IDENTIFYING THE TARGET BEHAVIOR

How can we apply the information derived from the learning theorists to an articulation treatment program? As a first step we must select a behavior that is important to change (Bailey & Lessen, 1984). We must ask whether the new behavior we have selected will make a difference to the individual. We also must ask if the behavior is age-appropriate and if the new behavior will make a difference in the individual's social interaction.

Describing the desired or *target behavior* is the second step. It is possible to describe /s/, for example, as having certain acoustic properties, a central airstream direction, and a specified position of tongue and teeth. When the production criteria for /s/ production are met, the listener perceives /s/. Our observations must be stated in objective terms:

we must observe a behavior or result of a behavior in such a way that it can be counted discretely. It must have a beginning and an ending. Subjective descriptions of articulation patterns such as "sloppy speech" or "slurred consonants" or "a lazy tongue" are not suitable because these impressions may mean different things to different people. Furthermore, it is impossible to count or objectively measure such vague impressions. Terms such as *interdental lisp, /ə/ for /ɚ/ substitution, lateral emission of the airstream,* and *omission of /s/* are features of the behavior that can be agreed upon and measured objectively.

Clinicians also are interested in the context and speaking situations in which the sound occurs. When articulation is sampled and described as it occurs in a variety of speaking situations over a period of several days, these data are called the *baseline*. Baseline data provide a description of the current state of the speech behavior. Often, clinicians sample a sound only in the initial, medial, and final positions using three test words to evoke responses. Such tests would be considered an inadequate baseline sample. McDonald's (1964) Deep Test of Articulation provides more complete information about how a sound is produced in a variety of phonemic contexts. It is also important to sample the sound as it occurs in conversational speech situations. Much of the information obtained from diagnostic testing can be used to describe the status of the behavior before treatment. A phonological process analysis such as the one derived from the Khan-Lewis Phonological Analysis (Khan and Lewis, 1986) can be an extremely useful part of a baseline measure. A baseline of the behavior is taken so that changes in behavior can be ascertained once the treatment program is initiated.

In summary, the first two steps are to select the client's present behavior (baseline) and to specify the type of behavior the client should exhibit when the treatment program has been completed (target behavior). In the next section, two of the most important aspects of the instructional process, antecedent and consequent events, will be presented.

ROLE OF ANTECEDENT EVENTS

Stimuli designed to evoke responses from the client are classified as *antecedent events*. They include the use of *cues* and *prompts*. Cues provide hints as to what the response should be, whereas prompts specify the exact response. The prompt, "Say /k/," specifically identifies the response that is expected. The cue, "Say it again," suggests what the response should be. Three types of cues and prompts can be used:

1. Auditory stimuli include spoken instructions and models of a sound.
2. Visual stimuli include visual models in which the clinician demonstrates certain tongue, lip, or teeth positions by using a hand cue, showing a diagram, presenting written material, or by actual demonstration of positions or movements.
3. Kinesthetic stimuli involve manipulation of part of the client's speech mechanism and may include touching the cheeks, holding the jaw open, using a tongue depressor to position the tongue, or pressing on the rib cage. Placing peanut butter on the alveolar ridge would be considered a kinesthetic cue.

These stimuli, cues, and prompts determine the nature of the response and serve to evoke the desired response. Skinner and his associates, however, have not had the advantage of using some of these explicit cues in their animal experiments. You cannot "tell" a rat to press the bar, nor can you show a pigeon how to peck the disk. In most animal research, a target behavior is chosen on the basis of the animal's ability to perform the task. If

it was likely the rat would press a bar when it was placed at a reachable level, then presence of the bar would be the antecedent stimulus event designed to evoke the response of pressing the bar. Visual cues are used in animal research almost exclusively, hence, we have limited knowledge concerning the effects of other types of cues and prompts.

ROLE OF CONSEQUENT EVENTS

Stimuli presented following a response are classified as the *consequent event*. Skinner and his associates focused on the effects of these events in much of their research with animals. The current emphasis on behavior modification techniques in education has drawn heavily from the information gained by meticulous observation of the effects of these events upon animal behavior. The core of behavioral research between the 1950s and 1960s centered around variables that affected rate of behavior, that is, the conditions that increased, decreased, or had no effect upon rate of behavior. We will now examine techniques used to increase and decrease behaviors.

Increasing Behavior Rate

Skinner identified two procedures that result in an increase in behavior rate. Only one procedure, *positive reinforcement,* will be presented here because it is used so extensively in human instructional settings. Positive reinforcement is said to occur when rate of behavior increases above the baseline behavior rate. Positive reinforcement immediately follows a response and satisfies a need of the organism. In most animal experiments, food pellets were chosen as the stimulus (positive reinforcer) that would most likely satisfy the animal's hunger drive. One can use body weight to quantify the state of an animal's hunger. By weighing a well-fed rat we can assume that the rat's weight defines a state of nonhunger. After depriving the rat of food for 3 days, body weight decreases a few ounces and this new lower weight defines a hunger condition for that rat. We can be assured that, when placed in a cage containing a lever, the rat will be very active in its search for food and will be likely to strike the lever. When a lever press occurs by chance, an automatic mechanism dispenses a food pellet that the hungry rat consumes. Within a short time, lever-pressing behaviors occur more frequently. The relationship that exists between the frequency of the response (lever pressing) and the presentation of the food pellet stimulus (the reinforcer) can be expressed by Graham's formula, $R = f(S)$ under c. The frequency of the rat's lever pressing behavior is controlled by the consequences of lever pressing behavior.

Although food is considered a primary reinforcer, soon just the click of the pellet-dispensing mechanism also becomes a reinforcer. The clicking sound, having been paired with the presentation of the food pellet, takes on the properties of a reinforcer. This new conditioned stimulus is called a *secondary reinforcer*. Pavlov (1927) demonstrated how an auditory stimulus (bell) when paired with a primary reinforcer (meat powder) could produce a similar response (salivation) when the two stimuli are presented in rapid succession. Humans quickly learn that money, a secondary reinforcer of little value in itself, can be used to procure food, shelter, and other types of reinforcers. Words such as *good, fine,* and *right* also serve as secondary reinforcers when paired with approval behaviors.

When we analyze the reinforcement paradigm, it is evident that two conditions are necessary for reinforcement to be effective. First, a state of need or desire must exist within the organism. This need can be manifested as thirst, hunger, desire for social recognition, or some similar state. Second, the experimenter must be able to control the presentation of a stimulus that satisfies this need. Skinner (1957) called such a stimulus a *positive reinforcer* when it resulted in an increase in rate of behavior.

One does not know whether a stimulus is a positive reinforcer until behavior rate increases. For example, if the researcher has conditioned a rat to

depress a lever by following each lever press with presentation of a food pellet, lever-pressing behavior will occur at a high rate until the rat is no longer hungry. When the rat becomes satiated with food pellets, lever-pressing behavior terminates. In this case, food no longer serves as a reinforcer.

Sometimes it is difficult to predict what stimulus might serve as an effective reinforcer for some children. I recall an instance of a teacher who was helping a 12-year-old boy with a reading problem. She used a hand tally counter to keep a record of each word the boy read correctly. This boy was told he could exchange points displayed on the hand counter for items of his choice like a flashlight battery, pen, knife, or similar item. But instead of exchanging his earned points at the end of each session, he preferred to save them for a more expensive item. This point-saving continued for several weeks until the tutoring was completed. He had earned several thousand points, enough to buy a radio or bicycle, which, by the way, his teacher could not afford to provide. But when asked what he wanted to buy with his accumulated points, he said, "The counter!"

The principle of positive reinforcement, when applied to human learning conditions, is one of the most effective means of controlling behavior. In spite of this, positive reinforcement has received scant attention from most authors who describe procedures for treating articulation problems. Many texts that describe articulation therapy recommend that an occasional friendly pat, smile, or positive verbal statement may be used as a reward for the client's efforts, but no explanations are provided regarding type, frequency, or schedule of these rewards. Clinicians are encouraged to use games as activities to capture the child's interest and maintain attention, but there is little reference to precise management of consequent events of the type Skinner described in his animal research. If human learning is governed by the same principles as is animal learning, and if lawful relationships exist between stimuli and response events, then clinicians could benefit by paying careful attention to the administration of consequent events.

Selecting Potential Reinforcers. Before we can modify behavior using positive reinforcement, we must first select stimuli that would serve as a reinforcer. Technically, one does not know if a stimulus will be a reinforcer until the target behavior has been observed to increase. Consequently, we must speak of selecting ''potential'' reinforcers: we will talk about selecting rewards instead of reinforcers because we cannot be sure these stimuli will result in increasing the frequency of the behavior.

The best way to ensure that food will serve as a reinforcer is to deprive the child of her meals for a day. This has been initiated in some institutional settings. But food deprivation is not a practical procedure for most speech clinicians. Of course, candy could be chosen (usually M&Ms) but use of candy may produce undesirable nutritional side effects and tooth decay. We should probably rule out food items as reinforcers, especially in public school settings.

The clinician must find potential reinforcers that do not wear out and have no undesirable side effects. Fortunately, certain words in our language have been paired with pleasant events and have thus taken on the properties of secondary reinforcement. Statements of praise such as ''Swell,'' ''You did a good job,'' and ''Great!'' can serve as effective reinforcers as long as they produce increases in behavior rates. Klotz and Shantz (1973) clearly demonstrated in their study of emotionally disturbed children how verbal praise alone was used to increase cooperative behaviors. Unfortunately, some populations such as autistic children do not respond to these common social pleasantries and so words of praise hold no reinforcing value.

Even if statements of verbal praise are found to serve as reinforcers, they may lose their effectiveness when used continually for long periods of time. After 20 minutes of listening to the clinician say, ''Good,'' ''Fine,'' ''Swell,'' Nice job,'' and

''Good going, Mary,'' the child has had enough and no longer finds these statements satisfying. Fortunately, other means have been found to maintain the child's interest for long periods of time. Of course, the most straightforward way to find out what might serve as effective reinforcers is simply to ask the individual what she would like to have. Tharp and Wetzel (1969) use a questionnaire to find out what children want. They ask what the child would like to do, what she would buy with $10, what the child likes to do at school, and similar questions.

Use of a Token Economy System. An alternative to the exclusive use of verbal praise statements is to pair verbal praise with the presentation of a visual stimulus such as pencil mark, bean, poker chip, or some similar marker. Thus, through association with the verbal praise, the child learns the value of yet another secondary reinforcer, the token. These markers or tokens acquire value when the child learns that she can exchange the tokens for material goods or activities that would interest the child. For example, colorful speech pencils[1] on which are printed a list of practice words containing the child's target sound can be used as potential reinforcers that can be purchased with tokens. If you choose to use toys as the redeemable item, the toys can be mounted on a large piece of cardboard, each toy with a price tag. A comb may cost 100 tokens, a plastic car 200 tokens, a bracelet 350 tokens, and so on. This is called a *reinforcement menu*. The child is told she can buy any desired toy on the menu with tokens that are earned. Activities can be purchased as well. It may cost 50 tokens to throw a dart, 40 tokens to toss a beanbag at a target, 100 tokens for being first in the cafeteria line at noon, 80 tokens for being allowed to use colored pens to color a picture, and so on. The activities children will work for are limited only by the clinician's imagination. Teenagers will work for tickets to plays and sporting activities, used phonograph records, cosmetics, and so on. Adults

---

[1]Speech pencils and toys are available from IDEAS, Box 1494, Tempe, Arizona 85281.

frequently will work just to know they are making progress as shown by a speech progress chart.

Wilson and O'Leary (1980) point out that a token economy system should include three ingredients: (a) a clearly defined behavior that will be rewarded, (b) presentation of a token immediately following the behavior, and (c) an agreement concerning how the tokens can be exchanged for prizes for special activities. Considerable evidence exists demonstrating the effectiveness of token economy systems when applied to classroom learning activities (O'Leary & Drabman, 1971; O'Leary, 1978).

Self-Reinforcement. To conclude that learning occurs only when someone reinforces a person for making certain responses would be naive. Learning can occur in many other ways. Skinner (1953) postulates that, if an individual knows she has produced a correct response, this knowledge alone may be sufficient to increase behavior rates. Perhaps you have enrolled in a course in which a programmed text was used. Typically, you read a statement and are asked to answer a question about the statement or fill in a missing word. Immediately after responding, you compare your answer with the correct answer printed on the next page of the text. If the two answers match, the knowledge that you were correct is presumed to be a reinforcer. If the material to be learned is presented in small sequential steps and you respond correctly throughout the program, the prescribed information is usually learned in accordance with the original intent of the program writer. In this situation, one literally rewards oneself.

Blount and Stokes (1984), in their review of studies in which children are taught to reinforce themselves, report that self-reinforcement often has been found to be more effective than externally administered reinforcement procedures. They conclude that children should gradually be given control over reinforcement procedures in order to assure desired treatment outcomes. In this procedure, the child scores her own responses as correct or incorrect and presents these data as points toward some desired reward. Procedures have been devised to check the child's response

monitoring to ensure that she is scoring correctly. Bandura (1976) set up the following guidelines for a self-reinforcement procedure: (a) individual cannot take rewards until the desired behavior is exhibited, (b) individual must exercise full control over rewards, and (c) standards must be set before rewards can be delivered.

A practical example of how self-reinforcement was observed in a treatment program may help clarify this concept. I administered an instructional program designed to correct lisping to 30 children (Mowrer, 1964). Children were divided into two equal groups. The program consisted of some 300 stimulus items, delivered during three 15-minute sessions. Children in one group were informed whether their responses were correct or incorrect immediately following each response and simultaneously given a redeemable token following each correct response. Those in the other group were given no information about the accuracy of their responses and no tokens were provided. A 30-item criterion test was given before and after the program to evaluate accuracy of /s/ production as taught in the program. Although children in the first group obtained scores that were significantly higher than those of the second group, inspection of individual scores revealed that a few children in the second group who received no information about the adequacy of their responses obtained near-perfect scores on the criterion test!

What could account for their learning correct /s/ production even though feedback was not provided? Some children may be very perceptive of subtle cues. For example, the fact that they were never told they made a mistake may have led them to assume they were performing the task correctly; their teacher was simply stingy with rewards. The learning histories of some children are such that they do not expect rewards during an instructional setting. They simply do what they are told to do. These children often are described as ''conscientious children.'' Thus, if the instructions are sufficient to enable the child to figure out what behaviors are expected, and if the child desires to please the teacher, then rewards such as tokens or verbal praise may not be required in order to change the behavior. If, on the other hand, the instructions alone are insufficient to help the child establish correct /s/ productions, it may be likely the child would not score well on the criterion test. Thus, antecedent events alone often play an important role during task acquisition.

Some Cautions. Clearly, it is difficult to establish a single set of reward procedures that will be effective with all children. Clinicians should view with considerable caution instructional procedures that demand a standard set of procedures be used for all children regardless of their educational histories or special needs. Although we have learned much from data gathered in research with animals, often it is not possible to apply simple solutions derived solely from this research directly to situations involving human learning. The child comes to us not as a *tabula rosa* but as a sophisticated learner whose behaviors have been shaped in many different ways. This might help explain the fact that even though a clinician seems to violate many of the principles of operant conditioning, some children learn the prescribed task because they have learned to be very perceptive in picking out salient characteristics of a learning task. On the other hand, some children may not be as perceptive and may require far more intensive instructional feedback.

An article published in a newsletter of the Harvard Center for Research and Development of Educational Differences (1964) pointed out that relatively little is known about the complex factors of aptitude, ability, interest, and motivation or their interactions on effects of learning. It is well known that differences exist among children in these areas, but educational research has seldom focused on them.

Schedules of Reinforcement. The frequency with which a reinforcer is presented contingent upon the correct response seems to influence how well the response is maintained once the reinforcement

is discontinued. Skinner (1957) investigated the effects of four different schedules of reinforcement upon animal behavior. He discovered that each schedule seemed to affect behavior frequencies differently. In one schedule, frequency of reinforcement depends upon a fixed number of responses called a *fixed ratio*. For example, one reinforcer may be delivered following two consecutive correct responses (FR-2) or after every six consecutive correct responses (FR-6). In a similar schedule called a *variable ratio*, the number of correct responses is used to determine when a reinforcer is administrated. For example, the following sequence of correct responses would reflect a VR-3 schedule: 2 correct → r+ (reinforcer), 4 correct → r+, 3 correct → r+, 5 correct → r+, 2 correct → r+, 2 correct → r+. From this sequence, a total of 18 correct responses were made in 6 groups. Eighteen divided by 6 equals 3, or the average number of correct responses contained in each group.

Examples of fixed and variable ratio schedules of reinforcement are relatively easy to identify as they occur in our daily lives. The strawberry picker who is paid 25 cents for every three baskets of berries picked is working according to a fixed ratio schedule (FR-3). On the other hand, the car salesman who averages one sale for every 10 people who inquire about cars is on a variable ratio schedule (VR-10). Both schedules result in high rates when used in experiments with animal behaviors.

Some important differences in the persistence of the response have been noted with regard to the frequency of reinforcement (Skinner & Ferster, 1957). If an FR-1 (continuous) schedule is used, once reinforcement is terminated, the response rate may increase briefly, but then it usually drops sharply and soon returns to its preconditioned rate. This is called *extinction*. If a reinforcement ratio such as FR or VR of 5 to 10 is selected, then the response is maintained at a high rate for a much longer period. However, if a very large ratio is selected early during the skill-learning period, the response may extinguish before the next reinforcement can be delivered. This condition is called *ratio strain*.

What type of schedule should the speech clinician use? It appears that, when a new task is being learned, the reinforcer should be delivered frequently, as often as FR-1. As the task is mastered, the ratio can be increased gradually to a variable ratio of perhaps 3, then 6, then 9, and more. Once the new behavior is firmly established, the reinforcer can be eliminated altogether, yet the behavior will not extinguish.

The practical application of this information to articulation learning seems obvious, although there is little research data to substantiate the effects of using various reinforcement schedules in articulation treatment programs. Undoubtedly, substantial individual differences exist among children so that it would be difficult to recommend one method of administering reinforcement schedules over another method.

In spite of the lack of empirical data, most authors who advocate behavior therapy for the treatment of articulation errors recommend using continuous reinforcement when a new skill is taught. Once the new behavior is produced many times without error, a variable ratio schedule is introduced beginning with a VR-2 followed by a VR-4 and later a VR-8 or -10 schedule. Boone and Prescott (1972) recommend a VR-4 once the treatment program is under way. Observations of the amount of verbal praise provided by their student clinicians in numerous treatment sessions indicated a VR-4 schedule was frequently used. We cannot, however, be certain this is the best possible schedule to use with all clients.

Two additional types of schedules were identified by Skinner (1959), but they seldom are used in articulation treatment programs. These schedules are based on time dimensions rather than rate of response. One schedule is fixed, the other is variable. If you provide a reinforcer every 3 minutes, this is called a *fixed interval* (FI-3) schedule. In the other schedule, *variable interval,* a reinforcer is delivered after an average time period, e.g., after 2 minutes, then 4 minutes, then 3 minutes, for an average of 3 minutes. Skinner (1959) found that both these schedules generate much lower response rates than the variable ratio schedules. The lowest rate occurred under a variable interval schedule.

There is still much to learn about the effects different reinforcement schedules have on learning articulation skills. We can extract some general principles from animal research and the few studies of human learning, but beyond that, we must rely upon the data we gather from working with individual children.

Wilson and O'Leary (1980) point out that attempts to produce human behavior patterns that follow patterns of animal behavior produced in the laboratory have not succeeded. Perhaps this discrepancy results because we often have such poor controls when working with humans. Factors other than reinforcement schedules may play a more important role in determining frequency of behavior.

Decreasing Behavior Rate

Extinction. Skinner was equally interested in stimulus conditions that decreased behavior rate. One technique, extinction, has already been mentioned. This principle was discovered by Skinner (1956) quite by accident when his food-dispensing apparatus jammed one night. He arrived in his laboratory early the next morning to discover a steady decrement in the rate of behavior on the cumulative recorder printout. Immediately after the apparatus stopped functioning, there was a burst of responses followed by a gradual decrement in response rate. Finally, response rate returned to its preconditioned rate. What Skinner discovered from countless repetitions of this experiment was that response rate decreases when reinforcement is removed. One can virtually eliminate a response by withholding reinforcement.

In subsequent studies, it was discovered that some behaviors persist in spite of the fact that reinforcement is eliminated. If the behavior has been practiced thousands of times and a "lean" variable ratio schedule was used, say, VR-100, then the behavior continues in spite of the fact that the reinforcer is eliminated. In this case, the behavior is said to be highly resistant to extinction. This is exactly what we want to happen during the articulation treatment program; that is, we want to make the correct speech response highly resistant to extinction. To do this, a "lean" schedule of intermittent reinforcement of the correct response is used, such as VR-20 or -30.

When a motor behavior is practiced thousands of times, changes occur in the neural pathways and the information is stored more or less permanently. Consequently, continual reinforcement may not be required to maintain a response. Suppose you are reinforced for hitting a tennis ball; you receive good instruction from a tennis coach. With continued practice you become a proficient tennis player. Then you move to Greenland for 10 years where there are no tennis courts. Upon return to your native country, you find you can still play a fair game in spite of the absence of any reinforcement or practice for 10 years. Extinction does not occur in one's *ability* to perform. On the other hand, suppose you didn't move to Greenland; you played tennis daily, but soon you felt no challenge in the game and you were making no progress. Due to lack of interest (lack of reinforcement) you took up another sport. You showed up less and less at the tennis court. Finally, you stopped playing tennis altogether. Extinction of the behavior occurred; you no longer play tennis.

It is uncommon for a person who has learned correct articulation to revert to the previous speech pattern with the exception of a few individuals who may have psychological problems associated with the speech problem. Of course, many children learn to discriminate between correct and incorrect articulation patterns but do not use the correct pattern in all situations. They are reinforced for using correct articulation in the speech clinic, but in the classroom, where they have not been reinforced for correct articulation, the error sound is likely to be used. This is not an example of extinction in the technical sense but a result of discrimination. The response class has not generalized from the speech clinic environment to other types of speaking situations.

Time-Out. A procedure that has been used to reduce the frequency of some behaviors is called time-out. In this case, all opportunities for obtaining reinforcers are eliminated; the child may be placed in another room or totally ignored for a certain time. Although this procedure has been used successfully in reducing disruptive behaviors (Patterson & White, 1969), as well as echolalia (Lovaas, 1966), stuttering (Costello, 1975), and similar deviant behaviors, it does not seem to be appropriate in treating misarticulations.

Punishment. A third procedure used to reduce unwanted behavior is punishment. Considerable research is available about the subject of punishment and its effects. Punishment exists when a stimulus is presented immediately following a response and a decrease in response rate is observed (Honig and Staddon, 1977). As in the case of reinforcement, a punisher is defined in terms of its effect upon response rate: it cannot be defined until behavior rate is observed to decrease.

The following example should clarify the concept of punishment. A child in Ms. Smith's classroom had the habit of leaving her seat frequently. Ms. Smith, tired of this behavior, decided to eliminate or at least reduce it by punishing the child for leaving her seat. Each time the child left her seat without permission, Ms. Smith told her to sit down. Ms. Smith's remarks became more emphatic. She threatened to send the child to the principal, force her to stay after school, or inform her parents of her misbehavior. In spite of Ms. Smith's reprimands and threats, the child was observed to leave her seat even more frequently than before. "I can't understand this," said Ms. Smith to her supervisor. "I keep punishing Terry for leaving her seat, but it doesn't seem to work." If the behavior increased as a consequence of Ms. Smith's remarks, then her reprimands acted as a reinforcer, not a punisher. Even though verbal threats would seem to be punishing events, they did not serve as punishers in this case. More likely, the child sought attention from the teacher. She received plenty of it when she left her seat!

Should we punish children for making the incorrect speech response? Here again, we have little empirical data regarding the role of punishment in suppressing misarticulations. I think most speech-language pathologists would agree that punishment in the form of aversive stimuli such as a threat, slap, or reprimand is not appropriate. Informing the child that a response is incorrect may be helpful, especially if this is followed by an instructive comment such as, "No, you forgot to close your teeth," or "No, your tongue stuck out," or "No, you didn't put your tongue high enough." Technically these comments would be classified as punishers if, as a result of using them, the incorrect response decreased.

Response Cost. Finally, a fourth type of consequent event found to be effective in decreasing behaviors is a procedure called response cost. In this case, a reinforcer is removed following an incorrect response. If you are giving tokens following correct responses and taking them away following incorrect responses, you are using this procedure. Mowrer and Conley (1987) used this procedure with one group of children who misarticulated /s/. They compared the performance of a group of children who lisped and were deprived of tokens contingent upon incorrect responses with another group of similar children who received no such punishment contingent upon their incorrect responses. They found that the group in which the response cost procedure was used produced significantly more correct /s/ responses in a storytelling speech situation than did those who did not receive punishment. McReynolds and Huston (1971) found token loss per se did not function as an effective punisher but they used only two subjects, one of whom was mentally retarded. Until more is known about the positive and negative effects of the response cost procedure, speech clinicians should view the use of response cost with caution.

USE OF ANTECEDENT AND CONSEQUENT EVENTS IN ARTICULATION TRAINING

Generally, antecedent events determine the type of response the child will produce, and consequent events serve to increase or decrease the likelihood a response will occur in the future. Often it is difficult to change articulation patterns using one event exclusively. Bruce Ryan and I attempted to

teach correct /ɝ/ production to children who distorted /ɝ/. The only antecedent information we provided was to request them to produce the sound differently. They were told to produce /ɝ/, but after that no instructions were provided regarding how to produce the sound. We thought we could control articulation by differential feedback at the consequent level. When the children made a sound that was close to /ɝ/, we would say "good" or "better." If the sound was unlike /ɝ/, we depressed a buzzer, and said, "No, make it different." We were unsuccessful in our attempts. Had we provided important antecedent events like, "Curl your tongue up and back," or "Make it sound like this, /ɝ/," we would have been able to evoke /ɝ/ with little difficulty. Sometimes it may be wise to ignore the incorrect response, especially during the initial treatment sessions. Some children react negatively to criticism. Following 10 consecutive "nos" they may burst into tears and refuse to continue.

Analyzing Effects of Antecedent and Consequent Events

Boone and Prescott (1972) outlined a procedure to help clinicians analyze their use of antecedent and consequent events. They classified antecedent events into two categories: (a) explaining and describing goals or procedures and (b) modeling the desired behavior or instructing the person how to produce it.

Consequent events were of two types: (a) good evaluations (clinician evaluates client response as correct and indicates verbal or nonverbal approval) and (b) bad evaluations. The last category was a neutral-social category that included the remarks made by the clinician that did not pertain to achieving the goals of the treatment program. Responses of the client were noted. After observing many clinicians, Boone and Prescott concluded that clinicians who were most effective followed rather consistent patterns in their use of antecedent and consequent events. First, the effective clinicians presented a model or instruction, which was followed by the client's response. The client was then informed whether the response was correct or incorrect. This was followed by another model or instruction, and the process was repeated. Poor clinicians provided insufficient cues and inappropriate consequences, and engaged in conversations that were unrelated to goals of the treatment program. Boone and Prescott present one of the few systems available to help clinicians analyze treatment sessions objectively by determining the relative importance to the client's progress of using antecedent and consequent events.

Observing and Recording Behaviors

There is no way of knowing whether one's use of antecedent and consequent events is effective unless accurate records of the client's behavior are kept. A clinician may have an elaborate system of cues designed to evoke correct responses, a well-planned schedule of reinforcement, plus highly desirable reinforcers, but unless behavioral change occurs, the treatment program is ineffective. The effectiveness of procedures is reflected in the client's performance. The chief value of recording responses is to provide guidance in the use of antecedent and/or consequent events.

The obvious way to evaluate behavior is to use a binary system; a response is either right or wrong. There are numerous ways of recording these responses. Many clinicians tabulate correct and incorrect responses using a score sheet similar to the one shown in Figure 6.1. Others use a hand tally counter or simply count up the number of tokens given plus number of wrong responses that have been tallied separately.

Computing Percentage of Correct Responses.
After tallying responses, the clinician can determine the percentage of correct responses. For example, if 220 responses are correct and 40 incorrect, the percentage correct would be 85% (220 ÷

260). Thus, it is possible to determine how accurately the client performed. By converting the number of correct responses into a percentage, we can make comparisons among treatment sessions that differ in time. Look at the data in Table 6.1. Although each session differed in length and number of responses, performance can be compared using correct response percentage figures.

These data can be recorded graphically. Letting the ordinate represent percentage correct in increments of 10% and the abscissa represent session, the percentage correct can be plotted for each session. Through connection of these points, the client's progress or lack of it can be portrayed. Figure 6.2 shows the percentage correct presented in Table 6.1 represented as a line graph.

Computing Rate of Response. Although calculating the percentage of correct responses provides us with important information about the accuracy of a client's performance, it ignores rate of behavior. Suppose the number of correct responses produced by clients A and B was 90%. Client A, however, produced 90 correct and 10 incorrect responses during a 5-minute session, whereas client B produced only 9 correct responses and 1 incorrect response during the same session. By calculating rate of response, we can determine how often the response occurred. In this example, rate of correct response per minute was 18 (90 responses ÷ 5 minutes) for client A, but only 1.8 (9 ÷ 5) for client B.

In order to obtain accuracy information, we also must compute either total response rate per minute (total number of responses divided by number of minutes) or error rate (number of errors divided by number of minutes) and compare one of these rates to the correct rate. Choosing total rate, we find that total rate is 20 (100 ÷ 5) for client A and 2 (10 ÷ 5) for client B. We conclude that although response accuracy was the same for both clients, client A produced 10 times as many responses in the same time period as did client B.

Rate information is important to clinicians who attempt to change articulation skills because the articulation of speech sounds involves motor acts (Milisen, 1954). Considerable practice is required

Name: _____

Date: _____

Task: _____

_____

_____

_____

Time (Min): _____

Key: X Correct
      O Incorrect

Response Summary Correct _____   Incorrect _____   Total Responses _____

FIGURE 6.1
Tally sheet for recording correct and incorrect speech responses.

TABLE 6.1
Data from Six Sessions Reflecting Accuracy of Response, Session Length, and Rate Information

Session	Number of Correct Responses	Number of Incorrect Responses	Duration of Session	Percent Correct	Correct Response Rate per Minute	Total Response Rate per Minute
1	58	8	10 min	87	5.8	6.6
2	30	9	15 min	77	2	2.6
3	180	10	20 min	95	9	9.5
4	48	0	8 min	100	6	6.0
5	20	1	20 min	95	1	1.05
6	160	72	32 min	69	5	7.25

to learn motor skills such as typing, playing a musical instrument, mastering sport activities, and so on. Hundreds of movement patterns must be practiced before the skill becomes automatic. Coordination of tongue and jaw movements required for precise articulation also requires considerable practice. The more a client practices a speech response in a variety of contexts, the more likely the

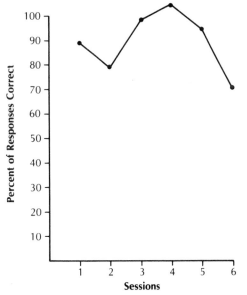

FIGURE 6.2
Percentage of responses produced correctly during each of six sessions, shown as a line graph.

response will become automatic. McDonald (1964) emphasized practicing certain speech patterns as an essential part of his sensory-motor approach to the treatment of articulation errors.

Not only the rate of responding but also the overtness of the response is important. In an attempt to evaluate the importance of making overt responses, I asked one group of lisping children to respond overtly to a series of instructional items (Mowrer, 1964). Another group of children who lisped simply listened to the instructions. Following completion of 45 minutes of instruction, most of the children who responded overtly were able to produce /s/ correctly on a criterion task, whereas none of the children who simply listened to the instructions produced /s/ correctly. This demonstrates the importance of making overt responses.

Theoretically, the clinician who provides many opportunities for the client to produce correct speech responses per unit of time should experience a greater success rate in terms of articulation change than the clinician who evokes but a few responses. A number of years ago I reported a study of the number of target responses seven public-school speech clinicians evoked from their clients (Mowrer, 1969a). I was amazed to find the average rate of response per minute was only 2.5. I also noted that some clinicians evoked an average of only .3 responses per minute, whereas others evoked as many as 16 per minute. The average rate of responses evoked using an instructional program to correct lisping (S-PACK) was 7.5 per minute, three times that of the average response rate evoked by traditional treatment methods (Mowrer, Baker, & Schutz, 1968).

The important point to be made here is that, unless we keep accurate records of response data and relate this information to behavioral change, we are unable to determine the effectiveness of specific treatment procedures. The careful observation and recording of events are a fundamental part of every science. If the treatment of communication problems is to become a science (as opposed to an art), then we must keep accurate accounts of our observations of the behavior we are attempting to modify. By analyzing correct and total response rate, we assess the accuracy and frequency of a client's response, two variables that reflect the effectiveness of our treatment procedure (Drash, Caldwell, & Liebowitz, 1970). Using data from Table 6.1, correct and total response rates plotted on the equal interval graph are shown in Figure 6.3.

It is readily apparent that some sessions were better than others with respect to rate of response.

If you compare sessions 3 and 5 shown in Figure 6.2, you might conclude that the two sessions were equal because accuracy was about 95% in both instances. But look at these same sessions as shown in Figure 6.3. It can be seen that the activities during session 3 resulted in a high rate of correct response. The client practiced the correct response often, and there were many opportunities for reinforcement to occur. But in session 5, the client produced few responses, and thus there was limited chance for reinforcement to occur. If practice makes perfect, then clearly session 3 was better than session 5.

Notations about Response Class. By making notations about what occurred during the session, we can summarize the nature of the responses. During session 3, the client was required to produce the sound in a variety of phonemic contexts in different words and phrases. In contrast, although most of the responses produced during session 5 were

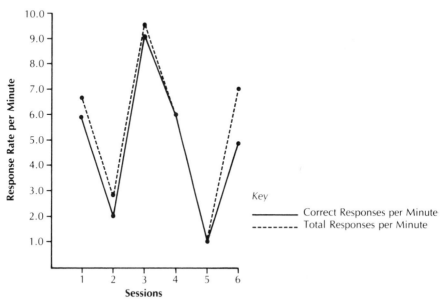

FIGURE 6.3
Response rate per minute plotted for six sessions on an equal-interval graph.

correct, the client received minimal practice saying the sound in a variety of contexts. The client repeatedly asked permission to spin an arrow mounted on a card. The single phrase *May I spin the spinner* was used as the carrier for the desired response, /ɚ/. Obviously, the type of response required in the two sessions differed greatly. Thus, in addition to rate and accuracy information, a third factor emerges as an important event to record: the type of response produced. The child who says the same word 50 times during one session with 90% accuracy has not made the same progress as the child who has used the target sound 50 times in a wide variety of phonemic contexts with 90% accuracy. Also, the child who practices saying the target sound only in the initial position of monosyllabic words has limited practice learning co-articulation skills that will help the response generalize to other words.

If the clinician is interested in changing articulation patterns, he or she must observe and record the accuracy of the client's response, the frequency of the correct and incorrect response, and the context in which the response occurs. If these data are not recorded, the clinician can only guess what is happening as a result of the treatment program. He or she cannot make effective changes in the treatment program because decisions are based only on intuition or feelings about the progress achieved by the client. One could hardly call such a procedure a science.

Behavioral Probes. Recording all responses may not always be practical. An alternative procedure is to sample the behavior periodically. Such samples are called *probes*. Both Diedrich (1971) and Elbert, Shelton, and Arndt (1967) describe procedures for assessing behavioral change based on an articulation test given at the end of a treatment session. The test items may include the target sound(s) embedded in many contexts or, in the case of the 10-item criterion test used in the S-PACK treatment program (Mowrer, Baker, &

Schutz, 1968), only in the phonemic contexts taught during a particular session.

The data from these behavioral probes are graphically recorded. These data provide a representative sample of progress being made during the treatment sessions.

Logarithmic Graphing Techniques. A more precise procedure for assessing behavioral change was introduced to educators by Lindsley (1964). Rather than divide the ordinate into equal intervals, he felt increments of behavior should be shown as equal ratios. The audiogram is an example of an equal-ratio-increment graph because sound intensity increases by logarithmic ratios, not by equal intervals. Behavior rates are recorded as points on this graph in the same manner as they are recorded on the equal-interval graph shown in Figure 6.3. The correct response rate from Figure 6.3 is plotted on a logarithmic graph in Figure 6.4.

The logarithmic graphing procedure offers several advantages over other graphing techniques. A greater range of behaviors of widely differing rates can be depicted, and several different behaviors can be recorded. Up to 140 calendar days can be included. The equal-ratio graph is more sensitive to behavioral change, and length of session also can be shown. Cooper, Heron, and Heward (1987), White and Haring (1976), and Mowrer (1969b) describe in detail how educators can use the logarithmic graphing technique to improve their teaching.

PREPARING INSTRUCTIONAL OBJECTIVES

Treatment programs based on vague, poorly stated objectives are often ineffective. Much valuable teaching time is lost if the clinician has no clear understanding of what must be accomplished during the brief time the client is seen for treatment. Supervisors of clinical training programs are well aware of the value of requiring student clinicians to write lesson plans. Students are usually asked to

SPEECH RESPONSE CHART

FIGURE 6.4
Correct response rate per minute plotted for six sessions on a logarithmic graph.

specify in detail planned activities for the treatment sessions. Once this careful planning is done, the execution of treatment programs can be more systematic and effective than if one has only a general idea of what should occur during the treatment process. In many states, speech clinicians are required by law to specify behavioral objectives for their teaching programs.

Mager (1962) wrote an easy-to-follow procedure for writing behavioral objectives. He specified three conditions that must be met for a goal to be considered a behavioral objective: (a) a do state-

ment, (b) a conditions statement, and (c) an accuracy statement.

The Do Statement. First, the clinician must describe objectively exactly what she wants the learner to *do* during the treatment period. It must be possible to count or measure the behavior. If it cannot be counted, there is no way to determine if the behavior has occurred or changed.

For example, if the objective is to make the client aware of the correct sound, how could the clinician count the number of times the client was aware? Awareness is a condition that is inferred to be present, but it cannot be counted. Instead, it is necessary to choose something countable that indicates that a person is aware. In this case, the indicator of a state of awareness becomes the do statement. Suppose the clinician asks the client to signal by raising her hand immediately after the clinician says /s/ in words. If the client signals by raising the hand immediately following each utterance of /s/, then the clinician infers the child is aware /s/ has been spoken. Hand raising serves as an indicator of awareness.

In the treatment of articulation, the desired behavior most often involves a speech response. The target behavior, a motor speech response, is the correct production of a sound or sounds in a variety of contexts; therefore, the verb *to say* frequently is used as the do statement.

The following verbs, used as do statements, may be the indicators of some other target or they may be the target behavior themselves:

to say	to produce	to describe
to put	to write	to vocalize
to repeat	to co-articulate	to name
to point	to read aloud	to count

The Conditions Statement. The second ingredient of a behavioral objective is a brief statement describing the *conditions* present when the behavior is to occur. Obviously, there is no need to specify all the conditions present, such as the color of the room, the construction of the table, or the hairstyle of the clinician. We need only specify the conditions relevant in evoking the response. If pictures are used to evoke the response, this needs to be stated, as well as whether the target sound will be articulated in the final position of words, in blends, or in various positions of polysyllabic words.

The client may be able to articulate /s/ correctly while the clinician shows a group of pictures that were used in the treatment program, but may be unable to do so when the parent asks him or her to name a group of unfamiliar pictures at home two weeks later. The relevant conditions are: the person showing the pictures, the familiarity of the pictures, the place where the pictures are displayed, and the time at which the pictures are shown. Some examples of conditions are:

when shown picture cards
in the presence of the teacher
in the classroom
5 times in a row

at home
during meal time
for 3 minutes
when modeled

The Accuracy Statement. A statement about *how well* the client is expected to perform comprises the third requirement that Mager listed as an important part of a behavior objective. This part of the statement deals with the accuracy of the client's response and is usually expressed in terms of a percentage correct or rate of correct response. Often, a time limit is specified as part of the accuracy statement; i.e., a certain number of correct responses are to be produced before a specific date. Accuracy statements may read as follows:

with 100% accuracy
80% correct
9 times out of 10

Types of Instructional Objectives

When an objective describes the client's articulation at the time of dismissal, it is called a *terminal objective*. These statements are broad in scope and usually specify an approximate date when the objective should be accomplished. An example of a terminal objective would be: "By May 1, 1988, Sue will correctly articulate /r/ and /l/ at all times as they occur in all positions in words in her spontaneous unmonitored speech." Individual segments of this objective can be identified as follows:

Do Statement: Articulate /r/ and /l/.

Conditions Statement: In all positions in words in spontaneous unmonitored speech.

Accuracy Statement: Correct at all times by May 1, 1988.

Another type of objective consists of day-to-day objectives written for each session or for small groups of sessions. These objectives have been called *short-range goals, subobjectives,* or *transitional objectives.* These objectives are very specific in describing the skill to be learned. The following example illustrates a subobjective one might write for a client who is beginning a treatment program for correction of /k/: ''Pat will say the /k/ in the final position of 10 words after being shown 10 pictures by the clinician. He will not be told whether his responses are right or wrong. /k/ must be produced correctly in 9 out of 10 words.'' A summary of the important statements of this subobjective is as follows:

Do statement: Say /k/.

Conditions Statement: In the final position of words. Ten pictures shown by the clinician. Not informed of results of response.

Accuracy Statement: 90% correctly articulated /k/ sound.

Task Analysis

Before writing behavioral objectives, the clinician must analyze the task to be learned. A series of skills are needed to perform complex tasks. For example, tying a bow in a shoelace involves numerous precise movements that must be performed in a proper sequence. First, the laces must be crossed. Then the overlapping lace is threaded through the lower /\\-shaped opening. The two ends are pulled in opposite directions to form a bow. A loop is formed in the left lace, and so it goes until the bow is completed. A behavioral objective can be written for each step in the series of movements. When teaching a child to tie a bow, a mother proceeds through these steps with her child until each step is learned in proper sequence. One

cannot skip steps or try to complete them out of order.

Similarly, if you need to change the front tire of your car, first you must take off the hubcap, loosen the wheel nuts or studs, lift the car with a jack, then remove the wheel nuts or studs. If you do not follow this sequence, that is, if you lift the car first, then try to loosen the wheel nuts, the wheel will simply spin and you will be unable to loosen the nuts. You must follow the correct sequence. The same is true for sequences involved in learning complex mathematical skills. Learning to divide requires prior mastery of skills such as addition and subtraction. One cannot learn multiplication and division until the basic skills are learned.

Most speech clinicians follow a similar procedure of sequencing skills in the remediation of articulation problems. Van Riper (1939) clearly identified the educational taxonomy of learning articulation skills when he specified that the client must be aware of the speech problem first. Then discrimination skills must be taught, followed by production of the target sound in isolation, in nonsense syllables, in words with the target sound in the initial position, final position, and medial position. Phrases that incorporate the target sound are then introduced. Polysyllabic words and blends are introduced, followed by sentence practice and using the sound in spontaneous speaking situations. This taxonomy follows an analytic approach to building a sequence of behaviors. The task, articulating a sound correctly in spontaneous speech, is broken into smaller components that are taught in a specific sequence.

Backus and Beasley (1951) devised a different sequence to teach articulation skills by presenting a complex task, a sentence, first. If the client is unable to produce the sound correctly in this context, a smaller segment of the task is presented, a word. If this proves to be too difficult, the client is encouraged to produce the sound in isolation. This synthetic approach can be broken into a series of tasks in much the same manner as the analytic technique. Similarly, behavioral objectives can be written for each step in the series.

An example of a task analysis of learning to produce /s/ in spontaneous speech is illustrated in the flowchart I devised for a lisp correction program (Mowrer, 1964). This flowchart, shown in Figure 6.5, depicts a sequential series of steps, each presumably more complex or difficult than the previous one. The effect of mastering each task is cumulative in that saying /i/ facilitates saying /is/, which in turn aids production of /s/ in isolation. Once the isolated sound is produced, a vowel is added, and when this is mastered a final consonant is added, yielding a monosyllabic word. Just as changing a tire requires following a prescribed sequence, the same holds true for learning articulation skills.

Numerous treatment sequences have been devised to change various aspects of articulation (see Baker & Ryan, 1971; Delbridge & Larrigan, 1973; McCabe & Bradley, 1975; Psaltis & Spallato, 1973; Weston & Irwin, 1971). Even though there is considerable variation among different treatment

FIGURE 6.5
Flowchart for three-part lisp correction program used in S-PACK. (*Source: Methods of Modifying Speech Behaviors,* 2nd ed. (p. 302) by Donald E. Mowrer, 1982, Columbus: Merrill Publishing Company. Copyright © 1982 by Merrill Publishing Company. Reprinted by permission.

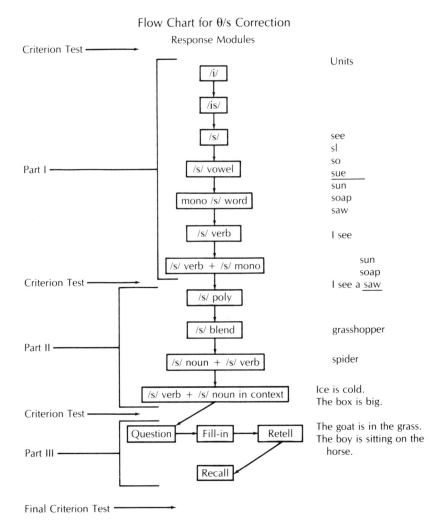

Flow Chart for θ/s Correction

sequences, the principles of behavior therapy apply. Deciding which sequence is most effective for a particular child is another matter. It is important that the clinician identify what seem to be the most important elements involved in acquiring a task. Only by clinically testing various aspects of the sequence can we determine which sequence of events results in the most effective treatment.

PROGRAMMED INSTRUCTION

During the late 1960s and early 1970s speech clinicians created instructional programs designed to change articulation. These programs were constructed following the format outlined by Fine (1962) as follows:

1. The client responds to a series of instructional items that the programmer has constructed beforehand.
2. The skill to be learned must be thoroughly mastered before the client can advance to the next task.
3. The client is presented with tasks he/she has been prepared to perform.
4. Cues and prompts are provided to help the client respond correctly.
5. The client is reinforced for producing correct responses.

Coolagan (1976) provides a simpler definition of *programmed instruction*. He says it is an interaction between student and instructional material wherein immediate feedback is provided about the adequacy of the student's response.

In order to write an instructional program, one must complete a task analysis. The next step is to decide how antecedent events will be managed.

Management of Antecedent Events

Once the task has been broken into smaller components and behavioral objectives have been written for each component, the activities that will lead to the attainment of each objective must be specified. The clinician will need to show or tell the client what to do. Hence, antecedent events will play an important role in the instructional process. If antecedent events, that is, the instructions for the client, are specified, as well as the consequent events following correct and incorrect responses, the result is an instructional program. The antecedent events may be so specific as to include everything the clinician says to the client. The S-PACK is an example of this type of program (Mowrer, Baker, & Schutz, 1968). On the other hand, the program may be written only to suggest what the clinician should say (See Baker & Ryan, 1971; McCabe & Bradley, 1975).

Usually, cues and prompts are used to introduce learning tasks. For example, a model of the target sound may be presented, followed by a request for the client to repeat the sound. Or the client may be given specific instructions concerning where to place the tongue to produce the sound correctly. Once the client is able to produce the sound correctly, cues and prompts are faded. For example, the prompt "Stick out your tongue and blow like this, [θ]" might be used early in the program, but several minutes later only cues such as "Say it each time I put my finger up" are provided. As new tasks are introduced, strong cues and prompts are introduced again and then weakened as the client masters task production. The procedure might follow this pattern:

Task 1
a. provide both prompts and cues
b. provide only position cues
c. provide nonverbal cues such as requesting responses to finger-raising signals

Task 2
a. provide both prompts and cues
b. provide only position cues
c. provide nonverbal cues

In this manner, supportive cues and prompts are provided when each new task is presented. Later, these cues and prompts are reduced as the client demonstrates mastery of the task.

Management of Consequent Events

Usually, every correct response is reinforced when the treatment program is begun and the client is learning to produce a new response. Once the client has practiced saying the correct response many times, the continuous schedule of reinforcement is changed to a variable ratio. The client may be given one token for saying *soap* correctly at the beginning of the program, but later, when asked to say *Sally has some soap,* only one token is given even though four correct responses were produced. As the client attains skill in producing /s/ and is able to use this sound correctly in conversational speech, perhaps 20 correct /s/ sounds must be produced before a token is provided. Soon it is not necessary to provide tokens for correct /s/ responses. The client uses the correct /s/ without thinking about it; the response has become automatic. In a carefully designed program, a changing schedule of reinforcement is built into the program with the aim of eventually eliminating reinforcement altogether.

Criterion Tests

Another feature of instructional programs is the frequent use of criterion tests or behavioral probes. The clinician needs to know how well the client has mastered a task because the succeeding task should not be presented until the prior task has been mastered. Criterion tests may consist of 3 or 4 items or as many as over 30 items. Data from these tests are usually transferred to graphs to provide a quick visual display of the client's performance.

Frequent measures of behavior are taken to provide the clinician with an ongoing account of behavioral change. If samples of behavior are not taken frequently, one is unable to make appropriate changes in the treatment plan that could lead to more effective instruction.

Editing and Validating Instructional Programs

An instructional program, unlike traditional instructional methods, is open to inspection and analysis. An expert, other than the person who wrote the program, should edit the program. This individual may see ways of improving the original program by changing the wording, the sequence of tasks, or schedule of reinforcement. At this stage of program construction, one is still operating from a theoretical framework because it is impossible to know how the client will respond until the program is administered.

After editing the program, the next step is to administer it to a small group of clients. An analysis is made of their responses, which aids in making decisions about changing certain items, rearranging task presentation, breaking tasks into smaller components, and so on. Usually, high error rates in certain parts indicate areas that should be changed. Sections that include a long series of correct responses might indicate that cues could be eliminated gradually or that the task is too easy. It might be decided to omit certain items entirely, resulting in a shortened version of the program.

The revised version of the program is then administered to a similar group of clients and revised again if necessary. This process is continued until a predetermined success rate is reached. If the program writer's intent is to produce a program that is effective with 85% of the target population for whom it was designed, then the testing and validation process is terminated when this criterion level is achieved.

It should be noted that a given instructional program might be validated for use with only one child. If a program is shown to be effective for that client, we can say that it is valid for him, but it is necessary to include more than one individual in the validation process if we want to say that it will be effective with other clients.

Dissemination of the program is the final step. It is published and marketed. An instruction manual should accompany the program so that the user can replicate the findings of the original work.

A large number of instructional programs designed to assist speech clinicians in modifying articulation patterns are currently available (see chapter 9 in Mowrer, 1982). Some of these programs have been validated through systematic analysis and field testing, whereas others have been placed on the market with little or no previous validation. Some programs provide only general guidelines for administration; others offer explicit directions. Some are designed to modify only one type of articulation response, such as a /θ/ for /s/ substitution (Mowrer, Baker, & Schutz, 1968). Other programs incorporate instructions for the correction of many consonant sounds (McCabe & Bradley, 1975).

The speech clinician has a variety of instructional programs from which to choose. Some are effective procedures for changing articulation patterns and others are less effective. Much depends upon the clinician's ability to follow instructions exactly. Many clinicians choose to use only parts of programs. The following list of criteria for helping speech clinicians choose or devise instructional programs is presented by Mowrer (1982):

1. clarity of instructions provided for the clinician
2. identification of target behavior and target population
3. cost of program and time required to administer it
4. field test data available
5. instructions provided for recording baseline, recording data, use of criterion tests, branching to other steps, rewarding client, and generalizing or maintaining the response

Costello (1977), Coolagan (1976), and McReynolds (1983) have also provided guidelines to help speech clinicians evaluate instructional programs.

Administering Instructional Programs

Once a program has been edited and field tested, the speech clinician can use it with clients. Some

programs are designed for individual instruction; others can be used with small groups of clients.

One of the values of using programmed instructions is that they can be administered by paraprofessionals. Many individuals who have had little or no teaching experience can be taught to administer these programs. For example, Dorothy Bokelmann, a supervisor of speech clinicians of the Clark County School District in Las Vegas, Nevada, organized a project that involved writing instructional programs to be used by paraprofessionals to aid speech clinicians in remediating articulation skills (Lundquist, 1972). Speech clinicians provided treatment for children who misarticulated consonants only until these children could produce the target sounds correctly in several words. Then the children were assigned to paraprofessionals who had been given training in administering the programs and discriminating between correct and incorrect sounds. The purpose of these programs was to help the children use newly learned articulation skills in a variety of contexts and speaking situations.

The programs Bokelmann and her colleagues wrote for the paraprofessionals consisted of a series of speaking activities that were to be practiced by the children. Each aide was provided with a workbook of activities for a specific target sound. The first activity was to name a series of pictures the speech clinician had used in previous treatment sessions. Other activities involved filling in words containing the target sounds in a sentence completion exercise, retelling short stories, asking directions, and so on. Situations were varied from the speech office to hallways, playground, classroom, and principal's office. Frequently, the speech clinician tested the children to monitor their progress. The aides provided the bulk of the instruction using the booklets they were provided.

Carrier (1970) reported results of a similar program in which he provided written instructions for mothers to use with their children who misarticulated /r/. The speech clinician provided a brief treatment program until the children could produce the target sound correctly and then the mothers were given six lessons written in program format. They were instructed to administer this treatment program to their children. Test results following completion of the program revealed that mothers served as effective supportive personnel who could greatly aid the speech clinician in bringing about changes in the articulation of their children.

I have also experienced success in using aides to administer instructional program material designed to correct misarticulation (Mowrer, 1967). Parents, teachers, siblings, and peers have been trained to administer programs designed to correct lisping. One speech clinician used fifth-grade children to administer S-PACK to second- and third-grade children who lisped and found they were as successful in changing lisping as she was.

Parents who are provided with materials that explain how consonants develop in the speech of their young child and explain what steps they can take to assist their child with articulation development (Mowrer, 1986) have experienced success in modifying the speech of their children (Sommers, Bradley, & Mowrer, 1987). The important point is that other individuals can perform many of the tasks speech clinicians provide if these individuals have adequate training and instructional materials.

TRANSFER AND MAINTENANCE

Although teaching children to produce sounds correctly in the clinic situation usually is an easy task, many speech clinicians find that children do not produce these sounds correctly while speaking in other situations. It is believed this problem, referred to as *lack of carryover,* exists because speech clinicians may not plan learning activities that foster generalization of the newly learned response to other speaking situations (Mowrer, 1982). There are several techniques that can be used to help clients articulate correctly in other speaking situations (Gerber, 1973; Griffiths & Craighead, 1972).

Stimulus Generalization

If we wish to improve carryover, it is important to understand the principle of *stimulus generalization.* Although many factors are involved in vocabulary development, the young child who identifies the mail carrier, the butcher, and the father as "daddy" may be used to illustrate this principle. In this case, the child may have originally been rewarded for saying "daddy" (the response) in the presence of the father (the stimulus). There are many other males who share the same stimulus properties as the father, such as pants, short hair, tall in stature, and so on. These common characteristics, taken together, represent the concept of maleness or "daddyness." Because the child is rewarded for saying "daddy" in the presence of one instance of this concept, the father, other instances sharing the same properties will be responded to in a similar way.

Soon the child learns to differentiate father from other males, namely, the mail carrier, the butcher, the fireman, and the truck driver, by using different verbal labels for each type of male. At first, young children may use only two words, *Daddy* for the father and *man* in the presence of all other males. Later, the child learns to use specific words to name familiar males, such as *Grandpa, Uncle Jim, Mr. Smith, the fireman,* etc. This example illustrates two different processes. First, stimulus generalization occurs when the same response is made to all stimuli that share characteristics with the original stimuli. Later, the process of discrimination is observed when a different response is made to two stimuli that have common characteristics. Sometimes, we want responses to generalize to similar situations, and at other times, we want the client to make accurate discriminations, as in the case of correct and incorrect sounds.

Stimulus Generalization in Phonemic Contexts. We can take advantage of stimulus generalization when teaching certain sounds. Elbert, Shelton, and Arndt (1967) demonstrated that once /s/ was learned, /z/ was learned even though clients received no training for /z/. We would expect generalization to occur from /s/ to /z/ because those sounds share many of the same acoustic and motoric characteristics. The clients in this study were also tested for /r/ production. They were unable to produce this sound correctly before treatment of the /s/, and were still unable to produce it correctly after its treatment. Learning /s/ had no effect upon learning /r/. This appeared to be the result of the differences in distinctive features between the /s/ and the /r/ sounds.

Generalization also occurs at the feature level. McReynolds and Bennett (1972) illustrated this fact in their study of three children who were taught specific sounds. They found that generalization occurred in other sounds that shared the same features. For example, if /s/ was taught, then all sounds sharing the [+stridency] feature were learned more quickly once /s/ was learned. I made use of this principle when teaching a young child fricative sounds (Mowrer & Case, 1982). Once the child learned /s/, the other fricatives were learned in less time. Learning to produce one fricative sound facilitated learning /θ/, /ʃ/, and eventually /tʃ/.

There are also instances in which generalization occurs across positions in a word. Weston and Irwin (1971) reported that once the sound was taught in the prevocalic position, the sound was learned more quickly in the postvocalic position. Powell and McReynolds (1969) also found this type of generalization occurring. When they taught sounds in syllables, they found that the child produced sounds correctly in all positions in words. Some investigators have not reported finding interposition generalization of sounds; consequently, more research is needed to verify these findings.

Stimulus Generalization in Situational Contexts. One of the areas speech clinicians report as their most difficult task is carryover outside the clinic. The client uses the correct sound while in the treatment situation but not when speaking in other situations, such as in the classroom, at home,

or on the playground. In many cases, this problem exists because the speech clinician has no strategy for enhancing transfer of the newly learned speech pattern to other speaking situations. It is possible to facilitate rapid transfer by incorporating procedures that maximize stimulus generalization from one context to another.

Numerous studies have demonstrated that positive transfer of training occurs when stimuli contained in the original learning task share features with some of the stimuli in the new situations (McGeoch & Irion, 1952). Holland and Skinner (1961) pointed out that if a subject has been reinforced for making a certain response under a specified stimulus condition, this same response will be produced in the presence of similar stimulus conditions even though the response is not reinforced. By keeping stimuli in the treatment situation similar to stimuli found in other speaking situations, the clinician is more likely to maximize generalization. For example, the words selected for practice should be those the client uses frequently in other speaking situations (McDonald, 1964). A strategy used by Mowrer, Baker, and Schutz (1968) to enhance generalization consisted of teaching the client to respond correctly to a small number of words containing /s/ or /z/. Following training in the clinical setting, parents were asked to provide further speech training in the home. They were given instructional materials containing the same picture stimuli that were used in the clinical training program. Also, many of the instructional items were identical or similar to those used in the original training sessions. They found that in 80% of the cases, parent interaction with their children was successful in that their children successfully produced correct /s/ sounds in conversational speech when tested three months later.

In addition to maintaining similarity of words and pictures, the speech clinician can provide training in other speaking situations, such as in the client's classroom or on the playground. The presence of the speech clinician serves as a reminder for the client to produce the sound correctly. If generalization is to occur, it is important to teach correct articulation in situations where the client frequently talks. It is also wise to involve significant others in the treatment program because the client frequently talks to those persons. Carrier (1970) found that children who were taught sounds by their parents obtained higher scores on an articulation test after treatment than did a similar group who were treated by speech clinicians only.

Teachers also have been asked to play roles in helping their students articulate correctly. One speech clinician conducted three half-hour training sessions for classroom teachers after school (Mowrer, 1967). Her objective was to help elementary classroom teachers (a) discriminate between correct and incorrect /s/ sounds, (b) provide appropriate instructions to children when lisping was observed, and (c) provide some group speaking activities that would foster correct use of the /s/. During the 3 weeks of training sessions, the speech clinician taught the children who lisped how to produce /s/ in words and phrases found in their school reading books.

The children were provided with speech books consisting of pages containing 25 dashes. They were instructed to give their speech books to the teacher as they came to their reading circle. Each time they said /s/ or /z/ correctly while reading aloud, the teacher placed a check above one dash in their speech book. If the child lisped, the teacher placed a zero above the dash and provided an appropriate cue such as, "Remember to close your teeth." At the end of the week, the children brought their speech books to the clinician to redeem points earned by saying /s/ correctly when reading. Small toys were provided as rewards. This is one example of how rapid carryover can be achieved by using the classroom teacher, daily speaking situations, and familiar materials from reading assignments.

Mowrer and Conley (1987) described a procedure they developed to study the effects of different types of reinforcement paradigms in which

peers were used to enhance carryover. The client was asked to invite four classmates to the speech class. The client was asked to tell stories containing many /s/ words. Both the client and the peers were rewarded for each of the client's correct productions of /s/. The important point of this activity was that peers, to whom the clients spoke daily, were included as part of the treatment program. Their presence and comments facilitated carryover.

Speech aides and peers have been used in numerous programs to aid in the generalization process. The program described by Lundquist (1972), and noted previously in this chapter, involved the speech clinician only to a minimal degree. Once the speech clinician had taught the client to produce the target sound correctly in several sentences, an aide was assigned to the client. The aide was provided with a book of exercises that the client was asked to practice in a wide variety of speaking situations. These situations included the places the child frequently visited during the day, such as the hallway, the playground, the cafeteria, and the classroom. The purpose of using these situations was to give the client practice in saying target sounds correctly in a number of speaking situations, not just in the clinic setting.

Although teachers, parents, and peers can be helpful in the carryover phase of therapy, it is important to consider certain factors before deciding to include them. Among these factors are (a) the ability of the helper to discriminate the correct production, (b) the relationship between the child and the teacher, parent, or peer, and (c) the child's feelings about involving a peer in the process.

Carryover also can be enhanced by teaching the client to produce the target sound correctly in idioms, slang expressions, and rapidly articulated sequences that are used frequently. For example, phrases to be used for clients learning the correct /s/ sound might include short speech sequences, such as *It's a* ———, *Here's a* ———, *What's a* ———, *That's a* ———, and so on. These sequences resemble nonsense syllables. Later, nouns are added to these rapidly articulated sequences to produce sentences, such as *It's a boy, He's a man, There's a bike, It's a car*, etc.

The purpose of repeating these sequences is to embed the correct sound in automatic speech (Mowrer, 1983). This type of speech repetition contrasts sharply with speech sequences found in many game activities that focus upon the child's occasional request to spin a spinner, draw a card, or roll dice. Sentences such as *May I please spin the spinner* or *Please can I take my turn* may provide practice saying the target sound correctly in context, but one cannot expect rapid generalization of /s/ to everyday speaking situations. The child needs to produce /s/ in speech sequences that are often used during daily conversations. In this way, the new response quickly becomes habituated.

Maintaining the Use of the Correct Response. There has been considerable research conducted by learning theorists regarding factors that enhance retention and use of newly learned responses (McGoech & Irion, 1952). Four factors are associated with increased retention. First, subjects retain information best when *meaningful material* is used. The early work by Ebbinghaus (1913) clearly demonstrated that nonsense material was quickly forgotten when compared with meaningful material. Hence, it seems unwise to use meaningless tongue twisters, nonsense syllables, and poetry as the chief source of words for practice. The clinician is more likely to achieve retention by choosing words that clients use daily than by presenting words chosen randomly from dictionaries. Names of family members, pets, favorite toys, frequently used household objects, and school supplies like a pencil, scissors, eraser, and so on, are good choices. Another source of useful words is verbs that are used often. Word lists containing words that children use frequently are available from several commercial publishers.

A second factor found to increase retention is *frequent instruction*. The client who receives practice three times daily is more likely to retain material than the client who receives instruction once a week. Backus and Dunn (1947) studied the effects of providing therapy daily to groups of children as compared with providing therapy twice weekly. They concluded that more progress was made in a 6-week intensive program than was

made during the school year when children were seen twice each week.

Studies by Sommers, Leiss, Fundrella, Manning, Johnson, Oerther, Sholly, and Siegel (1970) and Ausenheimer and Irwin (1971) confirm these findings that materials practiced more frequently are learned more effectively than those practiced infrequently. Speech clinicians should examine alternatives for delivery of service that will allow for more frequent instruction. In the public schools, it may be possible to schedule children to be seen several times a day, for example, on their way to the cafeteria, at the playground, during recess, immediately after school, and in some cases, before school begins.

Overlearning information has been found to improve retention greatly (Lawrence, 1954). But this is true only up to a certain point. Beyond a certain amount of overlearning, little benefit is derived from continued practice. One of the few studies reported in this area was conducted by Diedrich and Bangert (1976). They concluded that clinicians could dismiss children who have been working on /s/ and /r/ sounds when they could produce these sounds correctly 75% of the time. At present, it is not clear what amount of overlearning is needed in the treatment of articulation problems. The proverb "Practice makes perfect" may apply here in that the more one is exposed to saying the response, the better the task is learned. Just how much practice is necessary before further practice is unproductive is not known.

Finally, *motivational state* has been found to be an important factor with respect to retention of a response. The more highly motivated a person, the greater the retention of the material that has been learned. It has been suggested that high motivational states may result in an increased amount of rehearsal time. This, in turn, results in better retention. If this is the case, it would be beneficial to provide incentives for learning. Some speech clinicians argue that their clients do what they are asked to do and require little or no extrinsic motivation. This may be true in the speech class setting, but if increases in motivational states result in improved retention, then it is important that we provide some means of motivating clients to change certain behaviors outside the immediate clinical (speech class) setting.

APPLICATIONS

Beyond the work of my colleagues and me in the development of the S-PACK as a prototype of a behavioral approach to the correction of frontal lisping (Mowrer, 1964; Mowrer, 1967; Mowrer, Baker, & Schutz, 1968), a number of other researchers also have developed instructional programs of a similar nature aimed at correcting a variety of consonant sounds (Baker & Ryan, 1971; Carrier, 1970; Delbridge & Larrigan, 1973; Lundquist, 1972; McCabe & Bradley, 1975; Weston & Irwin, 1971).

A therapeutic approach must meet some important criteria to be considered a behavior modification program using operant conditioning: (a) A target behavior must be selected that is operationally defined, has a definite beginning and ending, and can be accurately measured. (b) An attempt must be made to establish a baseline of this behavior before therapy is initiated. (c) The antecedent events (what the clinician is supposed to do and say) must be specified clearly. (d) The target response must be capable of being evaluated objectively as either correct or incorrect. (e) A reinforcement schedule must be specified. (f) A series of tasks organized in a hierarchy from simple to more complex must be identified. (g) Criteria to be met must be established to determine when a task has been mastered and a new task introduced. (h) The exit behavior must be specified and usually consists of a specified performance on a final criterion test. (i) It must be possible to replicate the instructional program; that is, other clinicians should be able to administer the program in exactly

the same fashion as the author. (j) The instructional program should be field tested to establish its reliability.

Brief discussions follow of two programs that clearly demonstrate the use of behavioral approaches to the treatment of articulation disorders.

Paired-Stimuli Approach

Weston (1969) developed a structured approach to the treatment of articulation problems later to be published with Irwin as the Paired-Stimuli Therapy Kit (Irwin & Weston, 1981). First, the target behaviors or phonemes are identified through articulation testing. Once selected, the client must be able to say the target sound correctly 9 out of 10 times in two key words, one containing the target sound in the initial position, the other in a key word with the sound in the final position.

Once this entrance prerequisite is met, the authors present the first task of their program. The client is to say the key word (when presented with a picture of the word) to be followed immediately by presentation of another picture she is to name that also contains the target phoneme. These two words, one word that the child can say correctly using the target phoneme and one word that is likely to be misarticulated, constitute the paired stimuli for which the program is named. The clinician presents nine more different pictures, each containing the target phoneme in the initial or final position, to be paired with the key word until the child obtains a score of 80% correct out of at least 15 to 20 trials. The child is rewarded with a token following each correct response on a fixed ratio-1 reinforcement schedule. When the criterion is met, the next task, which is slightly more difficult, is presented. If the criterion is not met, the first step (or previous step) is presented.

Thus, the task is well defined, the response is specified operationally, the reinforcement schedule is established, and the criterion for advancing to the next task is stated. Fourteen more steps are presented culminating with a step that involves conversation with the child until she says 13 words containing the target phoneme, all of which must be correct to warrant dismissal. The reinforcement schedule is gradually leaned until, during the last four steps, tokens are no longer presented; only verbal reinforcement is used.

A rather sizable group of children who completed this program were studied by Irwin and his colleagues (unpublished studies reported in Weston & Irwin, 1985). Results indicated the paired-stimuli articulation program was an effective and efficient means of correcting misarticulations of young children.

Multiple-Phoneme Approach

A second program by McCabe and Bradley (1975), discussed at length in chapter 11 of this text, is designed to correct multiple articulation problems of young children. This Multiple-Phonemic approach differs from the Paired-Stimuli technique, yet it meets the criteria for the behavior modification model. The approach begins by establishing a baseline of articulation performance using a word accuracy articulation test involving conversational speech. Once the child's misarticulations are identified, the first phase of the program is begun. The child is asked to repeat each of 24 consonant sounds in isolation 5 times in succession in each of three different stimulus conditions. If the child is able to meet the criterion test, he or she is advanced to the next step using the sound with syllables, followed by its use in words, sentences, in reading (if applicable), and finally in conversational speech.

Each step of the three-phase program specifies the stimuli used to evoke the response, a description of the response, the schedule of reinforcement used, and the criterion level for each step. This program, as is true with most other well-written operant conditioning approaches, can be replicated easily because the instructions and criteria are stated in specific terms. Although field testing has not been carried out on large numbers of children, Bradley reported very positive results in a number of case studies she and her colleagues have con-

ducted using the program (Sommers, Bradley, & Mowrer, 1987).

GOLDEN RULES OF BEHAVIOR MODIFICATION

Speech clinicians can follow systematic procedures when adopting a behavior therapy approach for the treatment of articulation problems. Ten rules capture the essence of this approach (Mowrer, 1982):

RULES TO FOLLOW USING BEHAVIOR THERAPY

1. *Immediacy:* In order to help a child learn more efficiently, provide a reward immediately following the child's correct response. It may not be possible or even advisable to give a toy or food item, immediately, so provide a social reward, token, point, or some signal of immediate recognition.

2. *Attention:* Attention is a powerful social reward. Provide attention the way you would use a token, toy, or other form of recognition following a correct response. Be careful that you do not give attention to wrong or undesired behavior. This would only serve to reward the incorrect response. Attention can help children learn correct behaviors but it can also serve to reinforce undesired behavior if used inappropriately.

3. *Pairing Rewards:* Anything paired or associated with a reward also acquires rewarding properties. For example, if we talk to a child while feeding her, talk will become associated with food which is rewarding, and soon talk by itself will serve as a reward. Such a reward is called a secondary reinforcer.

4. *Continuous Reward:* At first when a behavior is being taught, reward each correct response. When the newly learned behavior is easier to produce, provide a reward every other time. Gradually decrease the frequency with which you provide a reward as learning progresses. This reduction in the schedule of reinforcement serves to maintain the behavior better than the continuous reward.

5. *Selective Reward:* Give a reward following the responses that are important for the child to learn. If a child is being taught to say /s/, use the reward for good /s/ productions, not for winning games or activities not related to /s/ production.

6. *Small Steps:* It is important to use small steps in establishing a complex behavior. At first, demand very little from the child. It may be necessary to model the desired behavior several times. By requiring small increases each day, the child can build a series of behaviors into a habit, providing rewards are presented following each bit of correct behavior.

7. *Chaining:* One behavior leads to another in a chain leading to a complex behavior. It is important that the reward follow the behavior that occurs at the end of the chain. Be careful that undesired behaviors are not included in the chain of desired behaviors.

8. *Getting the Child's Attention:* Be sure to get the child's attention (looking, listening or both) when giving directions. Looking and listening are important since children learn better when they are actively attending.

9. *Imitation:* Modeling desired behavior is important as a method of instruction. By rewarding the child for imitating correct models of behavior, we can improve learning.

10. *Relevant Cues:* It is important to use relevant cues when instructing children. For example, the cue "close your teeth when you say /s/" is important to children who lisp. Attention cues like "get ready" and "watch me" are also important. Cues provide children with a preparatory set to help them respond correctly.[1]

PRESENT STATUS OF BEHAVIOR MODIFICATION TECHNIQUES

Although the subject of behavior therapy and its implementation for the treatment of behavioral disorders remain very prominent in the literature deal-

[1]From *Methods of Modifying Speech Behaviors,* 2nd ed. (pp. 261–262) by Donald Mowrer, 1982, Columbus, Ohio: Merrill Publishing Company. Copyright © 1982 by Merrill Publishing Company. Reprinted by permission.

ing with deviant behavioral disorders such as anxiety disorders, sexual problems, adult psychotic behaviors, addictive disorders, autism, and hyperactivity, to name but a few areas (Franks, Wilson, Kendall, Brownell, 1984; Spiegler, 1983), one is hard-pressed to find current published articles about behavior therapy in speech and language journals. Certainly, there is nowhere near the number of articles and published programs that appeared during the 1960s and early 1970s. Does this mean that the speech clinician's interest in behavior modification as a therapeutic technique has terminated? Has the procedure gone out of style and become old-fashioned? Even though the newness has become somewhat worn, I believe that professionals in our field are employing the techniques.

Consider two presentations at the 1987 American Speech-Language-Hearing Association convention. One involved teaching socially deprived children how to communicate with each other (Sullivan & Hays, 1987). As the children conversed, the clinician reinforced each child for making appropriate statements and made suggestions when the topic came to a standstill. Data were kept regarding sentence length. In the other example, mentally handicapped children in a classroom situation were systematically reinforced or punished for specific behaviors following a behavior therapy technique (Rini, Hitt, & Soriano, 1987).

Perhaps some speech clinicians feel behavior therapy techniques are too powerful or inappropriate for articulation therapy involving the average normal child. Or perhaps they feel the rigors of this approach are too demanding. Many children make steady and persistent progress during widely differing articulation therapy programs. But to those interested in precision teaching and obtaining the greatest efficacy in learning, the data that have been reported clearly support the use of behavior modification techniques.

Most speech clinicians realize the benefits of behavior therapy techniques and use these techniques regularly during their therapy. They devise clear-cut behavioral objectives, present effective models, provide feedback to their clients, record pertinent data, and assist clients with generalization even though some may deny any outright attempt on their part to employ behavior modification techniques. Others have been trained in using these techniques and know of no better way to proceed in administering therapy. We needed the boost we received from the behaviorists during the

CHAPTER 6
The Behavioral Approach to Treatment

189

1960s and 1970s but, having learned these techniques, we perhaps are challenged to go on to other aspects of articulation.

SUMMARY

The major purpose of this chapter was to outline a strategy based upon principles of operant conditioning to change behaviors in an effective and efficient manner. The application of these principles frequently has been referred to as behavior modification or, more precisely, behavior therapy. This procedure involves two major elements: (1) effective management of consequent events and (2) careful organization of task sequences to be taught. The application of these two major elements can best be summarized in terms of the following seven steps.

First, select a target behavior that is observable and countable. Record the baseline behavior as it exists in the individual's repertoire.

Second, break down the learning tasks into their smallest components or steps.

Third, devise a set of behavioral objectives that define the learning tasks in terms of what it is you wish the person to do, the conditions under which it is to be done, and how well you want the person to perform. List the criterion the person must meet in order to advance to the next step.

Fourth, deliver the instructional program and include procedures that will maximize transfer and maintenance of the target behavior to environments outside the training setting.

Fifth, manage consequent events to ensure desired behaviors are increased and undesired behaviors are decreased. Use varying schedules of reinforcement to maximize high rates of the desired behavior.

Sixth, keep records of response rates and plot the correct and incorrect behaviors graphically. Make changes in therapy procedures according to results of the data.

Seventh, dismiss the individual from therapy when desired behavior is achieved. Execute a maintenance program if needed to make sure the undesired behavior does not return.

Through careful planning and execution of an instructional program designed to change a specific behavior, one can bring about desired behavioral changes in an efficient and practical manner. As stated at the beginning of this chapter, changing behavior is our principal job. When we learn to do this effectively our job becomes much easier and certainly much more enjoyable. The suggestions in this chapter should help in planning and executing instructional materials that are designed to bring about behavioral change.

REFERENCES

Ausenheimer, B., & Irwin, R. B. (1971). Effect of frequencies of speech therapy on several measures of articulatory proficiency. *Language, Speech and Hearing Services in Schools, 2,* 43–51.

Backus, O., & Beasley, J. (1951). *Speech therapy with children.* Boston: Houghton Mifflin.

Backus, O., & Dunn, H. M. (1947). Intensive group therapy in speech rehabilitation. *Journal of Speech and Hearing Disorders, 12,* 39–60.

Bailey, S. L., & Lessen, E. I. (1984). An analysis of target behaviors in education: Applied but how useful? In W. L. Heward, T. E. Heron, D. S. Hill, &

J. Trap-Porter (Eds.), *Focus on behavior analysis in education* (pp. 162–176). Columbus: Merrill.

Baker, R. D., & Ryan, B. P. (1971). *Programmed conditioning for articulation.* Monterey, CA: Monterey Learning Systems.

Bandura, A. (1976). Self-reinforcement: Theoretical and methodological considerations. *Behaviorism, 4,* 135–155.

Blount, R. L., & Stokes, T. F. (1984). Self-reinforcement by children. In M. Hersen, R. Eisler, and P. Miller (Eds.), *Progress in Behavior Modification* (pp. 195–225). New York: Academic Press.

Boone, D. R., & Prescott, T. E. (1972). Content and sequence analysis of speech and hearing therapy. *ASHA, 14,* 58–62.

Carrier, J., Jr. (1970). A program of articulation therapy administered by mothers. *Journal of Speech and Hearing Disorders, 35,* 344–353.

Coolagan, R. B. (1976). Programming primer. *School, Science and Mathematics, 76,* 381–391.

Cooper, J. D., Heron, T. E., & Heward, W. L. (1987). *Applied behavior analysis.* Columbus: Merrill.

Costello, J. (1975). The establishment of fluency with time-out procedures: Three case studies. *Journal of Speech and Hearing Disorders, 40,* 216–231.

Costello, J. (1977). Programmed instruction. *Journal of Speech and Hearing Disorders, 42,* 3–28.

Delbridge, L., & Larrigan, L. (1973). *Stimulus shift articulation kit.* Tempe, AZ: Ideas.

Diedrich, W. M. (1971). Procedures for counting and charting a target phoneme. *Language, Speech and Hearing Services in Schools, 55* (2), 18–32.

Diedrich, W. M., & Bangert, C. J. (1976). *Training speech clinicians in recording and analysis of articulatory behavior.* (Grant No. OEG-0-70-1689 and OEG-0-71-18-1689). Washington, D.C.: U.S. Office of Education, Dept. of Health, Education, and Welfare.

Drash, P., Caldwell, L., & Liebowitz, J. (1970). Correct and incorrect response rates as basic dependent variables in operant conditioning of speech in nonverbal subjects. *Psychological Aspects of Disability, 17,* 16–23.

Ebbinghaus, H. E., (1913). *Memory: A contribution of experimental psychology* (H. A. Ruger & C. E. Bussehius, Trans.). New York: Teachers College

Educational Reprint Services. (Original work published 1885).

Elbert, M., Shelton, R. L., & Arndt, W. B. (1967). A task for evaluation of articulation change. *Journal of Speech and Hearing Research, 10,* 281–288.

Fine, B. (1962). *The modern family guide to education.* New York: Doubleday.

Franks, C. M., Wilson, G. T., Kendall, P. C., & Brownell, K. D. (1984). *Annual review of behavior therapy: Theory and practice.* New York: Guilford Press.

Gerber, A. J. (1973). *Carryover.* Philadelphia: Temple University Press.

Graham, C. H. (1951). Visual perception. In S. Stevens (Ed.), *Handbook of experimental psychology* (pp. 868–920). New York: Wiley.

Griffiths, H., & Craighead, W. E. (1972). Generalization in operant speech therapy for misarticulation. *Journal of Speech and Hearing Disorders, 37,* 485–494.

Harvard Center for Research and Development on Educational Differences. (1964) *Newsletter.* Cambridge, MA: Harvard University.

Holland, J., & Skinner, B. F. (1961). *The analysis of behavior.* New York: McGraw-Hill.

Honig, W. K., & Staddon, F. E. R. (Eds.). (1977). *Handbook of operant behavior.* Englewood Cliffs, NJ: Prentice-Hall.

Irwin, J. V., & Weston, A. J. (1981). *Paired stimuli therapy kit.* Covina, CA: Fox Point.

Khan, L., & Lewis, N. (1986). *Khan-Lewis phonological analysis.* Circle Pines, MN: American Guidance Service.

Klotz, J., & Shantz, D. W. (1973). Cooperative behavior of emotionally disturbed boys as a function of contingent application of social approval. *Journal of Behavior Therapy and Experimental Psychiatry, 4,* 33–37.

Lawrence, D. (1954). The evaluation of training and transfer programs in terms of efficiency measures. *Psychology, 38,* 367–383.

Lindsley, O. R. (1964). Direct measurement and prosthesis of retarded children. *Journal of Education, 147,* 62–81.

Lovaas, O. I. (1966). A program for the establishment of speech in psychotic children. In J. K. King (Ed.), *Childhood autism.* Oxford: Pergamon Press.

Lundquist, R. L. (1972). *Speech therapy transfer program.* Las Vegas: Clark County School District.

Mager, R. F. (1962). *Preparing instructional objectives.* Palo Alto, CA: Fearon Publishers.

McCabe, R. B., & Bradley, D. (1975). Systematic multiple phonemic approach to articulation therapy. *Acta Symbolica, 6,* 1–18.

McDonald, E. (1964). *Articulation testing and treatment: A sensory-motor approach.* Pittsburgh, PA: Stanwix House.

McGeoch, J. A., & Irion, A. L. (1952). *The psychology of human learning.* New York: Longmans, Green.

McReynolds, L. V. (1983). Evaluation of treatment of children and adults with articulation disorders. In W. H. Perkins (Ed.), *Current therapy of communication disorders: Phonologic-articulatory disorders* (pp. 91–98). New York: Thieme-Stratton.

McReynolds, L. V., & Bennett, S. (1972). Distinctive feature generalization in articulation training. *Journal of Speech and Hearing Disorders, 37,* 462–470.

McReynolds, L. V., & Huston, K. (1971). Token loss in speech imitation training. *Journal of Speech and Hearing Disorders, 36,* 486–495.

Milisen, R. (1954). A rationale for articulation disorders [Monograph]. *Journal of Speech and Hearing Disorders, 4,* 5–18.

Mowrer, D. (1964). *An experimental analysis of variables controlling lisping responses of children.* Unpublished doctoral dissertation, Arizona State University, Tempe, AZ.

Mowrer, D. (1967). Programmed speech therapy—a field test. *ASHA, 9,* 369.

Mowrer, D. (1969a). *Modification of speech behaviors: Ideas and strategies for students.* Tempe, AZ: Ideas.

Mowrer, D. (1969b). Evaluating speech therapy through precision recording. *Journal of Speech and Hearing Disorders, 34,* 239–244.

Mowrer, D. (1982). *Methods of modifying speech behaviors* (2nd ed.). Columbus: Merrill.

Mowrer, D. E. (1983). Treatment of functional multiple phonologic problems. In W. H. Perkins (Ed.), Current therapy of communication disorders, *Phonologic-articulatory disorders* (pp. 23–35). New York: Thieme-Stratton.

Mowrer, D. E. (1986). *The parent's speech guide: Improving your child's articulation.* Tempe, AZ: Ideas.

Mowrer, D. E., Baker, R. L., & Schutz, R. E. (1968). Operant procedures in the control of speech articulation. In H. Sloane & B. MacAulay (Eds.), *Operant procedures in remedial speech and language training* (pp. 296–321). Boston: Houghton Mifflin.

Mowrer, D., & Case, J. (1982). *Clinical management of speech disorders.* Rockville, MD: Aspen Systems.

Mowrer, D. E., & Conley, D. (1987). Effect of peer administered consequences upon articulatory responses of speech-defective children. *Journal of Communication Disorders, 20,* 319–325.

O'Leary, K. D. (1978). Token reinforcement programs in the classroom. In A. C. Catania & T. A. Brigham (Eds.), *Handbook of applied behavior analysis: Social and instructional processes* (pp. 179–207). New York: Irvington.

O'Leary, K. D., & Drabman, R. (1971). Token reinforcement programs in the classroom: A review. *Psychological Bulletin, 75,* 379–398.

Patterson, G. R., & White, G. D. (1969). It's a small world: The application of "time-out for reinforcement." *Oregon Psychological Association Newsletter, 15,* Suppl. No. 2.

Pavlov, I. P. (1927). *Conditional reflexes.* London: Oxford University Press.

Powell, J., & McReynolds, L. (1969). A procedure for testing position generalization from articulation training. *Journal of Speech and Hearing Research, 12,* 629–645.

Psaltis, C. D., & Spallato, S. L. (1973). *Programmed articulation therapy: Time to modify.* Springfield, IL: Charles C. Thomas.

Rini, D. L., Hitt, K. M., & Soriano, D. (1987). Are you listening: Conversational strategies to enhance interpersonal communications. Video presentation at the 1987 American Speech-Language-Hearing Association Convention. *ASHA, 29,* 144.

Skinner, B. F. (1953). *Science and human behavior.* New York: Macmillan.

Skinner, B. F. (1956). A case history in scientific methods. *American Psychologist, 11,* 221–233.

Skinner, B. F. (1957). *Verbal behavior.* New York: Appleton-Century-Crofts.

Skinner, B. F. (1959). *Cumulative record.* New York: Appleton-Century-Crofts.

Skinner, B. F., & Ferster, C. (1957). *Schedules of reinforcement.* New York: Appleton-Century-Crofts.

Sommers, R. K., Bradley, D. P., & Mowrer, D. E. (1987). Contrasting multiple phonemic remedial approaches. Short course presented at 1987 American Speech-Language-Hearing Association Convention. *ASHA, 29,* 63.

Sommers, R. K., Leiss, R., Fundrella, D., Manning, W., Johnson, R., Oerther, P., Sholly, R., & Siegel, M. (1970). Factors in the effectiveness of articulation therapy with educable retarded children. *Journal of Speech and Hearing Research, 13,* 304–316.

Spiegler, M. D. (1983). *Contemporary behavioral therapy.* Palo Alto, CA: Mayfield.

Sullivan, J. P., & Hays, H. F. (1987). Teaming to facilitate language, social interaction, and functional behavioral change. Video presentation at the 1987 American Speech-Language-Hearing Association meeting. *ASHA, 29,* 144.

Tharp, R. G., & Wetzel, R. J. (1969). *Behavior modification in the natural environment.* New York: Academic Press.

Van Riper, C. (1939). *Speech correction: Principles and methods.* New York: Prentice-Hall.

Weston, A. J. (1969). The use of paired-stimuli in the modification of articulation (doctoral dissertation, University of Kansas, 1969). *Dissertation Abstracts International, 30B, 5738.*

Weston, A. J., & Irwin, J. V. (1971). Use of paired-stimuli in modification of articulation. *Perceptual Motor Skills, 32,* 947–957.

Weston, A. J., & Irwin, J. V. (1985). Paired-stimuli treatment. In P. W. Newman, N. A. Creaghead, & W. Secord (Eds.), *Assessment and remediation of articulatory and phonological disorders* (pp. 337–368). Columbus: Merrill.

White, O. R., & Haring, N. G. (1976). *Exceptional teaching.* Columbus: Merrill.

Wilson, G. T., & O'Leary, K. D. (1980). *Principles of behavior therapy.* Englewood Cliffs, NJ: Prentice-Hall.

CHAPTER 7 Linguistic Approaches to Treatment

The speech-language clinician frequently sees preschool and school-aged children who have so many articulation errors that their speech is very difficult to understand or is completely unintelligible. They are sometimes understood only by their parents, and even parents may fail to understand their more complex sentences. These children often exhibit limited communication characterized by short telegraphic sentences and an inclination to communicate as little information as possible. Children with such severe phonological disorders present many challenges.

GENERAL CONSIDERATIONS IN PHONOLOGICAL DISORDERS

Some clients will exhibit a severe articulation disorder as a result of organic causes such as hearing loss or a neuromotor deficit; however, most children with multiple errors do not have such identifiable etiologies. Current thinking suggests that an underlying linguistic deficit is the basis for severe phonological disorders in most cases. Just as the child with a language problem may have difficulty learning the *syntactic rules* of the language, a child

This chapter was written by **Nancy A. Creaghead.**

may have difficulty learning the *phonological rules*. Linguistic approaches to therapy are based on the assumption that what the child needs to learn is not how to produce all of the individual sounds of the language; rather he must learn the rules that delineate the set of phonemes of the language and how these phonemes can be combined into words.

This suggests that children with severe phonological disorders also have difficulty with other aspects of language, including syntax, semantics, and pragmatics (Gross, St. Louis, Ruscello, & Hull, 1985; Leonard, Camarata, Schwartz, Chapman, & Messick, 1985; Marquardt & Saxman, 1972; Menyuk, 1964; Panagos, 1974; Paul & Shriberg, 1982; Saxman & Miller, 1973; Schwartz, Leonard, Folger, & Wilcox, 1980; Smit & Bernthal, 1983). These sets of rules are closely related, and deficits in one area are often accompanied by deficits in another.

It is also possible that a child's limited language production is a result of poor articulation. This can happen in one of several ways. First, a child may reduce linguistic output as a strategy for being understood. Long sentences may be more difficult for the listener to interpret than key words accompanied by nonverbal clues. For example, a normal child might say, ''We were outside playing kickball, and Billy came up behind me and knocked me down.'' The child with a severe articulation disorder might produce that sentence as /wi wo aʊtaɪ pei tɪbɔ æ bɪɪ te ʌ biaɪ mi æ nɑ mi daʊ/. The listener would probably not understand that sentence, but might understand /bɪɪ ɪ mi/ to be ''Billy hit me,'' especially if it were accompanied by appropriate gesturing. In other words, there is no point in providing much information that no one will understand.

The second possible reason for a child's use of reduced language is embarrassment or self-consciousness stemming from previous unpleasant speaking experiences. Many children with language and/or articulation problems learn very early that they are not very good at talking. Therefore, they may give up trying, or at least restrict their output to essentials. This implies that an important objective of the speech-language pathologist may be to encourage the child to talk more.

The third possible reason for perceived language deficits among phonologically disordered children is that the articulation errors themselves may mask the child's language abilities. The child who omits final consonants will also omit many morphological markers, such as past tense verb endings (*walked, dragged, kissed*), third person present singular verb endings (*drives, hits*), plural markers (*flags, hats*), possessive markers (*John's, the cat's*). The child may know the rules for these grammatical forms but not use them because of the omission of final sounds.

Clinicians and researchers continually seek more effective methods of remediating speech disorders. Traditionally, articulation therapy methods have focused on the correction of one phoneme at a time, often beginning therapy by teaching a sound that usually develops early and moving to those that develop later as earlier ones are mastered. The rationale is that teaching one sound at a time is less likely to confuse a child. However, faced with children who exhibit multiple articulation errors like those described above, the clinician might reasonably look for strategies that would help such children learn several phonemes at one time in order to speed up the remedial process.

More important, if their problems are linguistically based, teaching children to produce isolated phonemes may not help them discover the phonological rules that will allow them to match the adult system. Linguistic approaches are designed to help the client learn the system. This usually means that phonemes are targeted in groups or by classes. In *multiphonemic approaches*, all error phonemes may be targeted for simultaneous correction as described in chapter 11, or the phonemes to be taught may be grouped according to feature similarities as described in chapter 14. Grouping sounds according to the phonological processes involved offers another avenue for multiphonemic correction.

MAJOR PRINCIPLES OF LINGUISTIC APPROACHES

Linguistic therapy approaches are based on two major principles. The first principle involves assumptions about the phonological system of the language and the child's own system. What the child must learn is the adult rule system. The child's system is patterned and rule governed, but different from the adult system. Therefore, the goal of therapy is to modify the child's rule system toward that of the standard. Teaching production of isolated phonemes will not enhance this rule discovery. The second principle is that the function of the phonological system is to support communication. Therefore, the end goal of therapy must be to establish an improved system for communication. Helping the child see the communicative relevance of his own speech patterns will be an important part of the therapy process.

Linguistic therapy approaches are based on phonological theory, as described in chapter 2. They can be described in two major groups: (a) distinctive-feature approaches and (b) phonological-process approaches. However, there is a great deal of overlap between the two groups. The point of both is to be able to make generalizations about the nature of the child's errors and to plan remediation based on these generalizations. In order to do this, a sample of the child's speech must be obtained and analyzed as described in chapter 4.

The task of distinctive-feature analysis or phonological-process analysis is valuable only if it leads to effective remediation techniques. McReynolds and Elbert (1981) emphasize the need to avoid using new procedures or terminology just because they are new. They suggest that without quantitative and qualitative criteria for assigning processes, we are just renaming what had been observed before. For example, we may now use the term *final consonant deletion* rather than *omission of final consonants*. Both refer to the same phenomenon. The difference in regard to treatment occurs when we target the inclusion of final consonants as a general rule to be learned rather than teach the child to produce /p/, for example, at the end of syllables.

It is only through careful observation regarding how often and in what contexts an error occurs that the clinician can determine whether a process or a pattern of error is manifest in the child's speech. In their study, McReynolds and Elbert (1981) used the following quantitative criteria for identifying phonological processes: (a) The error had at least four opportunities to occur and (b) the error occurred in at least 20% of the opportunities. Note that McReynolds and Elbert used only quantitative criteria for evaluation. Other authors (Hodson, 1980; Ingram, 1981; Shriberg & Kwiatkowski, 1980; Weiner, 1979) hold different views regarding the decision-making process. These may include different quantitative and/or qualitative criteria. Other quantitative criteria have been suggested (Hodson & Paden, 1983), and even one instance may be important, especially if it coincides with an overall pattern of error. This is an important consideration when only a small sample can be obtained.

The primary advantage of completing a feature or phonological-process analysis and using a multiphonemic approach to therapy is the potential efficiency in teaching a child a rule that may generalize and correct several phonemes at the same time. This of course applies only in instances of multiple misarticulations, so these techniques are not useful for all children.

Examples of clients who are not candidates for these approaches are individuals who exhibit only one or two errors, such as placement errors on /r/ or /s/, and individuals who exhibit a pattern that is due to a defined physiological/anatomical condition, such as "backing" in children with cleft palate or final consonant omissions and distortions resulting from dysarthria. Multiphonemic approaches seem to be most beneficial for children who exhibit multiple articulation errors in the absence of a definable organic cause. In many cases, the preferred therapy approach for individuals with diagnosed dysarthria, apraxia, or cleft palate may be based more on learning the production of individual sounds with auditory, visual, tactile, and kinesthetic stimulation than on learning phonological rules. In other words, production rather than rule learning may be the primary difficulty with these groups. However, attempts to use a phonological approach to describe errors of cleft-palate children (Hodson, Chin, Redmond, & Simpson, 1983; Lynch, Fox, & Brookshire, 1983) and cerebral-palsied children (McMahon, Hodson, & Allen, 1983) have suggested that this approach to therapy may be useful for at least some children in these groups. A third group of children who may not be candidates for a multiphonemic approach are those individuals who exhibit errors for which no pattern can be observed. These are usually considered phonetic errors and may be more amenable to a single-phoneme approach.

The remainder of the chapter will describe therapy approaches based on either a distinctive-feature or phonological-process model. It is important to remember that although authors generally describe their procedures according to one or the other model, in actual practice there is a great deal of overlap between the two.

DISTINCTIVE-FEATURE THERAPY APPROACHES

Distinctive-feature therapy approaches are based on a feature analysis that shows which features are present and absent in the child's phonological system. Several strategies for completing such an analysis were described in chapter 4, and feature systems were shown in Tables 2.4, 4.5, 4.7, and 4.8. No matter which feature system is used, the goal of therapy is to teach the child to include absent features in his own rule system.

One of two strategies is usually employed for remediating errors from a distinctive-feature base. In the most common approach, one or more target phonemes are used to establish the missing feature (Blache, 1982; Blache & Parsons, 1980; Blache, Parsons, & Humphreys, 1981; Costello & Onstine, 1976; Grunwell, 1985; McReynolds & Bennett, 1972). The second approach involves teaching all of the phonemes that have a given target feature at the same time.

In the first approach any phoneme or group of phonemes that illustrate the target feature may be taught with the idea that the feature will generalize to other phonemes. For example, any of the following phonemes could be used to teach the continuancy feature:

/f/ /v/
/θ/ /ð/
/s/ /z/
/ʃ/ /ʒ/

Other continuant sounds including /l/, /r/, and the nasals could also be used, but may be less effective for illustrating continuancy. This is because /l/ and /r/ are difficult to continue in a steady state, and the nasals might not be as likely to generalize to oral sounds. In fact, Chomsky and Halle (1968) do not consider the nasals to be continuants because the airstream is stopped from continuing through the oral cavity. Furthermore, children are likely to use nasals even in the absence of other oral continuants. However, if a child does not have nasals, these might be the easiest continuants to establish. Considerations such as these would be used in selecting the phoneme or phonemes to represent the missing feature. As noted above, a second approach would be to teach all of the above phonemes simultaneously to establish continuancy.

Phonemes that involve both the + and − contrast may also be used to illustrate the feature. Many phoneme pairs could be used for teaching the continuant/stop contrast including:

/d/ − /v/   /p/ − /f/
/t/ − /θ/   /b/ − /s/
/k/ − /ʃ/   /d/ − /s/

Some clinicians (Blache, Parsons and Humphreys, 1981; McReynolds and Bennett, 1972) choose two phonemes that differ by only the target feature. For example, the following choices might be made for teaching:

Unvoiced/Voiced
(Lax/Tense)
/p/ − /b/
/t/ − /d/
/k/ − /g/
/s/ − /z/
/f/ − /v/
Stop/Continuant
/t/ − /s/
/d/ − /z/
Front/Back
/t/ − /k/
/d/ − /g/

One such approach is described in detail by Blache in chapter 14.

Costello (1975) recommended training more than one error phoneme in conjunction with the substituted phoneme to demonstrate the contrastive function of distinctive features. Costello and Onstine (1976) trained two phonemes that illustrated the + value of the absent feature, and contrasted those with one phoneme that illustrated the − value of the feature. For example, to teach continuancy, they taught /θ/ and /s/ in contrast with /t/.

Ruder and Bunce (1981) used a slightly different strategy for training two children with severe articulation disorders that had been classified as phonetic rather than phonemic. These children had very small phonemic repertoires. One child consistently used only /m/, /b/, and /g/. The other used only /g/, /n/, /ŋ/, and /j/. Ruder and Bunce chose phonemes that the children had already produced on occasion to increase their repertoire. In the first case, the child had produced /p/, /s/, and /k/ in addition to the frequent /m/, /b/, and /g/. The authors chose to train /s/ and /k/ to encourage the use of the features +continuant, +strident, +coronal, −voice, +high. A primary research question was: Will training /s/ and /k/, which between them embody all features of /t/, cause /t/ to be produced? Following traditional training through the word level, the child could imitate /t/, /f/, /ŋ/, /z/, /tʃ/. On the basis of the generalization theory, /f/, /tʃ/, and /ʃ/ had also been predicted. Ruder and Bunce's research shows that careful selection of phonemes based on features missing from the child's system can encourage the use of new features and thus a larger repertoire of sounds.

Costello (1975, p. 69) outlined the following steps in designing a remediation plan based on distinctive-feature theory:

1. Administer traditional measures of articulation to determine error phonemes and stimulability.
2. Deep-test error phonemes for baseline data.
3. Complete distinctive-feature analysis using Singh and Polen's (1972) system (Table 4.5) and select target feature and three or four appropriate phonemes as vehicles for instruction.
4. Design a treatment program for these phonemes that includes steps for carryover in connected speech outside the clinical setting.
5. Following treatment, readminister articulation tests and obtain a spontaneous speech sample.

Although the target phonemes could be taught in isolation or in syllables, it has been suggested that features cannot be separated from the phonemes-in-words context (Costello, 1975; Parker, 1976). Parker suggests that features are not a component of speech production, but a component of the language, and hence inseparable from words. Therefore, Blache (chapter 14) recommends teaching the feature contrasts in minimal word pairs such as *big−pig, bass−bat, first−thirst* (Blache et al., 1981). Further details and advantages of the minimal-word-pair method will be discussed briefly in this chapter and more extensively in chapter 14.

Distinctive-feature approaches have been criticized on the basis of the time required to complete the analysis and the questionable articulatory va-

lidity of many feature systems (Parker, 1976; Walsh, 1974). However, Singh, Hayden, and Toombs (1981) showed that the Singh and Singh (1976) distinctive-feature system was useful in establishing a feature hierarchy for the articulation errors of 1,077 children in public-school speech therapy. Further, Toombs, Singh, and Hayden (1981) found that markedness theory provided a better explanation of 801 students' substitutions than did analysis of features per se. Markedness theory, as described in chapter 2, accounts for the relative complexity of phonemes on the basis of the number of features required for production and the physiological complexity of the particular features. However, McReynolds, Engmann, and Dimmitt (1974) found that the articulation errors of the children in their study did not always follow the direction that markedness theory would predict. Grunwell (1982) notes that the theory of markedness is not well developed, and its clinical relevance has not been clearly demonstrated. In regard to use of distinctive features in general, Grunwell states that use of ''a formalized distinctive feature analysis procedure'' is questionable, but the ''concept'' of distinctive features is valid and clinically applicable (p. 129).

It is important to remember that the casual application of distinctive-feature therapy without the kind of attention given to choice of target features and phonemes that is evident in research projects may not produce the same progress. Care in choosing therapy goals will be rewarded in efficient use of therapy time.

The advantages of distinctive-feature therapy can be obtained by use of articulatory-based feature systems that relate directly to speech production (see chapter 2). Further, the regularities captured by this approach are largely the same as those determined by phonological-process analysis. A phonological-process approach, however, has the advantage of exposing certain error patterns that are not revealed by distinctive-feature analysis, such as syllable and phoneme deletions and assimilatory processes.

THERAPY APPROACHES BASED ON PROCESS ELIMINATION

A phonological-process approach is based on several assumptions that give direction to the remedial program. First, as in distinctive-feature-based therapy, treatment of phonological processes will result in more efficient therapy than that produced by one-phoneme approaches. Treatment of one or a few processes can effect correction of groups of phonemes at one time. This means that therapy may be directed toward a group of phonemes simultaneously or that one representative phoneme may be taught with the expectation that generalization will occur. Second, this approach assumes that the child's problem is one of rule learning, and therefore the treatment program will entail discovery of rules by the child. Third, the child's problem is proposed to be a phonemic rather than phonetic problem, which suggests that therapy should begin at the word level so that phoneme contrasts are possible, although some work has been carried out at the syllable level, both in research and in clinical practice.

Following the identification of phonological processes in the child's speech (see chapter 4), the clinician must prioritize the processes for remediation. Ingram (1976) suggested the following three guiding principles from Edwards and Bernhardt (1973) for selection of processes for remediation:

1. Select processes that interfere most with intelligibility. Improvement of intelligibility is the primary goal of articulation therapy. Therefore, selection of target processes directed toward that end is therapeutically sound. The child's own perception of change in intelligibility can be motivating for future therapy.
2. Select less stable processes. It is likely that optional processes will be more amenable to change than those that are stable in the child's speech.

3. Select processes that are most common in young children. If we accept current thinking that phonologically disordered children are not totally unlike normally developing children, and that earlier learned phonemes or classes of phonemes may be easier than later ones, then it follows that in therapy the child may have an easier time learning the processes that are characteristic of younger children.

Edwards and Bernhardt (1973) advocated the application of these principles in the above order. In other words, the first process chosen should be the one that will produce the greatest change in intelligibility. If a clear-cut decision cannot be made on this basis, a process that is optional in the child's speech should be chosen. The normal acquisition sequence should be taken into account when the first two principles do not result in a clear choice.

These principles, although stated in linguistic terms, are really very like the criteria used in traditional therapy techniques (Van Riper, 1978). Traditionally, it was said that the target phoneme should be one that (a) interferes with intelligibility, (b) is stimulable, and (c) is early developing.

More recently, Edwards (1983) has given more detail to these principles. She suggests that it is not possible to define an order for remediation of processes because of the variability among children. However, it is important to have guiding principles. The principles are as follows:

1. "Choose processes that should result in early success" (p. 39). These would include processes that are optional in the child's speech (those that do not occur 100% of the time), processes that apply only in certain phonetic environments, and processes that affect sounds that are already in the child's phonetic inventory or sounds for which the child is stimulable. The principle is that the child will more easily and quickly eliminate a process if he has already demonstrated its suppression in some way.

2. ''Choose processes that are 'crucial' for the individual child'' (p. 39) in that they are especially deviant, call attention to the child's speech, interfere most with intelligibility, create a large number of homonyms, neutralize the distinction between sound contrasts, or apply consistently.
3. ''Choose 'early' processes or processes that affect early sounds'' (p. 41).
4. ''Choose processes that interact'' (p. 41) to create substitutions based on more than one rule change. First, work on the process that affects the greatest number of segments. Edwards gives the following example: If the child substitutes d/k, b/p, and d/t, work on prevocalic voicing before fronting because it affects all three substitutions.

Edwards suggests basically the same principles as guidelines in selecting phonemes to represent target processes. An additional consideration in selecting phonemes is the position in the word. The sound should be easy to produce in the target position. For example, voiceless sounds might be chosen as final-position targets and voiced as initial because prevocalic voicing and postvocalic devoicing are likely to occur.

Careful study of the principles will reveal some overlap. For example, some ''early'' processes, like final consonant deletion, are those that create homonymy and interfere most with intelligibility. On the other hand, there is also some contradiction. The clinician needs to choose processes that occur frequently enough to be important in the child's speech, but at the same time select optional processes for immediate success. For a given child, optional processes may not interfere most with intelligibility or be early developing. The important point, then, is that the clinician must have clear guidelines in mind, but apply them thoughtfully to each child. Edwards suggests targeting two processes at the same time in order to speed overall progress toward intelligibility.

The authors of published process analysis procedures have also suggested criteria for selecting

target processes after completing the analysis. Through describing case studies, Shriberg and Kwiatkowski (1980) suggest that final consonant deletion would be a priority process for elimination.

Hodson (1982) and Hodson and Paden (1983) present a formula for determining a phonological deviancy score that can be used to determine priority clients for therapy. The formula accounts for pervasiveness of the ten basic deficient patterns (syllable reduction, cluster reduction, prevocalic singleton consonant omission, postvocalic singleton consonant omission, stridency deletion, velar deviations, /l/ deviations, /r, ɜ˞/ deviations, nasal deviations, glide deviations), other deficient patterns, and age. Having determined which children should be seen for therapy, the authors go on to suggest strategies for determining target processes. They state that a target process should occur in at least 40% of the possible test contexts.

In Hodson and Paden's procedure, patterns are prioritized into four levels reflecting intelligibility. Level 0 patterns are characteristic of the most unintelligible children. Basically, these patterns consist of omissions of obstruents and liquids, and less frequently of glides and nasals. Children at this level have the highest priority for therapy. Level I patterns include cluster reduction and omission of syllables, prevocalic singletons, and postvocalic singletons. Substitutions at Level I include fronting of velars, backing, glottal replacement, and voicing alterations. Reduplication of syllables and vowel deviations also characterize Level I. Level II patterns include cluster reduction and omission of stridents as well as stopping, liquid gliding, and vowelization. Level III patterns do not significantly interfere with intelligibility; therefore, Hodson and Paden give them the lowest priority for remediation. They include nonphonemic alterations such as tongue protrusion and lateralization, affrication or deaffrication, minor place shifts, and devoicing of final obstruents. Children at Level I and at Level II will usually exhibit patterns from other levels.

Hodson and Paden suggest that therapy targets should be selected in accordance with the above levels; i.e., Level 0 processes should be selected first and Level III last. This order holds regardless of the percent of occurrence as long as it is above 40%. They focus on one phoneme that represents the pattern, with ease of elicitation the primary criterion for selection of the target phoneme. They recommend probing for a sound that the child can produce successfully, but based on their experience, they also provide a list of suggested target phonemes for each pattern and suggested words for each phoneme. Words are selected to facilitate correct production of the target phoneme. Careful attention should be given to phonetic contexts that will be most helpful. Table 7.1 presents suggested target words for facilitating selected patterns (Hodson & Paden, 1983). Hodson discusses selection of targets in greater detail in chapter 12.

Weiner (1979, pp. 3–6) recommends selecting a process from each of his three major categories to work on at the same time. He also provides a suggested order for remediation of the processes within each category. These categories and the order of processes are:

syllable structure processes
1. deletion of final consonants
2. glottal replacement
3. weak syllable deletion
4. cluster reduction

harmony processes
1. prevocalic voicing
2. final consonant devoicing
3. velar assimilation
4. labial assimilation
5. alveolar assimilation

feature contrast processes
1. stopping
2. affrication
3. gliding of fricatives
4. fronting
5. denasalization

TABLE 7.1
Two Suggested Target Words for Patterns Frequently Targeted in Cycle One. The Same Words May Serve for Probing.*

Final Obstruents:	
Final /p/	rope, soap
Final /t/	hat, boat
Final /k/	lock, bike
Consonant-Vowel-Consonant:	
/p/-vowel-/p/	pipe, pop
Syllableness:	
Two syllables	cowboy, baseball
Three syllables	cowboy hat, baseball bat
Velars:	
Final /k/	rock, lock
Initial /k/	car, cow
Final /s/-clusters:	
/ts/	boats, hats
/ps/	ropes, cups
/ks/	books, bikes
Initial /s/-cluster:	
/sp/	spoon, spot
/st/	star, stop
/sm/	smoke, smile
/sn/	snake, snow
/sk/	sky, school
Liquids:	
Initial /l/	lock, log
Initial /r/	rock, rug

*This list does not imply that there are no other words that are appropriate, nor that all of these words or patterns are routinely targeted, and no others, in Cycle One.
Source: Targeting Intelligible Speech (p. 65) by B. Hodson and E. Paden, 1983, San Diego: College-Hill Press. Copyright 1983 by College-Hill Press. Reprinted by permission.

6. gliding of liquids
7. vocalization

By selecting processes from the major categories, the child is learning about different aspects of the phonological system at the same time. There are two different strategies that might be used. One strategy would be to present new syllable structures and new feature contrasts together. For example, while learning new feature contrasts the child can also be learning about syllable structure by including newly learned sounds in the final position of words. Similarly, elimination of stopping and prevocalic voicing could be targeted at the same time by working on a voiceless continuant like /s/ in the initial position. However, task analysis as described in chapter 6 might suggest that this approach would be too difficult because the child would have to accomplish two new tasks at the same time. An alternative would be to include already-acquired phonemes in new syllable structures, and new phonemes in already-acquired syllable structures, both contexts excluding the likelihood of harmony. The first approach may be more efficient. The second may be necessary if the task seems difficult for the child.

A set of predictions provide the basis for Elbert and Gierut's (1986) selection of target sounds. These predictions are based on structural relationships within the phonological system and on the theory that teaching the marked member of a set will result in acquisition of the unmarked member. In general, these predictions have been described and researched in the literature on generalization. The predictions are:

- Teaching one member of a cognate sound pair will result in the use of the other sound in the pair.
- Teaching one allophone will result in the production of other related allophones.
- Teaching a distinctive feature in the context of one sound will result in the use of that feature in other untreated sounds.
- Teaching sounds in the final position of morphemes will result in more accurate production of the sounds in inflected intervocalic contexts.
- Teaching stops in word-final position will lead to more accurate production in word-initial position.
- Teaching fricatives in word-initial position will result in more accurate production of fricatives in word-final position.
- Teaching fricatives will result in more accurate production of stops.
- Teaching voiced obstruents (stops, fricatives, affricates) will result in accurate production of voiceless obstruents. (pp. 105–106)

Elbert and Gierut also consider the child's stimulability and consistency of production (what they call "phonological knowledge") in choosing target sounds. The authors state that the predictions

can be used individually or in combination for selecting targets for therapy.

Although the clinician should be aware of and consider certain guiding principles in selecting goals for therapy, the individual child and his environment must in the end determine specific goals. In some cases, idiosyncratic factors like the child's name or special concerns of parents or teachers can influence goal selection. This does not mean that the clinician should teach /r/ to a 2-year-old because his name is Roger and the parents want him to say it correctly. It is the clinician's responsibility to provide information for parents and to help them to set realistic goals. On the other hand, it is important to remember that therapy should not occur in the absence of interactions with the environment.

GENERALIZATION

Linguistic approaches including distinctive-feature and phonological process approaches are based on the assumption that when the child learns one or more exemplars of a phonological rule, this learning will generalize to other exemplars. In order for treatment to affect communication, generalization must occur.

Generalization occurs at a number of levels. First, unless all phonemes are being taught, generalization must occur from one phoneme in a sound class to others. For example, if the child stops fricatives, and /s/ was taught as an exemplar of fricatives, then this new manner of production must generalize to /z/, /ʃ/, /ʒ/, /f/, /v/, /θ/, and /ð. It has even been shown that generalization can extend to sounds in disparate classes (Elbert & Gierut, 1986; Weiner, 1981b). Second, generalization must always occur across words. It is never possible to teach the child all of the words in which a given phoneme occurs. As a matter of fact, some therapy techniques include only a few words in therapy with the assumption that generalization will extend to new words when the few are learned. The child must learn to include new phonemes in all the words in his vocabulary. Third, generalization may occur across word positions. It may not be necessary to teach a sound in the prevocalic, postvocalic, and intervocalic positions because the child may generalize from one position to another. Thus if we teach /f/ in words like *fat*, *far*, and *fine*, the child may learn to produce words like *knife*, *calf*, and *deaf*. Finally, generalization must occur across all listeners, situations, and contexts. This last consideration was discussed in chapter 5 under the heading "Transfer and Carryover."

Several studies have examined types of generalization. Researchers have shown that there is generalization from trained phonemes to other phonemes (Compton, 1970; Costello & Onstine, 1976; Dunn & Till, 1982; Ruder & Bunce, 1981; Tyler, Edwards & Saxman, 1987; Weiner, 1981b). As predicted by distinctive-feature theory, generalization seems to occur most effectively across phonemes that share features. Compton (1970) found that for one 4-year-old child, correction of /m/ resulted in correction of other nasals with no effect on any other defective consonants. As might be expected, Elbert, Shelton, and Arndt (1967) and McReynolds and Elbert (1981) found that training /s/ did not improve production of /r/. Further, Dunn and Till (1982) reported that in the training of fricatives, generalization occurred most frequently within place subclasses. For example, generalization occurred within the labiodental class (/f/ and /v/) and within the lingual class (/s/, /z/, /ʃ/), but not as readily between them.

Elbert and Gierut (1986) describe *implicational generalization*, which is defined as the predicted generalization within and across sound classes based on implicational relationships. These implicational relationships are determined by what is known about languages and language acquisition. For example in chapter 3, it was noted that Jakobson's (1968) theory predicts that children will not acquire a fricative until the homorganic (same

place of articulation) stop is acquired. Thus, if the child acquires /s/, it is "implied" that he has acquired /t/. Another way to look at such prediction is based on markedness theory, discussed in chapter 2. Acquisition of the marked member "implies" acquisition of the unmarked member of a pair. Based on the chart in Table 2.5, /s/ is more marked than /t/ for the feature under consideration. Dinnsen and Elbert (1984) showed that when children were trained to produce fricatives, they also learned to produce stops, but when they were trained to produce stops, they did not generalize to fricatives. This suggests that it may be more useful to teach the more marked sound of a feature set because generalization may extend to less marked sounds, but not vice versa. Similarly Gierut, Elbert, and Dinnsen (1987) found that when children were taught sounds of which they had least phonological knowledge, they showed wider generalization to other sounds throughout the sound system. However, when they were taught sounds of which they had greatest knowledge, the new learning did not extend to sounds of which they had least knowledge. This suggests that therapy should begin with the "harder" sounds rather than the "easier." This view is in opposition to other strategies for choosing target sounds that focus on a developmental pattern or on those sounds that are easier for the child to produce. Before this method is accepted, further research is needed to determine if there is a cause and effect relationship between the teaching of "harder" sounds and the learning of "easier" sounds. For example, assuming that teaching a "harder" sound requires more time, it is possible that "easier" sounds may meanwhile be learned spontaneously. It is important to consider which method will result in more efficient remediation of the child's entire system.

These studies have provided evidence to support the notion that generalization does occur; however, some researchers question the expectation that generalization will be complete and consistent (Blache et al., 1981; Dunn, 1983; Ingram, 1976; Weiner, 1981b; Weiner & Bankson, 1978; Winitz & Bellerose, 1978). These authors suggest training several examples of a feature or feature contrast rather than only one example in order to promote generalization. Weiner (1981b) stated that although he found training several examples to be effective, further research is needed to determine whether generalization will occur if only one phoneme contrast is used. Ingram (1976) concluded that the evidence for feature generalization is not sufficient to encourage use of a single-phoneme approach. He advocated a conservative view that features are learned in segments, not as features per se, and that all phonemes embodying a given feature should be trained. Hence, he recommended training all relevant phonemes at the same time.

In a further test of generalization, McReynolds and Bennett (1972) trained one phoneme example of an absent feature in nonsense syllables to determine if generalization would occur to words and to other phonemes with the same feature. For example, they trained /f/ in nonsense syllables to determine if the child would learn to produce /f/ in words and if he or she would also produce other stridents such as /s/ and /ʃ/. They did obtain generalization to words from nonsense syllables and to other phonemes from the example phoneme. There was, however, variation in degree of generalization based on the target feature and on word position. The findings regarding generalization from syllables to words are supported by Powell and McReynolds (1969).

It has been found that generalization does occur from trained to untrained words (Blache & Parsons, 1980; Blache, Parsons, & Humphreys, 1981; Costello & Bosler, 1976; Griffith, Irwin, & Weston, 1980; Pollack & Rees, 1972; Ruscello, 1975; Weiner, 1981b; Weiner & Bankson, 1978; Weston & Irwin, 1971; Young, 1987). Blache et al. (1981) found that generalization occurred from one word-pair example of the phonemes to other words. Weiner (1981b) trained two children using the method of minimal pairs. He found that the suppression of three phonological processes (final consonant deletion, stopping, and fronting) generalized from 4 training words to an untrained list of 20.

Generalization across word positions has also received attention (Powell & McReynolds, 1969; Ruscello, 1975; Weston & Irwin, 1971). Although generalization has been shown to occur, Dunn

(1983, p. 50) suggests that certain factors must be considered in determining whether to train sounds in all positions. These include the particular sound being trained, the individual child's abilities, and the treatment approach.

Dunn (1983) discussed two kinds of generalization: (a) stimulus generalization and (b) response generalization. She suggested that it is wise to plan for response generalization by providing diversity of material throughout the therapy program. Attention should be given to generalization across word positions, phonetic contexts, sounds, and linguistic levels, i.e., words, phrases, sentences. If the clinician begins early to measure generalization, it can be encouraged throughout the program. For example, consider the child who is taught one phoneme to represent a distinctive feature class but does not generalize the new production to other phonemes. A useful strategy might be to give the child limited experience with other phonemes in the same class in order to promote generalization.

The studies reviewed here indicate that there is value in examining features that are present and absent in the child's speech and using these features as a basis for expanding the child's repertoire of correctly used phonemes. The same principle applies to phonological processes. The potential for generalization when target phonemes are carefully chosen seems good, and valuable therapy time may thus be saved.

The linguistic approaches described in this chapter are based on the assumption that generalization will occur, but the clinician must always be aware of planning for it and testing success through periodic probes.

REMEDIATION STRATEGIES

A benchmark of linguistic therapy approaches is goal setting based on identification of patterns in the child's speech. Therefore, the choice of targets for therapy is the primary distinction between these approaches and the traditional ones. To some extent, any approach may be used for teaching the target sounds. However, the two principles noted at the beginning of the chapter direct the kind of therapy strategies employed by most clinicians who use this approach. The first is the principle of rule-governed knowledge. If the child is to discover the phonological rules of the language, he must be provided with opportunities that illustrate these rules and allowed to discover them. Second is the principle of communicative function. This principle demands that the therapy process allow the child to see the relevance of the phonological system for effective communication. Opportunities to demonstrate both success and failure in actual communication will be needed.

The following summarizes the therapy strategies that have been described by several authors and the rationale that they provide. Some authors have suggested general principles or methods for selecting therapy targets (Grunwell, 1985; Ingram, 1976), whereas others have outlined the actual procedures to use for remediation (Elbert, 1983; Elbert & Gierut, 1986; Grunwell, 1983; Hodson & Paden, 1983; Weiner, 1979). Each author's suggestions will be described briefly.

Ingram (1976) states that "the acquisition of phonology is concerned with the acquisition of the ability to use sounds contrastively" (p. 141). He outlines three goals for remediation:

1. Elimination of instability in the child's speech. Some children with articulation disorders demonstrate inconsistent production of words. The child who does not have firmly established phonemic contrasts may produce a given word in a variety of ways depending on the exact processes applied. Ingram (p. 142) gives the following example of a hearing-impaired child's productions of *pencil* from Oller and Eilers (1975).

1. bʌ'dɔ	3. pɛd	5. pʰad
2. pʌ'bə	4. pɛdə	6. pɪa

7. pɪtə	10. pɛdza	12. pɪt
8. ɛ'tə	11. pɛ'tə'	13. pʰɛ'ʔtu'
9. pɛ'ʔtəʔ		

Ingram states that establishing the form /pɛtə/ as a consistent production would eliminate some minor processes and isolate a stable form for further process elimination. Further, it would help the adults in the child's environment to learn the child's rule system and understand the child better.

2. Elimination of homonyms. The inclusion in a child's speech of many words that have the same phonetic form interferes greatly with intelligibility. For some children, an appropriate therapy strategy may be to teach the child contrastive productions of specific words that are homonyms in his speech. In this case, the selection of target processes will be based on their usefulness in eliminating specific homonyms in the child's speech.

3. Establishing contrasts within the child's system. Ingram explains that the first two methods approach remediation from the basis of specific words in the child's sample. With some children, it may be more appropriate to work on establishing certain contrasts throughout the child's system, which will mean working on a large number of different words. Selection of contrasts would be based on the principles of acquisition outlined in chapter 3 that suggest which consonants and contrasts are learned first. Generally, children learn larger or more general contrasts before finer distinctions.

Grunwell (1985, p. 96) presented basically the same general guidelines for remediation with one addition. She noted the importance of increasing the child's repertoire of consonant combinations to achieve greater communicative adequacy. She stresses communicative adequacy as the overriding principle for all remediation goals.

Weiner (1979) suggests that different remediation strategies may be applicable to different processes. He recommends two procedures for remediating syllable-structure processes. He calls the first a *sorting task,* in which the child hears pairs of words like *pool* and *spool* or *pill* and *spill* and sorts them into ''cluster'' and ''noncluster'' categories. Weiner states that this auditory sorting will improve production of the cluster.

The second approach is the *lexical approach,* in which the child must modify syllable structure in order to avoid producing homonyms for minimal pairs like *bow* and *boat.* In this approach, a game can be played in which the child names one of two pictures and the clinician chooses the picture that the child names (Weiner, 1981b). For example, a child with final consonant deletion will produce *bow* for *boat,* and the clinician will choose the bow picture each time until, with or without the help of the clinician, the child modifies production to include a final sound on *boat.*

For remediation of harmony or assimilation processes, Weiner suggests the paired stimuli approach (Weston & Irwin, 1971), in which a word like *dime* is paired with *dog* or *duck* for a child who shows velar assimilation. *Dime* is a word that will not show velar assimilation. By this pairing, the child may begin to produce *dog* or *duck* correctly. Weiner also recommends the use of facilitating contexts like *mad dog* for eliminating assimilation.

Weiner further suggests a distinctive-feature approach for eliminating feature contrast processes such as stopping, gliding, fronting, vocalization, denasalization, affrication, or neutralization. The use of minimally contrasting pairs of sounds like /t/ and /s/ or /t/ and /k/ may produce generalization to other phonemes. A second approach is to teach awareness of the feature characteristic, like blowing or flowing versus exploding or popping. This awareness can be used in both listening and production. Weiner and Bankson (1978) gave the following outline for teaching frication:

1. Introduce the stop-fricative concept by describing the fricative as running water and the stop as dripping water.
2. Present a 20 item probe test for fricatives in the initial position of CVC words. This probe test is repeated after each of the following steps.

3. Present 10 exaggerated fricative and 10 stop sounds in words for the child to identify. These words should be different from those used in the probe.
4. Ask the child to imitate the exaggerated productions and to identify the stop or fricative feature of the clinician's productions. The criterion for moving from this step is 18/20 correct identifications on two successive probes. Productions are not counted.
5. Repeat step 4, but omit exaggeration.
6. Ask the child to name pictures of the 10 fricative words used in the above steps and 10 additional words. Criterion is 18/20 correct productions on two consecutive trials.

Weiner and Bankson administered this program to 4 children and concluded that it was most useful with school-age children who had multiple errors and no attentional or behavioral problems.

Hodson and Paden (1983) present a treatment program for unintelligible children based on the following concepts:

1. Phonological acquisition is a gradual process. (p. 44)
2. Children with normal hearing typically acquire the adult sound system primarily by listening. (p. 46)
3. As the child acquires new speech patterns he associates kinesthetic with auditory sensations which enable later self-monitoring. (p. 47)
4. Phonetic environment can facilitate correct sound production. (p. 47)
5. Children tend to generalize new articulation skills to other targets. (p. 48)

Based on these concepts, Hodson and Paden's program includes (a) intensive auditory stimulation at the beginning and end of each session, (b) the use of auditory, tactual, and visual stimulation for correct production, (c) facilitation of correct production through the above means or through use of facilitating contexts or semantic cues, and (d) a cycle format that targets deficient phonological patterns for a few weeks and then allows time for the pattern to emerge.

This program differs from others in its cycle approach, which is based on the belief that children will progress on their own following a brief experience with correct production of the target pattern. In a cycle approach, unlike in traditional methods, a designated number of sessions are spent in training a given pattern. At the end of the cycle, probes are used to determine if the same patterns or new ones will be targeted in the next cycle. The method is described in detail in chapter 12.

Hodson (1982) reported performance data on 111 children who were seen for therapy using this approach. They were seen once a week for 75-minute sessions. Some children were also receiving therapy at school. Seventy children completed the program and were dismissed as intelligible. The average time in therapy was two semesters, with the longest being 18 months for the children with the most severe disorders. Thirteen children had progressed substantially, but were not dismissed by the end of the project. Twenty-three children were not in the program long enough to be counted.

Tyler et al. (1987) found the cycle approach to be effective with two subjects with multiple errors. Specifically, their study supported the notion of gradual acquisition, and they noted that the cycle approach takes advantage of this.

In their Clinician-Child Interaction Plan, Elbert and Gierut (1986), like other authors (Grunwell, 1985; Hodson, chapter 12 in this text) emphasize the active role of the child in the therapy process. The clinician's role includes the following major components that are characteristic of phonological approaches in general.

1. Characterization of what the child knows about the sound system. This is accomplished by obtaining a representative sample and completing a thorough analysis.
2. Helping the child reorganize his existing system by disrupting his current patterns and helping him develop new ways of or-

ganizing them. This can be accomplished by training only one or a few representative targets (training deep) or by training several sounds simultaneously (training broad). As was shown in the section on generalization, both strategies have been shown to produce generalization.

3. Selecting targets based on predictions of the changes that will occur in the child's sound system. These predictions were listed earlier in this chapter.
4. Monitoring progress and changes in the child's sound system during each session and over time.

When the clinician fulfills these roles effectively, the child is able to be successful in the following roles:

1. Practice of the articulatory gestures that will lead to acquisition of the target speech sound. Although drill is not looked upon with favor by many clinicians who use a linguistic approach, Elbert and Gierut (1986) observe that children practice sound production during normal acquisition. These normal children test out strategies for sound production during their practice. Phonologically disordered children can also be allowed to try out their own strategies during such practice. For example, the clinician might note what types of syllables or contexts facilitate correct production for this particular child and then allow practice in those contexts rather than in clinician-selected words. No matter what strategy is chosen, these authors assert that practice must occur for the child to learn to "produce" the sound.
2. Conceptualization of the sound's phonemic properties. After the child can produce the sound, he must realize its role in signaling phonemic differences. Elbert and Gierut suggest minimal pair treatment at this point. Therapy using minimal pairs will be described later in the chapter.
3. Integration of the new phonetic and phonemic knowledge into the sound system. Fi-

nally, the child must use the new phoneme(s) in everyday conversational speech. This will necessitate monitoring on the part of the child. The clinician can facilitate this integration by presenting naturalistic tasks during therapy so that transfer can occur.

It is, of course, the interaction between the clinician role and client role that results in successful change.

The procedures discussed thus far have used word-level material for remediation. Elbert (1983) reported using syllables for working on the phonological system of one child with a severely restricted phonetic inventory, consisting of only nine sounds including the glottal stop. The child received token reinforcement for correct imitation of contrasting syllables that illustrated more than one process. For example, the three pairs /ɑ–ɑb/, /ɑ–ɑt/, and /ɑ–ɑg/ illustrated final stops, voicing contrast, and a three-way place-of-articulation contrast. Elbert used words as probe items to evaluate generalization. Following 10 months of therapy the child had developed a full phonetic inventory and was highly intelligible. Pollack (1983) also reported using syllables, but found that words worked better for a child with a severe phonological preference for /d/ and /n/ in the initial position. She suggested modifying therapy plans for children with phonological preferences. For example, because of this child's strong preference in the initial position, it was necessary to work in the final position in order to expand his phonetic repertoire.

Grunwell (1983) reported the results of a program that is very different from the ones described above. The program was designed to allow the child to change her phonological system spontaneously through exposure to written English in a special education program, but with no direct articulation therapy. The child attended a preschool program with nine other children who had language-learning problems. The activities that were part of the general reading and writing program for all of the children included systematic exposure to the orthographic system, sound-symbol relationships, discriminating, classifying

and sequencing sounds, and sound blending to form words. The child under study followed a normal developmental order for phonological gains, but the changes occurred with much greater rapidity. Grunwell suggests that such a program ''facilitates the child's own development of a normal phonological system by providing him or her with direct access to the systematic and structural patterns in the adult system'' (p. 75).

Minimal Pair Therapy

One therapy strategy that is often associated with linguistic therapy approaches is the minimal pair method (Blache, 1982, and chapter 14 of this text; Cooper, 1985; Elbert & Gierut, 1986; Grunwell, 1985; Weiner, 1981b). Minimal pairs may be defined in two ways by linguists and clinicians. A minimal pair can be defined as two different words (i.e., different meanings) that differ by only one phoneme. Thus the following are minimal pairs:

tan—pan	calf—cat
fat—cat	bit—big
bird—heard	his—hid
could—wood	rid—rig
tick—sick	rack—rag
bat—pat	move—mood

A finer definition of minimal pairs would state that the two phonemes must differ by only one feature. By this definition only the following pairs from the above list would be selected:

tan—pan	rid—rig
tick—sick	his—hid
bat—pat	rack—rag

The pairs in the first line differ only by front/back place of articulation. The pairs in the second line differ by stop/continuant manner, and the pairs in the third line differ by voicing alone.

Both kinds of minimal pairs can be useful in therapy. At least two aspects of this method make it fit particularly well with linguistic approaches.

First, minimal pairs can clearly illustrate distinctive features as will be shown by Blache in chapter 14. The examples just given show how only one feature can change the meaning of the word. Pairs that differ by only one feature are especially useful for demonstrating distinctive features. A second way in which minimal pairs are useful is that they can demonstrate communication failure resulting from incorrect phonological patterns. Choosing from the examples, if the aspiring actor asks for a ''bit part'' when he really wants a ''big part,'' his communication will be unsuccessful.

In actual practice, clinicians often use pairs that consist of the child's error paired with the correct production. This may result in single-feature minimal pairs if the child has a single-feature error or it may result in pairs that differ by more than one feature.

Elbert and Gierut (1986) describe yet another strategy for choosing minimal pairs. They suggest using minimal pairs that represent maximal oppositions so that the child can see the full range of sound possibilities. For example if the child omitted final consonants, we would typically use the following kinds of minimal pairs in therapy to show the presence and absence of the final sound.

see — seat
pen — pens
be — beat
Kay — cake

However, using the Elbert and Gierut model, if the child ever used any sound in the final position (for example, /m/), then we would pair /m/ with a very different sound like /k/ to show that different sounds can be used in that position. Elbert and Gierut suggest that when the child begins to use these disparate sounds, the other missing contrasts will come in without treatment.

Minimal pairs can be used in a number of ways within the therapy session. They can be used for discrimination by having the child identify which picture the clinician names. They can be used for drill by having the child name the two members of the pair until he is able to distinguish their production. More importantly, they can be used meaningfully in game or play situations where the child must request or name the correct or desired item in order to communicate a request or command. For example, a game could be designed in which there is a choice to ''tell a story'' or ''sell a story'' or to ''see a monster'' or ''be a monster.'' Stories can also be designed that include minimal pairs as key words. For example, ''A girl named Carrie and a boy named Terry were searching for the cook who took the cake. But where did she take the cake?''

Fokes (1982) also recommends use of contrast pairs in therapy, but she states that the word pairs do not have to be minimal. She advocates using the pairs in a variety of ways to promote the contrast — dividing them into two categories, imitating them, playing games, and telling stories with them. She suggests using eight to ten different pairs for a given contrast.

Sometimes it may be difficult to think of minimal pairs to fit a given child's errors. There are a number of strategies for developing appropriate pairs. First there are several published sources (Elbert, Rockman, & Saltzman, 1980, 1982). Second, the clinician would be wise to begin keeping a list of minimal pairs used in therapy and the activities or stories that are associated with them. These pairs may be used again with future clients. Elbert and Gierut (1986) suggest a third way to expand the repertoire of minimal pairs. They recommend the use of *near minimal pairs* where the vowel adjacent to the target sound is the same, but another sound in the word may differ. Examples are *toe* and *soap*, *shame* and *chain*, *bee* and *feet*. Allowing a second difference between the pairs can greatly expand the available words to use in pairs. A fourth way to increase the number of minimal pairs is to assign meaning to nonsense words. Cooper (1985) suggested using the child's incorrect production of any real word as a nonsense word and assigning meaning to it. Thus *sand* could be used as a real word with the child's production *tand* denoted as something else; for example, a Play-Doh® shape. These two words can now be used in a game or other communication activity. It is easy to use nonsense words in stories. They can be the names of characters, including monsters, or of places. Science-fiction objects can also be named in stories.

If nonsense words are to be used, it is important to first establish the assigned meaning for the child. After the temporary meaning has been established, they can be used in any way.

Minimal pairs can be a powerful tool in therapy for phonologically disordered children when the pairs are carefully chosen to match the goals of therapy. They are useful for drill activities, but can be even more powerful when they are used communicatively to demonstrate to the child that the production of a phoneme can determine whether communication succeeds or fails. This is done by including the words in activities where the child must produce the correct phoneme to control the clinician or the activity.

Example Therapy Plan

The following example of a therapy program for one child illustrates the kinds of information that the clinician needs to obtain prior to therapy planning. This section also contains a description of therapy goals based on the information gathered and an overview of the remediation process.

Assume that the spontaneous speech sample in Table 7.2 was obtained from a 5-year-old child and analyzed according to the procedures in chapter 4. (This analysis is shown in Table 7.3.) After analyzing the child's speech, the clinician must identify remediation goals. Hodson and Paden (1983) list the following processes as being characteristic of the speech of the most unintelligible children: backing, final consonant deletion, syllable reduction, prevocalic voicing, glottal replacement, and reduplication. Of these, this child exhibits final consonant deletion. Backing consistently occurs for /t/ and /k/, which become /h/. Other major processes are stopping of fricatives, cluster reduction, velar fronting, and liquid simplification. Hodson and Paden also note these as being characteristic of unintelligible children.

Priority processes for remediation for this child would be:

1. final consonant deletion
2. stopping of fricatives

There are a number of reasons for choosing these two processes as targets for remediation. First, they both have a significant effect on intelligibility. Together, they create many homonymous forms in the child's speech. A few examples are:

$$
\begin{array}{l}
\text{man} \\
\text{Max} \\
\text{mask}
\end{array} \!\rightarrow\! [\text{mæ}] \qquad
\begin{array}{l}
\text{ball} \\
\text{fox}
\end{array} \!\rangle\! [\text{bɑ}] \qquad
\begin{array}{l}
\text{six} \\
\text{this}
\end{array} \!\rangle\! [\text{dɪ}] \qquad
\begin{array}{l}
\text{it} \\
\text{is}
\end{array} \!\rangle\! [\text{ɪ}]
$$

In addition, these processes are widespread in the child's speech. Each of them affects a large number of phonemes. The two phonemes /ʃ/ and /tʃ/ account for a large portion of both the fricatives and the final consonants used. Like the two processes targeted, velar fronting creates homonymous forms (/dɑ/ = *got, dog*), but its remediation would change only one phoneme. Another reason for choosing these processes is that developmentally they take precedence over others that might also increase intelligibility. For example, cluster reduction is widespread in the sample, but its suppression is developmentally more sophisticated. A final rationale for targeting these two processes is the observation that the child does use both fricatives and final consonants on a very limited basis. He uses /ʃ/ correctly and as a substitution for /tʃ/ in the initial and final position. This suggests that remediation of these processes is likely to be successful.

The therapy plan might focus on the use of minimal pairs to illustrate the contrast between stops and fricatives and between open and closed syllables. The starting point might be the inclusion of other fricatives besides /ʃ/ in the final position. Words that can be pictured or for which objects are available could be used to illustrate to the child that the target distinctions are important in being understood. One obvious distinction that depends on final fricatives is the singular/plural contrast. It can be very important to the child whether he gets the *car* or *cars* or the *block* or *blocks*. The following

TABLE 7.2
Spontaneous Speech Sample for a 5-Year-Old Child

zipper	bɪbɚ	feet	bi	cow	hoʊ
baby	bebi	fishing	bɪi	fish	bɪ
blue	bu	five	baɪ	bed	bɛ
feather	bebɚ	birthday	bɝde	fox	bɑ
bathtub	bæə	big	bɪ	finger	bɪdo
ball	bɑ	busy	bɪi	boat	boʊ
soap	bop	pencil	pɛdə	pumpkin	pʌɪ
pretty	pɝni	milk	mɪo	monster	mɑɚ
pipe	paɪ	me	mi	pig	pɪ
P. Mooney	pipume	mouth	maʊ	smoking	moi
Poland	poʊwɪ	moon	mu	pants	pæ
Stanley	pæwi	miss	mɪ	Maye	me
picture	pɪpɚ	wagon	weɪ	lamp	wæm
matches	mæʃə	what	wʌ	window	naɪno
water	wɑdɚ	snowman	nomæ	squirrel	wɝu
one	wə	sit	ni	tooth	hu
witch	wɪʃ	that	dæ	lady	weni
where	wer	scissors	dibɚ	six	dɪ
walking	wɑi	shovel	dʌu	lay	we
lap	wæ	thumb	dʌm	dog	dɑ
seven	dɛbə	carrot	herə	down	daʊ
door	dor	ten	hɪə	tail	heə
get	dɛ	Halloween	hæoʊwi	this	dɪ
daddy	dædi	cook	hʊ	Carla	hɑrə
donkey	dɔi	Connie	hɑni	car	hɑr
hammer	hæmɚ	cake	he	help	hɛ
turtle	hɝdə	hill	hi	Terry	heri
taken	heɪ	rabbit	ræbɪ	scratch	ræʃ
homework	hoʊwɝ	trip	rɪp	chicken	ʃɪi
shirt	ʃɝ	throw	ro	britches	rɪʃɪ
church	ʃɝʃ	Roundtree	raʊri	yellow	jɛwo
Charlie	ʃɑri	telephone	ɛwɪbo	vacuum	æu
you	ju	orange	or	airplane	eɪrpe
two	u	stove	o	got	dɑ
eight	eɪ	eating	iə	outside	aʊdaɪ
eleven	ɛbɪ	Santa	ræ	Claus	rɑ
mask	mæ	Christmas	rɪ	ugly	ʌwi
break	re	tree	rɪ	face	be
flag	be	Max	mæ	man	mæ
white	waɪ	wipe	waɪ	have	hæ
cat	hæ	have	hæ	light	waɪ
hat	hæ	knife	naɪ	drum	rʌ
nine	naɪ	brush	rʌ	gun	dʌ
cup	dʌ	floor	bor	four	bor
duck	dʌ	three	ri	go	do
ghost	do	tree	ri	off	ɔ
scare	deɪr	on	ɔ	house	hoʊ
there	deɪr	it	ɪ	is	ɪ

TABLE 7.3
Phonological Analysis of the Speech Sample

Word Structures	Substitutions			Omissions		
	Initial	Medial	Final	Initial	Medial	Final
V	p/m	b/p	ʃ/tʃ	t	m	p
CV	n/w	b/f		v	v	m
VC	b/f	b/v		st	θ	θ
VV	d/ð	b/ð			t	f
CVCV	h/t	n/t			d	v
CVV	n/s	n/d			z	t
VCV	b/z	d/s			n	d
CVCV	w/l	w/l			l	s
VCCV	d/ʃ	p/t			ʃ	z
VCVCV	ʃ/tʃ	ʃ/tʃ			k	n
CVVCV	d/k	d/g			g	l
CVCVCV	h/k	p/pl			mp	ʃ
	d/g	r/tr			st	k
	p/pr				nt	g
	b/bl				nk	ŋ
	r/br				lk	st
	b/fl				kj	sk
	r/θr					ts
	r/tr					ks
	r/dr					nd
	m/sm					
	p/st					
	n/sn					
	w/sl					
	d/sk					
	w/skw					
	r/skr					
	r/kr					
	r/kl					

Phonemic Repertoire:
1. Always used correctly: b, m, w, r, h
2. Used correctly in some context: p, b, m, w, d, n, r, j, h, ʃ
3. Appears, but never correct: none
4. Never appears: f, v, θ, ð, t, s, z, l, ʒ, tʃ, dʒ, k, g, ŋ
5. Not represented in sample words: none

Processes:
1. Final consonant deletion: 93 of 113 opportunities; all phonemes except m, r, tʃ, ʃ
2. Stopping of fricatives: all phonemes except h, final ʃ, tʃ
3. Cluster reduction: all clusters
4. Velar fronting: 6 of 14 opportunities; all opportunities for g
5. Unstressed syllable deletion: 3 of 57 opportunities
6. Liquid simplification: 1 only
7. Backing: h/k, h/t
8. Frication: h/k, h/t
9. Assimilation: 5 examples

are examples of appropriate words for minimal pairs:

eye	baby	bee	boy
eyes	babies	bees	boys
ice		beef	

no	my	two	tea
nose	mice	tooth	teeth
			teach

door	row	car	purr
doors	rose	cars	purse

bear	hoe	night	bow
bears	hose	knife	bows
		nine	boat
			both

A variety of game-like activities involving these pairs could be used. For example, the child could request one of the two objects or pictures, or he could tell the clinician which one to point to or move or find. Inclusion of words ending in /ʃ/ or /tʃ/ would provide an opportunity for immediate success.

It is important to remember that therapy planning is not over when initial goals and an initial therapy plan have been established. One of the most crucial and yet most difficult tasks is the continuing modification of goals, target phonemes, and remediation strategies. Suppose that as this child progressed, he began to include final consonants, and did not stop fricatives as they were acquired in the final position. After the child had begun to use /f/, /s/, and /z/ in the final position, similar therapeutic strategies might be used to target fricatives in the initial position and additional classes of phonemes in the final. Examples of minimal pairs for the initial position are:

two	bun	bat	toe
Sue	fun	fat	sew

passed	bear	tie	tanned
fast	fair	sigh	sand

It is possible that it would be difficult to eliminate stopping in the initial position, but let us assume that /f/ and /s/ can be elicited through modeling and the minimal-pair method. The next target might be the substitutions of /h/ for /t/ and /k/ because of the bizarre nature of the processes involved. The final process to receive remediation could be cluster reduction. As the child progresses through the remediation program, it is not always necessary to work on the elimination of every process. Some processes may be eliminated without therapy as the child begins to make more sense of the phonological system.

SUMMARY

This chapter has presented an overview of current therapy methods based on phonological theory. The guiding principle is that the child's faulty articulatory patterns may be a result of a phonological system that is different from the standard adult model and that thorough analysis of the child's rule system will lead to efficient management based on remediation of error patterns.

Therapy based on distinctive-feature theory generally involves one of two procedures. The clinician either groups the phonemes that represent a target feature or teaches one or a few phonemes that exemplify that feature in anticipation that correct production will generalize to other phonemes. In therapy based on phonological processes, the clinician helps the child eliminate those processes that cause groups of phonemes to be different from the standard model.

A mandatory facet of both approaches, as well as any teaching program, is generalization to other sounds, contexts, situations and listeners. It is important that planning for generalization be an integral part of the entire remediation process.

Although procedures based on distinctive features and those based on phonological processes were described separately, they are both directed by the same principles and in that sense cannot be separated. The ingenious clinician will select elements from each and integrate them to deal effectively with each child's problem. In part III of this text, specific therapy techniques are described that

are based on these principles or combine them with traditional, behavioral, or communication-centered techniques.

REFERENCES

Blache, S. E. (1982). Minimal word pairs and distinctive feature training. In M. Crary (Ed.), *Phonological intervention: Concepts and procedures*. San Diego: College Hill Press.

Blache, S. E., & Parsons, C. L. (1980). A linguistic approach to distinctive feature training. *Language, Speech and Hearing Services in Schools, 11,* 203–207.

Blache, S. E., Parsons, C. L., & Humphreys, J. M. (1981). A minimal-word pair model for teaching the linguistic significance of distinctive feature properties. *Journal of Speech and Hearing Disorders, 46,* 291–296.

Chomsky, N., & Halle, M. (1968). *The sound pattern of English*. New York: Harper & Row.

Compton, A. (1970). Generative studies of children's phonological disorders. *Journal of Speech and Hearing Disorders, 35,* 315–339.

Cooper, R. (1985). The method of meaningful contrasts. In P. W. Newman, N. A. Creaghead, & W. A. Secord (Eds.), *Assessment and remediation of articulatory and phonological disorders*. Columbus, OH: Merrill.

Costello, J. (1975). Articulation instruction based on distinctive features theory. *Language, Speech and Hearing Services in Schools, 6,* 61–71.

Costello, J., & Bosler, S. (1976). Generalization and articulation instruction. *Journal of Speech and Hearing Disorders, 35,* 344–353.

Costello, J., & Onstine, J. (1976). The modification of multiple articulation errors based on distinctive feature theory. *Journal of Speech and Hearing Disorders, 41,* 199–215.

Dinnsen, D. A., & Elbert, M. (1984). On the relationship between phonology and learning. In M. Elbert, D. A. Dinnsen, & G. Weismer (Eds.), *Phonological theory and the misarticulating child* (ASHA Monograph no. 22). Rockville, MD: American Speech-Language-Hearing Association.

Dunn, C. (1983). A framework for generalization in disordered phonology. *Journal of Childhood Communication Disorders, 7,* 46–58.

Dunn, C., & Till, J. A. (1982). Morphophonemic rule learning in normal and articulation-disordered children. *Journal of Speech and Hearing Research, 25,* 322–332.

Edwards, M. L. (1983). Selection criteria for developing therapy goals. *Journal of Childhood Communication Disorders, 7,* 36–45.

Edwards, M. L., & Bernhardt, B. (1973). *Phonological analyses of the speech of four children with language disorders*. Unpublished paper, Stanford University, Palo Alto.

Elbert, M. (1983). A case of phonological acquisition. *Topics in Language Disorders, 3,* 1–9.

Elbert, M., and Gierut, J. (1986). *Handbook of clinical phonology: Approaches to assessment and treatment*. San Diego: College Hill Press.

Elbert, M., Rockman, B., & Saltzman, D. (1980). *Contrasts: The use of minimal pairs in articulation training*. Austin, TX: Exceptional Resources.

Elbert, M., Rockman, B., & Saltzman, D. (1982). *The source book: A phonemic guide to monosyllabic English words*. Austin, TX: Exceptional Resources.

Elbert, M. A., Shelton, R., & Arndt, W. (1967). A task for evaluation of articulation change: I. Development of methodology. *Journal of Speech and Hearing Research, 10,* 281–288.

Fokes, J. (1982). Problems confronting the theorist and practitioner in child phonology. In M. Crary (Ed.), *Phonological intervention: Concepts and procedures*. San Diego: College Hill Press.

Gierut, J. A., Elbert M., & Dinnsen, D. A. (1987). A functional analysis of phonological knowledge and generalization learning in misarticulating children. *Journal of Speech and Hearing Research, 30,* 462–479.

Griffith, F. A., Irwin, J. V., & Weston, A. J. (1980). A historical overview and critical assessment of the paired-stimuli technique for the modification of articulatory disorders. In W. D. Wolfe & D. J. Goulding (Eds.), *Articulation and learning*. Springfield, IL: Charles C. Thomas.

Gross, G. H., St. Louis, K. O., Ruscello, D. M., & Hull, F. M. (1985). Language abilities of articulatory-disordered school children with multiple or residual errors. *Language, Speech and Hearing Services in Schools, 16,* 171–186.

Grunwell, P. (1982). *Clinical phonology*. Rockville, MD: Aspen Systems.

Grunwell, P. (1983). Phonological development in phonological disability. *Topics in Language Disorders, 3,* 62–76.

Grunwell, P. (1985). *Phonological assessment of child speech*. San Diego: College Hill Press.

Hodson, B. W. (1980). *The assessment of phonological processes*. Danville, IL: Interstate.

Hodson, B. W. (1982). Remediation of speech patterns associated with low levels of phonological performance. In M. Crary (Ed.), *Phonological intervention: Concepts and procedures*. San Diego: College Hill Press.

Hodson, B. W., Chin, L., Redmond, B., & Simpson, R. (1983). Phonological evaluation and remediation of speech deviations of a child with a repaired cleft palate: A case study. *Journal of Speech and Hearing Disorders, 48,* 93–97.

Hodson, B. W., & Paden, E. (1983). *Targeting intelligible speech*. San Diego: College Hill Press.

Ingram, D. (1976). *Phonological disability in children*. New York: Elsevier.

Ingram, D. (1981). *Procedures for the phonological analysis of children's language*. Baltimore: University Park Press.

Jakobson, R. (1968). Child language, aphasia and phonological universals. The Hague, The Netherlands: Mouton.

Leonard, L. B., Camarata, S., Schwartz, R. G., Chapman, K., & Messick, C. (1985). Homonymy and the voiced-voiceless distinction in the speech of children with specific language impairment. *Journal of Speech and Hearing Research, 28,* 215–224.

Lynch, J. I., Fox, D. R., & Brookshire, B. L. (1983). Phonological proficiency of two cleft palate toddlers with school-age follow-up. *Journal of Speech and Hearing Disorders, 48,* 274–285.

Marquardt, T., & Saxman, J. (1972). Language comprehension and auditory discrimination in articulation deficient kindergarten children. *Journal of Speech and Hearing Research, 15,* 382–390.

McMahon, K., Hodson, B. W., & Allen, E. (1983). Phonological analysis of cerebral palsied children's utterances. *Journal of Childhood Communication Disorders, 7,* 28–35.

McReynolds, L. V., & Bennett, S. (1972). Distinctive feature generalization in articulation training. *Journal of Speech and Hearing Disorders, 37,* 462–470.

McReynolds, L. V., & Elbert, M. (1981). Criteria for phonological process analysis. *Journal of Speech and Hearing Disorders, 46,* 197–204.

McReynolds, L. V., Engmann, D., & Dimmitt, K. (1974). Markedness theory and articulation errors. *Journal of Speech and Hearing Disorders, 39,* 93–103.

Menyuk, P. (1964). Comparison of grammar of children with functionally deviant and normal speech. *Journal of Speech and Hearing Research, 7,* 105–108.

Oller, D. K., & Eilers, R. E. (1975). Phonetic expectation and transcription validity. *Phonetica, 31,* 288–304.

Panagos, J. M. (1974). Persistence of the open syllable reinterpreted as a symptom of language disorder. *Journal of Speech and Hearing Disorders, 39,* 23–31.

Parker, F. (1976). Distinctive features in speech pathology: Phonology or phonemics? *Journal of Speech and Hearing Disorders, 41,* 23–29.

Paul, R., & Shriberg, L. D. (1982). Associations between phonology and syntax in speech-delayed children. *Journal of Speech and Hearing Research, 25,* 536–546.

Pollack, K. E. (1983). Individual preferences: Case study of a phonologically delayed child. *Topics in Language Disorders, 3,* 10–23.

Pollack, E., & Rees, N. (1972). Disorders of articulation: Some clinical applications of distinctive feature theory. *Journal of Speech and Hearing Disorders, 37,* 451–461.

Powell, J., & McReynolds, L. (1969). A procedure for testing position generalization from articulation training. *Journal of Speech and Hearing Research, 12,* 629–645.

Ruder, K. F., & Bunce, B. H. (1981). Articulation therapy using distinctive feature analysis to structure the training program: Two case studies. *Journal of Speech and Hearing Disorders, 46,* 59–65.

Ruscello, D. M. (1975). The importance of word position in articulation therapy. *Language, Speech and Hearing Services in Schools, 6,* 190–195.

Saxman, J. H., & Miller, J. F. (1973). Short term memory and language skills in articulation deficient children. *Journal of Speech and Hearing Research, 16,* 721–730.

Schwartz, R. G., Leonard, L. B., Folger, M. K., & Wilcox, M. J. (1980). Early phonological behavior in normal-speaking and language disordered children: Evidence for a synergistic view of linguistic disorders. *Journal of Speech and Hearing Disorders, 45,* 357–377.

Shriberg, L. D., & Kwiatkowski, J. (1980). *Natural process analysis.* New York: Wiley.

Singh, S., Hayden, M. E., & Toombs, M. S. (1981). The role of distinctive features in articulation errors. *Journal of Speech and Hearing Disorders, 46,* 174–183.

Singh, S., & Polen, S. (1972). The use of a distinctive feature model in speech pathology. *Acta Symbolica, 3,* 17–25.

Singh, S., & Singh, K. (1976). *Distinctive features: Principles and practices.* Baltimore: University Park Press.

Smit, A. B., & Bernthal, J. E. (1983). Performance of articulation-disordered children on language and perception measures. *Journal of Speech and Hearing Research, 26,* 124–136.

Toombs, M. S., Singh, S., & Hayden, M. E. (1981). Markedness of features in the articulatory substitutions of children. *Journal of Speech and Hearing Disorders, 46,* 184–190.

Tyler, A. A., Edwards, M. L., & Saxman, J. H. (1987). Application of two phonologically based treatment procedures. *Journal of Speech and Hearing Disorders, 52,* 393–409.

Van Riper, C. (1978). *Speech correction: Principles and methods* (6th ed.). Englewood Cliffs, NJ: Prentice-Hall.

Walsh, H. H. (1974). On certain practical inadequacies of distinctive feature systems. *Journal of Speech and Hearing Disorders, 39,* 32–43.

Weiner, F. F. (1979). *Phonological process analysis.* Baltimore: University Park Press.

Weiner, F. F. (1981a). Systematic sound preference as a characteristic of phonological disability. *Journal of Speech and Hearing Disorders, 46,* 281–286.

Weiner, F. F. (1981b). Treatment of phonological disability using the method of meaningful minimal contrast: Two case studies. *Journal of Speech and Hearing Disorders, 46,* 97–103.

Weiner, F. F., & Bankson, N. (1978). Teaching features. *Language, Speech and Hearing Services in Schools, 9,* 29–34.

Weston, A., & Irwin, J. (1971). Use of paired stimuli in modification of articulation. *Perceptual and Motor Skills, 32,* 947–957.

Winitz, H., & Bellerose, B. (1978). Interference and the persistence of articulatory responses. *Journal of Speech and Hearing Research, 21,* 715–721.

Young, E. C. (1987). The effects of treatment of consonant cluster and weak syllable reduction processes in misarticulating children. *Language, Speech and Hearing Services in Schools, 18,* 23–33.

CHAPTER 8 Pragmatic Considerations in Treatment: Communication-Centered Instruction

Pragmatics deals with the use of language in social and communicative contexts. Thus a procedure that treats articulatory and phonological disorders in a social and communicative context is a pragmatic approach. Communication-centered instruction (CCI) is just such an approach. CCI consists of practicing speech sounds in prosocial, communicative activities in which correct responses are reinforced by natural consequences. For example, an activity used by one communication-oriented school clinician was a plastic bubble basketball game. The players pulled a plunger, which shot the ball into one of several concentric circles to score 2, 4, 6, 8, or 10. Those who had an /r/ deviation said, "I want a turn"; if the problem was /ʃ/, the child said, "I want to shoot"; whatever the target sound, the response gave the child a chance to practice. Keeping score also provided opportunities for children in the group to use responses that fit their articulation needs; for example, "My score is six" for /s/ or /r/ problems or "Last time my score was five" for /l/, /r/, or /v/ problems.

Gordon M. Low, Ph.D., is a professor emeritus of communication disorders in the Department of Educational Psychology at Brigham Young University, Provo, Utah. Parley W. Newman coauthored Chapters 2 and 4 of this text. Mildred T. Ravsten is assistant professor of educational psychology and member of the core faculty of the Comprehensive Clinic at Brigham Young University, Provo, Utah.

The clinician made this game a privilege. It was used only briefly in each lesson; thus it remained an activity of high interest. On occasion, the children played in the school gymnasium with a real ball and backboard. Some also played basketball in their neighborhoods; hence the activity gave useful rehearsal for real-life speech and resulted in significant articulation improvement, not only during therapy but in daily communication as well.

This communication-centered activity illustrates essential conditions of language pragmatics as the context within which speech articulation may most efficiently be improved. In a relatively early study of a communication-centered approach to articulation therapy, a total of 84 mentally retarded children were studied. Of these, 30 received communication-centered therapy; 16 received traditional therapy; and 38 received no therapy as a control group. The communication-centered group made significantly greater improvement (Lassers & Low, 1960).

CCI has been attempted in some form or other for many years. Early efforts to embed articulation improvement in a pragmatic or communication-centered context include those of Backus and Dunn (1947), Backus and Beasley (1951), and Low, Crerar, and Lassers (1959). More recently Wulz, Hall, and Klein (1983) described similar procedures for home-centered communication training.

CCI is effective in the home and in both individual and group instruction in the clinic. However, it is especially useful in school programs of articulation and language treatment where group instruction is a common practice. Instructing clients in a group provides the ideal opportunity to develop a pragmatic, communicative learning situation. Individual CCI is effective as clinician and client or parent and child communicate with each other, with puppets or dolls, etc., but communication among a group of peers in natural communicative activities is the ideal situation.

Increased emphasis on communication pragmatics has given new impetus to CCI, not only for the improvement of phonological aspects of language but in the acquisition of all aspects of language and in all other communication-based learning. In the interest of explaining CCI in terms of contemporary principles of learning, pragmatics, and other theories of human behavior, a brief rationale is presented for the kind of communication-centered instruction we have been using and refining since 1959. Further discussion of principles of pragmatic or communication-centered instruction follows in subsequent sections.

RATIONALE FOR COMMUNICATION-CENTERED (PRAGMATIC) INSTRUCTION

"Communication is the social matrix of psychiatry," according to Ruesch and Bateson (1951). They further suggest that communication is the "one single system for the understanding of the multiple aspects of human behavior" (p. 5).

Validation for this position is found in (a) the interactive conceptions of child development of Piaget (1952a, 1952b) and others (Bruner, 1966, 1975; Sharan, 1980); (b) the interactive concept of language acquisition (Snow, Midkiff-Borunda, Small, & Proctor, 1984); (c) the concepts of schemata (Piaget, 1952a; Rumelhart, 1980) and scripts (Minsky, 1975; Nelson, 1981); (d) the logical representation of learning as sign behavior, of which language is the chief example (Osgood, 1957); (e) the coincidence of the problems, instructional approaches, and disciplines of learning disabilities and communication disorders (Lerner, 1981); (f) the acknowledgment by language specialists that communication, i.e., the pragmatic situation in which language is used and has meaning, is the natural and ideal context for language acquisition (Bloom & Lahey, 1978; Holland, 1975; Muma, 1978; Rees, 1978), and "the ultimate goal of any language therapy for language disordered children" (Lucas, 1980, p. 223); (g) the apparent relationship of communicative intent and phonological production, as suggested by Leonard's (1971) finding that the speech of a 6-year-old child was characterized by more deviant articulations of /z/ in utterances carrying the least information, and Menyuk's (1980) finding that children with misarticulations, when attempting to communicate information that is important to them, modify their utterance so that it more closely approximates normal speech.

These validations appear to be ample justification for Ruesch and Bateson's (1951) view about the place of communication in relation to other aspects of human behavior. We also believe that they justify a companion premise to Ruesch and Bateson's assumption that "communication is the social matrix of psychiatry," namely, that *communication is the matrix of human learning.* We believe that optimum learning takes place only under optimum communicative conditions, with the implication that "language is acquired in a social context, through a process made possible by the communication that occurs during social interaction" (Snow et al., 1984, p. 72). Psycholinguistic research in the 1970s led us to the awareness of pragmatics, i.e., the functional use of language in a context. Phonology deals with the units that make up a language; thus a CCI approach treats phonological disorders with consideration for the pragmatics, or the use of sounds, in conversation.

PRINCIPLES OF COMMUNICATION-CENTERED INSTRUCTION

Communication-centered instruction (CCI) for articulation improvement generally consists of instruction and practice of speech articulation in oral communicative interchange among two or more people. We must look to this communicative interchange in our efforts to effect remediation of articulation disorders. CCI suggests that therapy should address the broader context of communication (Kemp, 1983; Spinelli & Terrell, 1984) with emphasis on pragmatics or the social use of language. All language is, after all, pragmatically based (Bates, 1976). CCI uses the pragmatics of communication by focusing not on the isolated phoneme but on the phoneme in a word that is part of a socially useful communicative utterance. Thus the phoneme is practiced in the context in which it will be used in real life. CCI does not postpone the carryover, or generalization, stage of usual speech therapy. Instead, CCI uses procedures of carryover during each instructional period and thus also during the normal communication experiences the client has between instructional sessions.

Principles of CCI can be stated in various ways. The first CCI principle will be stated in terms of communication and learning as a system. *System* here refers to the interdependence of all processes and events in the sequence of receiving and sending messages, so that a disturbance at any point can affect other points in the system. Because a learning formula that includes *stimulus, response,* and *reinforcement* has already been explained (chapter 6), other CCI principles will be described under these three headings.

Principles Related to Communication-Learning as a System

A system instructional approach should be used to ensure that the interdependent processes of communication-learning, in which speech articulation, language, and other communication behavior are embedded, are used to enhance improvement of communication skills, including speech articulation.

This principle can be explained using a variety of theories and their terminology. The first explanation uses *communication-learning* terms, the second uses *linguistic* terms, the third uses terms from *cognitive theory*. All three explanations imply that a communicative context provides the optimum set of conditions for learning language, including speech articulation.

Communication-Learning. In speaking, a person uses not only speech articulation movements but, at the same time, a highly complex system of interdependent communication-learning processes. Some of these processes are *intrapersonal,* including the receptive, organizational, and output processes of communication. Some are *interpersonal,* including the relationships of those communicative and other pragmatic features of a communicative interchange.

The importance of intrapersonal processes in speech production has been recognized for many years. An example is ear training (sensory-perceptual training). It is assumed that auditory precepts serve as patterns for motor production of speech sounds, and auditory feedback serves as a monitor in guiding speech production to those patterns (Winitz, 1969). At the same time, tactile-kinesthetic monitoring also accompanies and guides the neuromotor patterning that determines movement of the articulatory mechanism. But this is only the phonetic or articulatory aspect of speech production. In addition to dependence on the peripheral processes of perception, speech sound production depends on the central processes of cognition. Were it not so, speech sounds would be phonetic utterances, not phonemic signs. Meaningful speech involves utterance of phonemes chained to produce morphemes, words, and sentences having appropriate language structure, all of which are selected through cognitive processes to express ideas or concepts.

In addition to the influence of cognitive and language elements, interpersonal social and affective elements exert their influence on speech production. How those communicating feel about each other, what previous experiences they have had with each other, their role expectations, etc., also influence speech articulation as well as other elements of language expression (Leonard, 1971; Menyuk, 1980).

This complex of communication elements and communicative relationships is the context of speech articulation. All these elements are associated with speech sound production. All influence how speech sounds will be produced as well as what language is chosen and what ideas are formulated to be expressed. Thus, when efforts are made to improve production of a particular speech sound, consideration must be given to the influence of these associated cues on articulation of the sound. A system approach is required that takes into account the interdependence of intrapersonal and interpersonal processes of communication. Using communication as the matrix for learning communication behavior fulfills this requirement.

In CCI the communicative interchange of the client with others provides the communicative context within which these elements—words, language, communicative intentions, communicative relationships, etc.—are most naturally associated with the target speech sound. With this provision, the client learns a set of natural language associations, along with the target sound, in a communicative setting. When other natural language opportunities occur in the client's daily life, this set of associations prompts the use of the communicatively learned target sound. On the other hand, having learned the target sound in a noncommunicative setting, the client may have to unlearn a set of unnatural associations in order to generalize her improved articulation to real-life communication.

This explanation of the principle of speech learning in a communicative context may become clearer when stated in terms of several other contemporary concepts related to human communication: communication pragmatics, schema, and scripts.

Communication Pragmatics. As language specialists extended their purview from syntactic elements of language to include semantic language features, it became inevitable that attention would be given to the context within which language is used, for without considering context, language meaning—its semantics—cannot be fully understood (Arwood, 1983). This context is the communicative interchange between two or more people—the act of communication. The term *pragmatics* has been used to designate the conditions of a communicative interchange, including the language itself, that determine the use and significance of a language unit. It has to do with the *intent, use,* and *effects* of language rather than with the dictionary definition (semantics) of a language unit or of its grammatic or morphologic (syntactic) structure.

A major implication of pragmatic theory for treatment of articulation disorders is that all language processes, including phonological, are naturally developed in the pragmatic context of communicative interaction. Theoretically, then, *target speech sounds are learned best in a remediation program that takes into account pragmatic features of the language in which speech sounds are naturally developed.* CCI provides a learning situation that is communicative in nature; thus the *intentions* of the client and of those with whom she interacts are communicative in nature, the language being practiced is *used* in communicative ways, and the result of the client's communicative efforts are natural communicative *effects.* For example, clients make requests, instruct others, give information, etc. As they communicate they use appropriate language that contains the target sound being learned. The pragmatic context for improving speech sounds is the communicative context that, as already explained, provides for natural association of the target sound with other elements of the pragmatic situation so that in subsequent communicative situations the newly learned target sound is naturally evoked.

Schemata and Scripts. The use of Bartlett's (1932), Piaget's (1952a), and Rumelhart's (1980) concepts of schemata in describing language acquisition is another way of illustrating the essential significance of communication in treatment of language disorders and articulation.

Schemata are structured memories of related perceptual, conceptual, social, emotional, and other elements of information; they are derived from interactions with the environment and change their structure in the ongoing experience in which they are used (Piaget, 1952a). For example, young children may develop a perceptual schema of *dog* that they use to classify all four-footed animals until they experience some differences between dog and cat. They then change their schema of dog and develop a new schema for *cat*.

Language, of course, becomes associated with the many perceptual, conceptual, social, and emotional elements of a schema. In fact, language itself becomes a set of phonemic, syntactic, semantic, and pragmatic features of schemata. Schemata in communicative interchange include elements of past communicative experiences and elements of the present communicative experience including the intentions of the communicants, their expectations of each other, the total physical setting, the reactions of the communicants to the situation, to each other, and to the communicated messages, etc. Snyder and Downey (1983) suggest: ''The use of schemata in processing is integral to the development and use of pragmatics. Appropriate interpretation and use of the contextual elements of any communicative interaction requires an elegant system of flexible and efficient schemata'' (p. 83).

Among the important insights provided by the theory of schemata in cognitive development is the explanation of the difficulty learners have in generalizing from one situation to another. For example, if a client's improved articulation is learned in relation to a schema in which *imitating* a target speech sound is a major element, the client may not produce the newly learned speech sound when the schema required is one of *communicating* ideas, even though words containing the target sound are part of the dialogue. A further explanation of this failure to generalize is described in a

subsequent section on communicative stimulus conditions.

Scripts are schemata in which a series of actions or events occur; for example, buying something in which asking is involved. This activity consists of a sequence of actions and expressions that become a schema for use in other similar situations, such as asking for a certain kind of paper in a stationery store. When language is involved in the schema, it becomes a predictable part of the experience when the schema is used. The language therefore becomes a useful vehicle for improving the articulation of a speech sound contained in that language. Those schemata, including the language used, that occur in natural communicative situations become the natural facilitators for learning all aspects of language including speech production.

Following are descriptions of three principles of CCI stated in the familiar learning terms of stimulus, response, and reinforcement. Because these principles are based on the assumption that both learning and communication are system processes, the reader may expect that each of these learning conditions will be described in terms of their place in a pragmatic context.

Principles of Communicative Stimulus

The practice situation should be like the performance situation.

The principles regarding stimulus conditions outlined in chapter 6 are important considerations in communication-centered instruction. Stimulus conditions in learning generally include all those elements of the learning situation or schemata of which the learner is aware. Hence, these conditions constitute a context or complex of stimuli, not just a single stimulus. As clinicians, we may think that we are offering a client a single stimulus when we ask her to imitate a particular speech sound. The fact is that the speech sound presented for imitation is only part of the total context. Other elements in the stimulus complex are the clinician's dress, grooming, looks, mannerisms, gestures, etc.; the instructions the clinician gives the client; the seating arrangement; the room situation; the expectations both the clinician and the client have developed in prior speech-imitation episodes; the generality of client-clinician relationship; and other elements of the situation that may justly be called the *pragmatic elements of interpersonal exchange*.

Kemp (1983) supports this concept that the traditional view of context needs to be broadened to include the pragmatic elements necessary for the acquisition of social, affective, and cognitive behaviors. Although his conclusion relates specifically to language, it appears relevant to articulation learning because there appears to be no real use for articulation outside of language and communication.

The goal of CCI is to assist the client in developing schemata, scripts, and frames that provide information not only about correct phoneme production but also about expectations of given situations and how to respond appropriately. The real-life activities or scripts of CCI provide the client with "a framework of shared knowledge about events" (Nelson, 1981) with roles, dialogue, and sequelae of events that enable clients to interpret contextual cues and respond with appropriate phrases and sentences once they are in their own natural environment.

An important implication of context learning is that what is learned by the client is not only the speech sound, but its association with all other elements of the stimulus complex or schema. Herein lies an important explanation of the too-frequent failure of carryover of new speech learning to the client's daily speech usage. One possible reason for this failure of generalization is the difference between the clinic situation and the client's communicative world (Costello, 1983). This explanation is found in studies of learning transfer, learning retention, and carryover.

Some years ago, Osgood (1949) concluded that "where stimuli are varied and responses are func-tionally identical, positive transfer and retroactive facilitation are obtained, the magnitude of both increasing as the similarity among the stimulus members increases" (p. 135). Other similar educational principles are stated by Ellis (1965): (a) "Transfer of training is greatest when the training conditions are highly similar to those of the ultimate testing conditions," and (b) "When a task requires the learner to make the same response to new but similar stimuli, positive transfer increases with increasing stimulus similarity" (pp. 72–73). Hulse, Deese, and Egeth (1975) explain problems of learning carryover as "cue-dependent forgetting." They suggest that "when we forget something, it does not necessarily mean that the memory trace is lost; it may merely be inaccessible because the current context does not permit retrieval schemes that are congruent with the encoding schemes employed at the time of original learning" (p. 359).

One of the authors of this chapter (GML) recalls a vivid experience as a student clinician with an aphasic client whose speech was unintelligible jargon even after numerous careful attempts at imitation. Together they worked on words that appeared to have some communicative use to the client, including the words "come in." Finally, out of desperation, and with a subsequent insight that has remained primary in this clinician's understanding of remedial instruction, the clinician had the client rehearse the words "come in" in preparation for the daily visits of her friends. She grumbled as she forced herself out of her chair in response to the housekeeper's knock on the door. The clinician asked her to repeat the words "come in" before she crossed the room to the door. She said /ʃemba/, /ʃemba/, but when she took hold of the doorknob and pulled the door open, a smile came over her face and she said, /kʌm ɪn/ with perfectly acceptable articulation.

Many clinicians have had this same kind of experience with aphasic and other clients and have realized that clients may demonstrate remarkable success when the stimulus conditions of the testing or performance situation are similar to those of the original learning situation. To use an earlier explanation, these instances of remarkable recall occur because the performance situation permits ''retrieval schemes that are congruent with the encoding schemes employed at the time of original learning'' (Hulse, Deese, & Egeth, 1975, p. 359).

From this rationale we infer the principle of CCI related to stimulus context that *the practice situation should be similar to the performance situation* (Costello, 1983; Spinelli & Terrell, 1984). Implied in this principle is the concept of *rehearsal*, in which speech practice simulates daily communication much more than does imitative speech practice. Conditions of clients' daily communication often consist of communicative interaction with other individuals and groups in various activities, including classroom instruction, play at home and school, family activities, encounters with the mail carrier and other community helpers, etc. Practice situations simulate these settings and activities, most often in group instruction where pragmatic skills are so vital. An illustration of the principle as applied to improvement of articulation follows.

Ms. Jones, a speech clinician, engages in a non-communication-centered instructional program for

improvement of Gary's /t/k/ substitutions. She has the child practice /k/ in various ways, including repeating a list of /k/-words, such as *car, cake, call, cat, coat, come, pick, tack,* and *talk*. With almost 100% /k/ accuracy in the word list in the clinic, the clinician is pleased to go on to carryover or generalization activities. She next practices the /k/ in word combinations including such sentences as *Pick a number, Talk to the parrot, Come in, Call the cat,* again achieving a high degree of /k/ accuracy. Then Ms. Jones has occasion to visit Gary's home. She knocks on the door. Gary opens it and says /tʌmɪn/. Ms. Jones is so discouraged she has thoughts of leaving the field of speech-language pathology.

Why has this well-learned correct use of /k/ in the clinic not generalized to the home situation? Figures 8.1 and 8.2 illustrate the stimulus complex explanation of the problem. In imitative speech practice (Figure 8.1a), the stimulus cues include a,

Clinic

FIGURE 8.1a
Stimulus cues in practice situation: (a) clinician, (b) child, (c) come, (d) word list, (e) clinician seated, (f) child seated, (g) chairs.

Home

FIGURE 8.1b
Stimulus cues in performance situation: (a) clinician, (b) child, (c) come, (h) clinician standing, (i) child standing, (j) door, (k) reaching for door.

224
     PART TWO
   General Considerations in Treatment

b, c, d, e, f, g, whereas in the life performance situation (Figure 8.1b), the stimulus complex consists of the cues a, b, c, h, i, j, k.

To increase the probability of carryover, the clinician should make the practice situation like the performance situation, which would result in the conditions of Figures 8.2a and 8.2b. In the CCI situation (Figure 8.2a), the stimulus cues are a, b, c, h, i, j, k, and in the life performance situation (Figure 8.2b), they are essentially the same.

On the basis of this similarity of stimulus cues in practice and real life, it is safe to predict that a correct utterance in the therapy session will carry over to correct production in the classroom and at home. Of course, making the practice and performance conditions alike is best achieved by making the clinic situation like the client's daily life, not trying to make the client's daily life like the clinic. It is much easier and more effective to ask the

family to help the client at home or the teacher to help in the classroom if the help they are expected to give fits the client's daily communication opportunities, instead of involving them in contrived speech practice totally unrelated to family or classroom communication activities.

Principles of Communicative Response

The response should (1) include the targeted phoneme in a communicative utterance, (2) be at the child's level of functioning, (3) be useful to the client and frequently occurring in the child's daily communication, and (4) be powerful in controlling the environment.

Having established a context for therapy that is similar to the natural environment, the clinician looks to the targeted phoneme to determine what kind of practice materials should be used to help clients improve their articulation.

Clinic

FIGURE 8.2a
Stimulus cues in practice situation: (a) clinician, (b) child, (c) come, (h) clinician standing, (i) child standing, (j) door, (k) reaching for door.

Home

FIGURE 8.2b
Stimulus cues in performance situation: (a) clinician, (b) child, (c) come, (h) clinician standing, (i) child standing, (j) door, (k) reaching for door.

Target Phoneme in a Communicative Context. More often than not spoken words consist of several speech sounds. The clinician using a CCI approach must look then at (a) the relation of the error speech sound to the rest of the practice word in which it is uttered and (b) the relation of the practice word to the client's lexicon and communicative reality. Pragmatics, of course, requires that practice of the target speech sound be done in words used in a communicative utterance. This is a chief feature of CCI. At the same time, the experience of the authors of this chapter is that articulation improvement can be hastened through practicing speech sounds in isolation from the words, sentences, communicative intentions, and communicative interactions in which they may subsequently be used, providing that practice of isolated speech sounds is done only as part of the whole learning experience. CCI includes what may be called *whole-part-whole practice* (Backus & Beasley, 1951).

In whole-part-whole procedures, *whole practice* consists of using the target sound in real communication. The whole context includes all the elements of the communicative situation—the pragmatic elements, the semantic, syntactic, and morphological elements, the schemata of the communicative episode—with which the target sound is associated. *Part practice* is practice of the target sound apart from the communicative use of the language within which the sound is embedded. Both whole and part practice are used in a single therapy session in CCI. Part practice of a specific speech sound usually is not necessary after a few periods of instruction. Whole-part-whole procedures may be used in group or individual instruction.

The key to effective use of such part practice is to precede and follow it with whole practice, that is, the practice of the target sound in the whole pragmatic schema of communication-centered activities, including the appropriate language response. Thus, in a communicative game situation where a child says, "I want a turn" in order to improve her /r/, the /r/ may be practiced in isolation, in syllables, or in words and phrases in a noncommunicative way. The whole practice—the

communicative interchange of the game—is interrupted for a few moments for part practice of the target sound. Then, even though completely accurate production is not achieved, whole practice is resumed by continuing the game with its communicative response, or by engaging in other similar activities.

Part practice of the targeted phoneme may utilize any of a number of techniques, some as simple as modeling and imitation. Others that are more structured might include multiple phoneme (chapter 11), paired stimuli, distinctive feature (chapter 14), etc. Any approach that is most helpful with the individual client can be effective in the part practice as long as the sound and word are also practiced in communicative discourse in each therapy session and the phoneme is learned as part of that schema or script to facilitate carryover into the client's daily communication.

Client's Level of Functioning. An additional feature of communicative response is that of requiring a response whose difficulty is a challenge to the learner but not so difficult as to be discouraging. In other words, *the response should be at the client's level of functioning.*

Obviously, if a client has deviant articulation, she usually will not be able to produce the sound accurately in conversation, even when given a model to imitate. Often, however, after two or three attempts to say the sound correctly in a word, a client may improve the error sound ever so slightly and begin to use the improved sound in communication and communication practice. Both Leonard (1971) and Menyuk (1980) found that a child tried to make her articulation clearer in a communicatively important situation.

One might believe that permitting the client to speak the target sound incorrectly in conversation may interfere with the eventual acquisition of the correct sound. Our experience has demonstrated otherwise, as might be expected in the light of the process of normal speech-sound development in children. Ingram (1976), in his discussion of speech-articulation therapy, suggests that training in gradual acquisition of a sound is preferred. He criticizes therapy in which the goal is correct production as compared with the adult model. He refers to this as the "fell-swoop principle" and argues that the transition from the child's utterance to adult pronunciation in one step is based on an unjustified assumption. He gives several reasons why this approach is unsound, and he proposes adoption of the "gradualness principle" based on the assumption that a child will progress more rapidly to the next stage of development than to one several stages ahead. He even suggests that a fell-swoop approach may actually retard development.

As mentioned in chapter 4 on assessment, Olmsted (1971) too, in his analysis of the speech of 100 children ranging in age from 15 to 54 months, found that children do not acquire individual speech sounds suddenly, but gradually over time, with extended periods during which any particular sound is produced both correctly and incorrectly. There are gradual increases in the percentage of successes and decreases in the relative numbers of errors. Coexistence of success and error, then, is the most frequent pattern of developing use of phones.

An explanation can also be given that is consistent with what is known about learning. First of all, in non-communication-centered articulation therapy, the client may continue to use the incorrect sound in daily communication while learning to produce the sound correctly in therapy. Surely this can be at least as harmful as practicing a gradually improving but not completely accurate speech sound. Secondly, we believe that the conditions of successive approximation are as much at work in this gradual improvement, while the client actually uses his newly developing sound, as they are in those other shaping procedures in which the client must be able to produce the sound correctly before being allowed to use it in communication.

Useful and Frequently Occurring. An important condition of communicative response is that the response should be *useful* to the learner, occurring frequently in her daily communication. Because words are the natural contexts of articulated speech sounds, practice words used in articulation improvement should be words that are communicatively useful to the client. Snow et al. (1984) state that "the value of an utterance lies in its usefulness to the child" and that the clinician needs to select material that will help the child be a more effective communicator. Obviously, this is not a very different requirement from that of providing a natural, real-life learning context for response practice. However, in this instance, the response as well as the stimulus is drawn from the client's daily life. Coupling real-life responses with real-life communicative stimulus conditions ensures maximum carryover of the newly acquired speech sound that is embedded in the context of a frequently recurring word. Indeed, it ensures natural reinforcement of the generalized new behavior outside the clinic even though the clinician is not present, thus extending the therapy experience to the daily life of the client.

Communicatively Powerful. The response that is chosen in CCI should have one other quality. To be appropriately communicative in nature, *the response should be communicatively powerful*. That is, the result of the utterance should in one way or another be satisfying to the person who speaks it. The fact is that most responses used in communication are communicatively powerful, but some are more powerful than others. The literature on language acquisition is replete with observations and explanations of the kinds of communicative responses children develop. Antinucci and Parisi (1975) suggest that language may be "descriptive" on the one hand and "requestive" on the other or, as Snyder (1975) suggests, "declarative" and "imperative." The implication of these classifications is that declaring and describing are sharing acts and may require less reaction than requesting and commanding. "Manding" (Skinner, 1957) or commanding or requesting may be more powerful than naming and thus more useful in therapy.

In relation to articulation improvement, the purpose in choosing responses that have power is not only to fulfill the client's need for successful communicative interaction, as important as that may be, but also to establish a condition of learning that no instruction should overlook, and that is a meaningful and satisfying consequence of the practice response. Obviously, a powerful response is one that causes something to happen. As we shall see in the next section on reinforcement, the degree of reinforcement of a communicative consequence is directly related to the degree of the communicative response.

In pragmatic activities for children, such responses as "May I have a _____?" "What do you want?" "Ready, aim, fire." "May I look?" "Sit down." "I want to run." "I want the red one." are chosen to provide communicatively powerful responses in which target speech sounds may be practiced. These responses are rehearsed in activities that present the need for the client to say the response in order to obtain the communicative result that the activity calls for.

One young first grader, who had been ridiculed by peers for his misarticulation of /r/, behaved in the classroom as a conversationally responsive but nonassertive child. We recall our efforts to get him to speak by setting up a Ping-Pong-ball cannon that required stepping heavily on a rubber bellows to shoot it. Each child in turn became (a) the retriever of the ball, (b) the marksman who aimed the cannon, (c) the one who jumped on the bellows, and finally (d) the commander who said, "Ready, aim, shoot." It was with considerable interest that the clinician and observers waited as Johnny took his turn to give the command. What could he do with peer expectations so high? He spoke, right on cue, and, having spoken in the group, continued to do so in subsequent therapy sessions. For Johnny, this was an experience in which his deviant /r/ was being improved in a pragmatic context. For other children with misarticulations of /r/ and /ɝ/, the response was also an opportunity for articulation practice in a communicatively powerful activity.

Principles of Communicative Reinforcement

Communicative reinforcement in communication-centered instruction is the fulfillment of the purpose of the communicative response.

Having argued that establishing communicative stimulus conditions and using communicative responses is highly advantageous in improving articulation, we introduce what should be a rather clinching conclusion to our case for communication-centered articulation therapy, i.e., *communicative reinforcement*. We have already referred to "mand"-type communicative language as having particular value as a vehicle in articulation improvement. It was pointed out that all communicative efforts are intended to influence others, but that some efforts are more demanding than others. Imperative language—i.e., requests and commands—has more power than describing or naming, so it is capable of more powerful reinforcement. Among its benefits is the natural, communicative reinforcement that follows mand responses in the home, school, and elsewhere in the absence of the clinician.

In a parent group in our clinic one day, we explained reinforcement in the learning formula. The following account was given to introduce the topic.

Mrs. Smith walked into her kitchen with an armful of laundry. She noticed Jimmy, her mentally retarded child, standing in front of the kitchen sink. Jimmy had never uttered anything that sounded like words. But today he said, "Wa, wa." Mrs. Smith dropped her jaw, and her laundry, and thought very quickly, "This is Jimmy's first word. What can I do to be sure he says it again? I know—reinforcement. I studied that in child psychology."

"Let's see. I could give him a token reinforcer—a tally mark on the bulletin board or a piece of candy. No, maybe I should let him choose from a reinforcement menu—a look at the kaleidoscope, a swing on the top bar of the bunk bed a chance to feed the fish. Oh, but how about using the probability principle? I could use the high-probability behavior (HPB) to reinforce the low-probability behavior (LPB). Hmm, the low-probability behavior (LPB) is saying "wa, wa"—but what is the HPB? Well, it could be his favorite mealtime activity: smearing peanut butter on the table. Oh, what to do?"

By this time the parents' worst fears were confirmed: These people at the university really are in their ivory tower.

"What would you do as parents to reinforce Jimmy's response?" we asked.

"Give him a drink of water," they replied in unison.

"Yes," we assured them, "the fulfillment of the purpose of Jimmy's communicative effort."

How strange that such a simple concept could be so distorted in the giant step from the shaping of pigeons' behavior to the reinforcement of human learning responses. The reinforcement aspects of this situation included controlling an adult, receiving the water upon requesting it, and the approbation of the mother.

PROCEDURES OF COMMUNICATION-CENTERED ARTICULATION THERAPY

Diagnosis in Communication-Centered Instruction

The usual initial procedure in improving most communication disorders is that of diagnosis with the intent of arriving at a prescription for improvement of the disorder. Diagnosis of articulation disorders may consist of several steps or phases, most of which are universally used by speech clinicians. Some diagnostic procedures, on the other hand, are specifically designed for use with a particular instructional approach. Some of these are described in chapter 4 and in such other reviews as

those by Darley (1979). CCI uses many of the usual procedures but adds some that are necessary for effective communication-centered instruction. Only these additional procedures are described in detail in this chapter.

Case History. Assessment of conditions relevant to CCI is approached as evaluation of the total communication system. Thus information about both the client and those who communicate with the client is relevant. In addition to this information usually assembled from case history interviews and referral reports, information is obtained that is particularly related to the conditions of stimulus, response, and reinforcement as defined in communication-centered articulation therapy. For example, with respect to communicative *stimulus* conditions, making the practice situation like the performance situation requires the clinician to know something about the client's performance situation—home, play, and school activities, particularly communication activities and opportunities. Parents are asked to report on the opportunities their child has for communication. This information may encourage the parents to arrange more communication experiences for the child at home, but it will also be useful to the clinician in planning to simulate the client's daily communication experiences. If the child attends school, similar information can be obtained from the child's teacher so the clinician can plan school-type activities that will be like those the child will experience with her own teacher and classmates.

In reviewing the home and school situations it is useful to obtain names of family members, classmates, friends, pets, etc., and information about the kinds of communicative *responses* the child has opportunity to use. There are specific expressions families, classmates, and teachers use, and it may be far more fruitful for the clinician to rehearse the client in commonly occurring responses expected at home and school than to require the parents and teacher to use responses that the clinician decides might be useful. The clinician's familiarity with curricula and textbooks at various grade levels is a decided advantage in understanding teacher information about daily communication responses used in classroom activities. Whether in group or individual instruction, the client benefits little from the use of words from articulation practice whose probability of occurring in home or school is less than optimal.

Parent and teacher information about the client's communication opportunities may also include information as to the opportunity for powerful *reinforcement*, i.e., for the client to use mand responses that make something happen, that influence someone else with direct observable consequences. There are frequent opportunities for use of such responses at the dinner table, in parent-child discussions, in play, in classroom participation, etc. The clinician needs to know about these in order to simulate like experiences.

If, in assessment of communicative stimulus, response, and reinforcement conditions in the home and school, the clinician finds these conditions to be inadequate, she may profitably train parents and teachers in arranging better communication circumstances for the client. We remember a mother who couldn't think of a way to involve her child in communicatively powerful experiences. Another mother said, ''You drive all the way to the clinic past many stop lights. Why don't you have Bobby tell you 'red-stop' and 'green-go'?'' Subsequent trips to the clinic were probably as beneficial to the mother and child as the daily clinic experience itself, both in mother-child relationships and language and articulation development.

Assessment. In CCI, assessment may include many traditional procedures for evaluating articulation, auditory processing, language, and other features of the communication system. In addition, because CCI is a system approach, assessments must be made of the various elements of the communication system, and their functioning within that total system, that are not usually included in articulation diagnosis.

From earlier descriptions of the communication-learning context in CCI, it should be apparent that evaluation related to articulation disorders must also include assessment of the communication-learning situation itself, both the client's

daily relationships in the home and school and in the therapy situation. Some of the factors that contribute to a child's articulation deviation are very likely in the relationships with his family and classmates. Certainly it is not unusual to find immaturities of speech articulation associated with the client's social-emotional immaturity, much of which may be attributed to the child's communication failures in the home and school.

One of the first diagnostic concerns in CCI is the degree of success and failure the client has in daily communication experiences in the home. Parents are asked to report on the family interactions when the child gets up in the morning, at the breakfast table, when getting off to school, at lunch time, during play with peers or family members, when speaking with father and mother, etc. Parents are helped to understand what constitutes a successful communication experience and also what characterizes a failure experience. They are then asked to report about their child in these terms.

Successful communication experiences for children include (a) the child's being able to speak spontaneously, make requests, help others, etc., and (b) parents and siblings giving the child encouragement to participate, showing approval, and providing for the child to take the lead.

Parent reports of their child's communication experience include instances of success as well as some negative experiences of communication interaction. Unfavorable sibling competition is often identified. Parent overindulgence, perfectionistic expectations, and other personally depreciating conditions come to light in this approach. Because the focus is on communication, not on what bad things mothers or fathers do or on the emotional status of the family, parents are more apt to approach these difficulties as problems in communication rather than as psychological threats to themselves as parents.

The total communication-learning system includes more than the client and the client's family. It also includes the clinician and other children with whom the client relates in therapy. Thus the system approach calls for evaluation of the communication-learning context in the clinic as well. This is somewhat unusual in speech therapy—to evaluate the learning situation as well as the learner's behavior. It leads to the peculiar notion that clinicians and what they do may not only be a solution to the client's problems but indeed may be part of the problem. We know of junior-high-aged children whose years of speech therapy have netted them little improvement of deviant /r/ and /s/ and a seriously negative attitude about their speech, themselves, school, and speech therapy in particular. We are reminded of the observations of Bateman (1974) and Cohen (1971) that poor teaching may be a major cause of poor learning. Bateman suggests that the term *teaching disabilities* be used instead of *learning disabilities* to emphasize the significance of poor teaching in children's learning problems. Because communicative interaction among learners and teachers is the context in which learning takes place, diagnosis in CCI must include assessment of the quality of that communicative interaction.

In CCI, the clinician designs and conducts a group activity in which there are opportunities for attending, imitating, cooperating, self-initiating, leading, and other pragmatic behaviors. The activity may be videotaped for later analysis or another observer may evaluate the children's communication performance and identify communication-learning needs of the individual or the group. We have found it helpful to use two rating scales, the Communication Competence Scale and the Developing Communication Competence Scale, which will be described under "Objectives" in the section on "Instructional Procedures in Communication-Centered Articulation Therapy."

Concurrent Diagnostic Teaching. One other aspect of diagnosis that deserves additional consideration is concurrent diagnostic teaching: *the adjustment of teaching objectives and procedures* that are suggested by information from concurrent, ongoing diagnosis.

The ideal concurrent-diagnostic-teaching situation is one in which diagnosis and teaching occur simultaneously, where teaching decisions are made from moment to moment depending on the present evaluation of client performance and awareness of the client's present need. For example, concurrent diagnostic teaching occurs each time a clinician hears a client's target sound and suggests a retrial. In treatment of articulation, CCI provides not only for monitoring articulation behavior and making appropriate adjustments in teaching the client correct sound production, it also provides for monitoring the language used and other features of the pragmatic context so it can be made optimally conducive to use of correct articulation in the client's communicative interaction with others. This total contextual monitoring provides the necessary database for guiding instruction toward effective and efficient articulation improvement, the procedures of which will be described later in this chapter.

Exit Evaluation. The ultimate measure in any instructional program—the dependent variable—is the learner's performance in the main task. In articulation therapy, the dependent variable is the client's correct use of the target sound in daily communication. The place to measure the client's production of corrected articulation thus becomes daily communication. Indexes to permanent improvement include performance on articulation tests, ability to read word lists or paragraphs, and performance in conversation in the clinical setting. A more sure index, however, is the client's performance in clinic activities that are highly similar to communication activities of the home and school. The best test is actual performance in communication with family and in classroom and playground activities. Training parents and teachers to evaluate the client's articulation accuracy makes it possible for them to provide useful information about the child's postinstruction articulation competence. Communication-centered articulation therapy would not be complete without confirmation of articulation improvement in the client's real-life communication.

Instructional Procedures in Communication-Centered Articulation Therapy

The several examples of communication-centered articulation therapy procedures sprinkled through earlier sections of this chapter illustrate relatively well the application of principles of CCI in articulation therapy. In this section additional examples are given and specific organizing and therapy techniques are described. The organization is probably presented best in the typical outline of a communication-centered therapy lesson plan.

Lesson Plan for Group Communication-Centered Instruction. The outline of a typical CCI group lesson plan includes objectives, activities, and recommendations, as represented in Table 8.1. These main features are described here and illustrated with references to a specific lesson theme, namely, *what-is-missing,* an activity that young children may experience at home and play and in prereading perceptual training at school.

Objectives. Consistent with the system nature of CCI, instruction is designed to take account of the

TABLE 8.1
Outline of a CCI Group Lesson Plan

Categories of objectives
  Communication competence
  Language
  Speech production
  Diagnostic

Activities
  Introduction
  Rehearsal
  Activity #1
  Activity #2
  Activity #3

Recommendations

various elements of the communication-learning system. Objectives reflect this system orientation, as seen in Table 8.1, where communication competence and the processes involved in the production of speech and language are represented.

Communicative competence objectives are a major consideration of the clinician in CCI. They have to do with establishing an optimum communicative-learning context in which pragmatic behaviors are encouraged and opportunities to improve a client's communicative competence are provided. That context should include *intrapersonal variables,* both psychological and cognitive, and *interpersonal variables,* both situational and participant (Spinelli & Terrell 1984). Before describing specific communication competence objectives, we will discuss briefly two rating scales that we have found useful.

For the past several years, we have studied client and clinician behaviors, particularly in relation to their communicative interaction. Our efforts resulted in the development of two rating scales: (1) the Communication Competence Scale (CCS) for assessing the clients' communication behaviors that are necessary for an optimum communication-learning context and (2) the Developing Communication Competence Scale (DCCS) for assessing clinician behaviors that encourage specific pupil behavior and that provide conditions necessary for optimum communication in CCI. The scales were refined through factor analysis of rating data. They are reproduced in Appendixes 8.1 and 8.2.

The CCS identifies the client behaviors that we found to be important pragmatically: (1) communication-learning readiness behaviors including attending, imitating, and cooperating; (2) communicative relationship behaviors including caring, helping, and sharing; and (3) communicative intentions including self-initiating, trying to cause, and leading.

Our analysis of clinician behaviors in using the DCCS focuses on these areas: (1) what the clinician does to establish a pragmatic learning context and (2) what the clinician does to enhance the client's communicative competence.

Our goal, then, is to create an environment in which (a) clients pay attention, imitate expected behavior, demonstrate prosocial behaviors, act and speak spontaneously, try to influence and lead others and (b) the clinician explains, demonstrates, encourages, and reinforces those behaviors. The clinician also provides a practice situation and activities like the clients' daily communication activities. These activities provide for practice of appropriate responses so that articulation skills are learned in relation to whole schemata and so that natural consequences follow these and other communication efforts of the clients.

The scales are presented in the appendixes so that a clinician might use them as a guide to identify the pragmatic behaviors of clinician and client that would create the most effective communicative environment for developing schemata and facilitating generalization. We have found this to be an efficient method the clinician can use without paper and pencil in *concurrent diagnostic teaching*.

Specific goals for communicative competence are selected for each child and incorporated into the next day's lesson plan, such as:

> Activities will be chosen that allow Dawn, Jimmy, and Sue practice in answering ''wh'' questions: *What is missing? Whose turn?* Given two bottles of glue, the six children will ask for the glue, using a phrase containing each child's target phoneme as in *I want—, Please pass—, My turn* (as modeled by the clinician), and glue in a missing piece on the picture. The clinician will present at least one opportunity for both John and Jimmy to lead others by giving directions for the activity.

Language objectives are frequently as important to clients in an articulation improvement program as are speech production objectives. Significant articulation disorders are often accompanied by language difficulties, as might be expected in light of the interdependent nature of the communication-learning system and the fact that even phonemes by definition have semantic value as well as direct association with lexical, morphological, and syntactic elements of language. Furthermore, language responses clearly constitute the chief vehicle for articulation improvement.

Language objectives should fit the language needs of the client as determined by appropriate language tests, diagnostic teaching, the types of expressions used in the client's home and school, and the concepts that are objectives of the lesson, and they should fit the articulation needs of the client as well. Thus, if the client has /s/ distortions in speech, language responses should be chosen that contain /s/. In our clinic, when the phoneme to be remediated is identified, clinicians select four or five words from the child's lexicon that contain the target phoneme (usually in initial position) and a language unit (word category, syntactic form, speech act) containing the same phoneme. This affords practice of the target sound in words useful to the child and in communicative use from the very beginning of instruction, thus eliminating the need for a separate program of carryover and maintenance. The preschool lesson being represented here might have the following language objective:

> In the appropriate context, each client will express completely, with or without model: *I want a turn. What is missing? The big one. The little one. That's right. That's wrong.*

Included with the language objectives are those having to do with the concepts, ideas, and the semantics or meaning of communication. The significance of concepts to children depends upon their opportunities and requirements. Preschool children benefit from schemata related to play activities, home interactions, and perhaps to other concepts at appropriate developmental levels identified by Piaget and his interpreters. School-age children benefit from learning schemata related to play and home and also to their daily experiences in the various curricular areas of their classroom instruction. Problem-solving and creative-thinking tasks are valid activities for conceptual and cognitive development, particularly if they are borrowed from the clients' frequently occurring classroom activities.

Semantic activities are, like the language that accompanies them, an integral part of the total communication context and may provide opportunity for practice of specific speech sounds. In planning semantic activities, the clinician should provide for a degree of spontaneous interaction and for language elaborations beyond the specific planned responses. Bloom and Lahey (1978), Muma (1978), and Fey (1986) discuss language elaboration, expansion, expatiation, etc., as ways to expand language form and content in communicative interchange. An example of a semantic objective is:

> Given a display or sequence of items, each child will ask, *What is missing?* The child will then correctly name the item that is missing and describe it as either *big* or *little*.

Speech production objectives may include improvement of voice, stuttering, and other speech behaviors as well as articulation. The same pragmatic experiences, the same system procedures, that are beneficial in language improvement may also serve in the improvement of speech. This has been one of the premises of this discussion of CCI. Another basic claim is that procedures for improving specific speech sounds, including speech sounds in isolation, may be incorporated as part practice within the whole context of this system approach. Articulation objectives are, of course, specific for each client and appear much like speech objectives in other instructional approaches. Examples of speech production objectives are:

☐ Shawn, Jimmy, and Sue will produce improved /s/ 80% of the time as they practice /s/ in isolation, then in *missing* and in the phrase *What is missing?*

☐ Shawn, Jimmy, and Sue will produce improved /s/ 80% of the time as they use the word *missing* and in the phrase *What is missing?*

☐ Jimmy, Richard, and John will produce improved /r/ 80% of the time as they use

the words *turn, right,* and *wrong* and in the phrases *My turn, That's right, That's wrong.*

☐ Dawn, Sue, and Jimmy will produce improved /l/ 80% of the time as they practice /l/ in isolation and in the word *little* and in the phrase *Let me have—.*

☐ Dawn, Sue, and Jimmy will produce improved /l/ 80% of the time as they use the word *little* and the phrase *Let me have—.*

We include within our speech production objectives activities that heighten and improve auditory, haptic, and perceptual-motor skills, particularly those that are involved in articulation production. An example of an auditory and haptic perceptual objective that would enhance a client's perception of a phoneme follows.

☐ As the clinician or client produces the word *missing,* Shawn, Jimmy, and Sue will indicate correctly, 80% of the time, whether /s/ is right or wrong.

☐ During their practice of the word *missing,* Shawn, Jimmy, and Sue will indicate correctly, 80% of the time, whether the tongue position for /s/ is right or wrong.

☐ As the clinician or client produces the word *little,* Dawn, Sue, and Jimmy will indicate correctly, 80% of the time, whether /l/ is right or wrong.

☐ During their practice of the word *little,* Dawn, Sue, and Jimmy will indicate correctly, 80% of the time, whether the tongue position for /l/ is right or wrong.

Where considerable perceptual-motor abnormality appears, it is not unreasonable to involve young clients in sequential learning activities, laterality discrimination, etc. These same activities may also enhance conceptual growth in the cognitive abilities described by Piaget, such as conservation and spatiality.

The contribution of perceptual-motor learning other than that involved in speech production may not be obvious. However, the integrated performance of fine and gross body movements in meaningful tasks may well be helpful in strengthening the cues that evoke learned responses as part of the total schema. For example, we recall the adult aphasic client who was unable to produce the words "come in" until she stood at the door, opened it, and addressed the person waiting to come in. This same accompaniment of speech with appropriate body activity in meaningful communication acts has been noticeably effective with mentally retarded clients.

Diagnostic objectives have to do with the ongoing evaluation of client and clinician behavior. As explained earlier, concurrent diagnostic teaching is an essential feature of CCI. The summary of the clinician's impressions during the therapy session becomes the basis for next-lesson objectives and planning. How well the clients performed in relation to the day's lesson objective suggests their needs. How well the clients performed and what the clinician did to achieve or fail to achieve good client performance suggests the clinician's needs. As with the objectives already described, diagnostic objectives include many more expected results than are explicitly stated in the lesson plan. Usually diagnostic objectives are stated in terms of most urgent improvements that the clients and clinician have been working to achieve.

Activities. Most of the guidelines for planning activities of CCI have been described earlier in this chapter as principles of system-type instruction and communicative stimulus, response, and reinforcement. These principles suggest that activities be designed to simulate the clients' daily communication experiences. The simulation is not an exact duplication of life experiences for any of the clients. Instead, it is intended to be an ideal representation of the several types of communicative interaction experienced by the clients during their daily life at home, play, and school. They then are able to participate more effectively in these daily experiences as they bring newly learned skills to their daily communication.

Another guideline that is followed in designing CCI activities is that of arranging circumstances more than arranging children. Generally, activities in communication-centered group instruction are arranged to encourage various client behaviors more than to teach them directly. This is a natural feature of communication-centered activities because the communicative interaction of clients with each other, as well as with the clinician, naturally provides opportunity for attending, imitating, self-initiating, cooperating, etc. At the same time, the clinician may explain, demonstrate, wait for, encourage, require, and approve specific client behaviors as well as arrange situations that naturally call for these behaviors.

Positive group interaction is essential to effective CCI. With it come all the benefits of group work, small-group instruction, and cooperation in education (Sharan, 1980). Group unity or cohesiveness is a necessary condition of group instruction and often requires emphasis on activities that unify the group by requiring all children to work together to complete a task. For instance, six children may be given two puzzles to assemble rather than provide a separate puzzle for each child. The children then are given opportunities to practice sharing and other social and communicative skills while learning to use language effectively in an interactive environment.

Another important guideline in planning communication-centered activities is based on principles of generalization. Ellis (1965) suggests that in addition to the benefits of making the practice situation like the performance situation, transfer of learning increases (a) with increase in the amount of time spent on learning the original task and (b) with a few different experiences in tasks that are variations of the original. Similarly, Gagne (1977) suggests that to enhance retention and transfer of learning "provision needs to be made for encouraging the learner to apply the learning in as great a variety of new situations as can be devised" (p. 296). The activities in CCI are thus designed to follow these recommendations. Practice of target behaviors is repeated in several communication-centered activities, all of which provide for use of the target responses, but all of which are slightly different. For example, activities that provide practice of /s/ in *May I see?* may consist of clients asking the clinician and other clients (a) *May I see the picture?* when the picture is in a book, a Viewmaster, a dime-store viewer, a diorama, a photo album, etc., or (b) *May I see?* when an object is in another person's hand, in a box, out the window, etc.

The activities that constitute the usual communication-centered therapy session are an introduction, a rehearsal, and several practice activities.

The *introduction* usually includes greetings and roll call, in which each child participates in greeting the teacher or teacher's helper and each responds to name with *I am here* or some other response, such as putting a name tag or picture on the bulletin board.

The *rehearsal* at the beginning of each group lesson introduces (a) the concepts of the lesson, (b) the specific language form or function to be emphasized that day, (c) the speech sounds to be improved, and (d) the kind of communicative interchange in which the language unit may be used. The rehearsal consists of a communication activity or a story and activity illustrating the story, in which the concepts, language unit, and speech sounds are rehearsed. The rehearsal activity is similar to the rest of the communication activities in the lesson, but with time for whatever practice is necessary to obtain the client's best performance of target behaviors. It is chiefly in the rehearsal that the target speech sound is practiced. In the rehearsal, the target sound in the language response may be isolated for practice in sound discrimination, phonetic placement, or many of the other procedures described in other chapters. This part practice is immediately followed by use of the sound in the target words of the lesson, and finally restored to its whole context of communicative use of the response in the rehearsal activity.

For example, in a what-is-missing activity, the clinician demonstrates the use of *What is missing?*

by telling the clients, "Look at the things on the table. Now close your eyes. I took one thing away. Open your eyes. What is missing? Jimmy?"

Jimmy: The big dog.
Clinician: The big dog is there or the big dog is missing, Jimmy?
Jimmy: The big dog is missing.
Clinician: Right. Did you hear how Jimmy said *missing*? Let's all try—*missing*. Listen to /s/ and watch where I put my tongue and teeth. Let's try /s/. Good. Now, *missing*. Jimmy, you be the leader. Everyone close your eyes. Jimmy, take something away. O.K., open your eyes. You ask them, Jimmy.
Jimmy: What is missing?

The children respond, and the action is repeated as each child takes the turn of the leader. Several times a brief moment may be spent practicing /s/ in *missing*, /l/ in *little,* and /r/ in *right* and *wrong*.

Activity #1 is a near-replication of the rehearsal activity, as are the rest of the activities in the session. They are all designed to provide a communicative exchange among the group, including the clinician, in which the day's target responses are used naturally. The activities are different enough to provide new, but similar, stimulus cues in each activity while at the same time repeating the same responses.

In the sample lesson, Activity #1 may consist of the clinician's displaying a quarter and a penny in outstretched hand. Then one of the coins is removed without letting the children see which one, and the clinician's fist is closed around the remaining coin. The question is then asked, "What is missing?" or "Which one is missing, Sue, the big one or the little one?"

Sue guesses, "The big one."

The clinician opens her hand and asks, "John, was she right or wrong?"

"All right, Sue, you hold the penny and the quarter. We'll close our eyes while you take one away."

Each child has a turn being the leader and a turn guessing which coin is missing and telling whether the guess was right or wrong.

Activity #2 uses the same responses as the rehearsal and Activity #1 in a different setting. For example, the clinician has prepared a picture of a carnival in which there are two clowns, one selling balloons of different sizes and one juggling some balls of different sizes. Colored paper discs are lightly stuck on the balloon and ball outlines in the picture. The children close their eyes while another child removes a ball or a balloon and then asks what is missing; appropriate responses are given.

Activity #3 uses the same responses as in the other activities. This time a cloth or paper bag is used to conceal big and little paired objects, such as toys, coins, and balls. The children take turns removing one of the paired objects and asking another child to feel in the bag and tell what is missing.

Several other activities may follow, in each of which the target responses are practiced in relation to what-is-missing situations.

Recommendations are the last feature of the lesson plan; these are not formulated until the day's lesson is over. Then, having been aware throughout the lesson of the behaviors of the individual clients in relation to the lesson objectives and of her own effectiveness as a clinician, the clinician may summarize progress and present needs. We find the CCS and DCCS useful in this evaluation. The needs that have been identified, along with the long-term communication goals of each client, provide the basis for objectives of the next therapy session. Recommendations may be summarized, as illustrated here, or they may be stated as new objectives for the next group or individual therapy session.

- ☐ Shawn and Jimmy need more practice on /s/ discrimination and placement in both individual and group therapy.
- ☐ Jimmy, Richard, and John are more nearly approximating /r/. John and Richard should

have more /r/ discrimination and placement during individual therapy. Jimmy has enough to do with /s/ practice.

- ☐ Dawn, Sue, and Jimmy are beginning to produce a good /l/. The inclusion of /l/ in whole responses in group and individual lessons will likely be sufficient to remediate /l/.
- ☐ CCS strengths were the increased cooperation of Jimmy, Dawn, and Sue and Jimmy's willingness to take the lead. CCS weaknesses were John's frequent lack of attention and reluctance to be the leader in an activity.
- ☐ DCCS strengths were the involvement of all clients in the various roles of each activity, including their making something happen with the language they used to practice their specific target articulation. DCCS weaknesses were too many failures to commend John for his occasional spontaneous behavior and not introducing the language response in a clear way so the children would use it naturally.

Lesson Plan for Individual Communication-Centered Instruction. The objectives and activities of individual instruction are much the same as those for group instruction. The key to planning individual therapy is the performance of the client in group therapy as well as in home, school, and play activity. Remedial instruction, i.e., group therapy, is a supplement to and rehearsal for both school and daily life. Individual instruction as a resource to group instruction thus becomes a supplement to and rehearsal for the client's group, school, and life activities.

As the clinician rehearses the individual client in the responses that have been or will be used in the group, there is more opportunity than in the group for isolating the target sound from the whole response for phonemic and phonetic discrimination and for practice in articulatory placement and movement. Further contextual testing (chapter 4) and other useful articulation evaluation and therapy procedures may be pursued as part of the individual lesson, always accompanied by whole practice of the target sound in communicative responses and communicative activities, some of which are rehearsal for subsequent group lessons and experiences in the classroom and school.

Communication between clinician and client in individual instruction may still be a meaningful and powerful communication experience, although not usually as effective, in our experience, as such communication among peers. Having the client use communicative mand responses that direct the adult or a puppet to act in various ways, such as *throw the ball, drop the ring, give me the little one,* is a communicatively reinforcing use of language. To enhance the communicative value of individual therapy, another client may be involved in the communicative interchange. We recall a clinician's efforts to involve a male child who was listless and unresponsive until the clinician brought a little girl into the activity. Little boys, of course, will stand on their heads for little girls. Immediately the activity came alive as the interaction included three instead of two people, peer-peer-clinician relationships instead of child-clinician only.

Individual therapy is considered a supplement to group therapy in a communication-centered articulation therapy program. The influence of the group on individual clients is so essential in establishing pragmatic skills that it may be assumed that instruction without client interaction achieved in small groups is not optimally communication-centered. At best, individual instruction provides an opportunity for a child to rehearse behaviors that can be used effectively in group activities.

Home Instruction. As indicated throughout the description of CCI, the clinician must be aware of communication activities from the clients' home, classroom, and play situations so that simulations of these activities are the basis of the intervention. The simulation, thus planned, is generally the best guarantee of carryover of clinic learning to daily life. The involvement of the parent and family routines in the therapy plan extends the therapeutic efforts. CCI also suggests that parents, teachers, and friends can hasten a client's articulation improvement if they are given some understanding of the instruction the client receives and specific instruction as to how they can create situations in which the client may be expected to use newly acquired speech behavior. We train parents in the use of CCS and DCCS to help them become aware of opportunities for communication and facilitate better interaction in the home. Costello (1983) supports the idea of adjunct home therapy as a method of increasing generalization of learning and further suggests that the addition of training of additional exemplars is still another plus for stimulus generalization. An important feature of communication-centered articulation therapy is sharing with parents and teachers information that allows and expects them to encourage the use of their child's new articulation skills, particularly in language units practiced in the school and home environment.

SUMMARY

In this chapter we have described communication-centered instruction (CCI), which we believe to be a logical, integrated, pragmatic approach to articulation therapy. The eclectic nature of this approach allows the integration of many new and used techniques within its whole-part-whole learning contexts. CCI uses procedures of carryover during each instructional period, making additional procedures of generalization and maintenance unnecessary. In fact, CCI is a generalization program in itself. CCI is applicable not only to articulation therapy, but also to stuttering, voice problems, and language disorders in particular. In general, CCI is effective in improving the communication and learning of the mentally retarded, learning disabled, aphasic, autistic, and other handicapped children and adults. CCI provides an optimal learning context for most kinds of learning, helps clients learn behaviors of significance among their peers, and improves clients' interpersonal skills and feelings of worth, not only among those in the clinic but with those at home, at school, and at play.

The ability to adjust to new interpersonal communicative situations generalizes from CCI to clients' daily lives along with their improved communication and learning skills, and in that process many of the unfavorable learning and psychogenic conditions contributing to the communication disorder are greatly reduced. As a child's confidence in speech and language skills increases, the child interacts more with others, which provides more opportunity for practice and improvement in speech-language and social-emotional relations.

As a closing comment, let us consider an often-repeated concern of clinicians who are unsure of using CCI. "But I only have 15 minutes with each client," the clinician says. "I can't have the client repeat the response enough times for adequate practice if I make the activity communication-centered." Usually this observation changes when consideration is given to the relative importance in learning of repetition, on the one hand, and communicativeness of the learning situation, on the other.

Clinicians should approach remediation of communication disorders, including articulation deviations, as problems in communication that need communication solutions. CCI, as described here, may be one way for clinicians to make their therapy more pragmatic, as they center their instruction in communication.

REFERENCES

Antinucci, F., & Parisi, D. (1975). Early semantic development in child language. In E. H. Lenneberg & E. Lenneberg (Eds.), *Foundations of language development: a multi-disciplinary approach* (Vol. 1). New York: Academic Press.

Arwood, E. L. (1983). *Pragmaticism*. Rockville, MD: Aspen Systems.

Backus, O., & Beasley, J. (1951). *Journal of speech therapy with children*. Cambridge, MA: Houghton Mifflin.

Backus, O., & Dunn, H. (1947). Use of conversational speech patterns to promote speed and retention of learning. *Journal of Speech and Hearing Disorders, 12,* 135–142.

Bartlett, F. C. (1932). *Remembering*. Cambridge, England: Cambridge University Press.

Bateman, B. (1974). Educational implications of minimal brain dysfunction. *Reading Teacher, 27,* 662–668.

Bates, E. (1976). Pragmatics and sociolinguistics in child language. In D. M. Morehead & A. E. Morehead (Eds.), *Normal and deficient child language*. Baltimore: University Park Press.

Bloom, L., & Lahey, M. (1978). *Language development and language disorders*. New York: Wiley.

Bruner, J. S. (1966). On cognitive growth: II. In J. S. Bruner, R. R. Olver, & P. M. Greenfield (Eds.), *Studies in cognitive growth*. New York: Wiley.

Bruner, V. S. (1975). The ontogenesis of speech acts. *Journal of Child Language, 2,* 1–19.

Cohen, S. A. (1971). Dyspedagogia as a cause of reading retardation in learning disorders. In B. Bateman (Ed.), *Learning disorders—reading* (Vol. 4). Seattle: Special Child Publications.

Costello, J. M. (1983). Generalization across settings: Language intervention with children. In J. Miller, D. E. Yoder, & R. Schiefelbusch (Eds.), *Contemporary issues in language intervention* (1983 ASHA Reports). Rockville, MD: American Speech-Language-Hearing Association.

Darley, F. L. (1979). *Evaluation and appraisal techniques in speech and language pathology*. Reading, MA: Addison-Wesley.

Ellis, H. C. (1965). *The transfer of learning*. New York: Macmillan.

Fey, M. E. (1986). *Language intervention with young children*. San Diego, CA: College Hill Press.

Gagne, R. M. (1977). *The conditions of learning* (3rd ed.). New York: Holt, Rinehart, & Winston.

Holland, A. R. (1975). Language therapy for children: Some thoughts on context and content. *Journal of Speech and Hearing Disorders, 40,* 514–523.

Hulse, S. H., Deese, J., & Egeth, H. (1975). *The psychology of learning* (4th ed.). New York: McGraw-Hill.

Ingram, D. (1976). *Phonological disability in children.* New York: Elsevier.

Kemp, J. C. (1983). The timing of language intervention for the pediatric population. In J. Miller, D. E. Yoder, & R. Schiefelbusch (Eds.), *Contemporary issues in language interaction* (ASHA Reports 12). Rockville, MD: American Speech-Language-Hearing Association.

Lassers, L., & Low, G. M. (1960). *A study of the relative effectiveness of different approaches to speech training of mentally retarded children.* San Francisco: San Francisco State College.

Leonard, L. B. (1971). A preliminary review of information theory on articulatory omissions. *Journal of Speech and Hearing Disorders, 36,* 511–517.

Lerner, J. W. (1981). *Learning disabilities* (3rd ed.). Boston: Houghton Mifflin.

Low, G. M., Crerar, M., & Lassers, L. (1959). Communication-centered speech therapy. *Journal of Speech and Hearing Disorders, 24,* 361–368.

Lucas, E. V. (1980). *Semantic and pragmatic language disorders.* Rockville, MD: Aspen Systems.

Menyuk, P. (1980). The role of context in misarticulations. In G. H. Yeni-Komshian, J. F. Kavanagh, & C. A. Ferguson (Eds.), *Child phonology: Vol. I. Production* (pp. 211–226). New York: Academic Press.

Minsky, M. (1975). A framework for representing knowledge. In P. H. Winston (Ed.), *The psychology of computer vision.* New York: McGraw-Hill.

Muma, J. R. (1978). *Language handbook: Concepts, assessment, intervention.* Englewood Cliffs, NJ: Prentice-Hall.

Nelson, K. (1981). Social cognition in a script framework. In L. Ross & J. Flavell (Eds.), *The development of social cognition in children.* Cambridge, MA: Cambridge University Press.

Olmsted, D. L. (1971). *Out of the mouths of babes: Earliest stages in language learning.* The Hague: Mouton.

Osgood, C. E. (1949). The similarity paradox in human learning: A resolution. *Psychology Review, 56,* 132–143.

Osgood, C. E. (1957). A behavioristic analysis of perception and language as cognitive phenomena. In C. E. Osgood (Ed.), *Contemporary approaches to cognition.* Cambridge, MA: Harvard University Press.

Piaget, J. (1952a). *The origins of intelligence in children.* New York: International Universities Press. (Originally published in 1936.)

Piaget, J. (1952b). *The construction of reality in the child.* New York: Basic Books. (Originally published 1937.)

Rees, N. S. (1978). Pragmatics of language. In R. L. Schiefelbusch (Ed.), *Basis of language intervention.* Baltimore, MD: University Park Press.

Ruesch, J., & Bateson, G. (1951). *Communication: The social matrix of psychiatry.* New York: Norton.

Rumelhart, D. E. (1980). Schemata: The building blocks of cognition. In R. J. Spiro, B. C. Bruce, & W. F. Brewer (Eds.), *Theoretical issues in reading comprehension.* Hillsdale, NJ: Erlbaum.

Sharan, S. (1980). Cooperative learning in small groups: A review of recent methods and effects on achievement, attitudes, and ethnic relations. *Review in Educational Research, 50,* 241–271.

Skinner, B. F. (1957). *Verbal behavior.* New York: Appleton-Century-Crofts.

Snow, C., Midkiff-Borunda, S., Small, A., & Proctor, A. (1984). Therapy as social interaction: Analyzing the contexts for language remediation. *Topics in Language Disorders, 4,* 72–85.

Snyder, L. S. (1975). *Pragmatics in language disabled children: Their prelinguistic and early verbal performatives and presuppositions.* Unpublished doctoral dissertation. Denver: University of Colorado.

Snyder, L. S. & Downey, D. C. (1983). Pragmatics and information processing. *Topics in Language Disorders, 4,* 75–86.

Spinelli, F. M., & Terrell, B. (1984). Remediation in context. *Topics in Language Disorders, 5,* 29–40.

Winitz, H. (1969). *Articulatory acquisition and behavior.* New York: Appleton-Century-Crofts.

Wulz, S. V., Hall, M. K., & Klein, M. D. (1983). A home-centered instructional communication strategy for severely handicapped children. *Journal of Speech and Hearing Disorders, 48,* 2–10.

APPENDIX 8.1 Attributes of Communication Competence (CCS)

I. Communication-Learning Readiness

Attending
1. Makes eye contact with central person or object
2. Maintains interest
3. Pays attention

Imitating
4. Imitates actions of others
5. Imitates words of others
6. Imitates others

Cooperating
7. Willingly does what others expect
8. Accepts help from others
9. Cooperates with others

II. Communicative Relationships

Caring
10. Acts positively toward others: listens to, directs comments to, touches, smiles, etc.
11. Looks out for the interests of others: shows concern for others' well being
12. Shows caring behavior toward others

Helping
13. Helps others with tasks
14. Encourages others to participate
15. Helps others

Sharing
16. Gives material or information to others
17. Accepts material from others
18. Shares with others

III. Communicative Intentions

Self-Initiating
19. *Acts without being prompted*
20. *Expresses ideas spontaneously*
21. *Shows initiative*

Trying to Cause
22. *Makes requests*
23. *Sets example for others to follow*
24. *Tries to make something happen*

Leading
25. *Gets others to follow his or her directions or example*
26. *Influences others to look to him or her for ideas or help*
27. *Leads others*

APPENDIX 8.2 Attributes of Developing Communication Competence (DCCS)

What Clinician Does in General to Enhance Children's Communication Competence

1. Explains or has child explain expected language and/or action
2. Models or has child model expected language and/or action
3. Structures materials and sequence of events to encourage children to perform expected language and/or action with minimal teacher direction
4. Requires language that is natural for the situation in which it is used
5. Encourages every child to participate
6. Encourages child's best effort to perform expected language and/or action
7. Allows time for children to perform expected language and/or action
8. Has children practice part of the expected language and/or action when whole is difficult
9. Plans situation that provides natural consequences for expected language and/or action
10. Encourages children to perform expected language and/or action willingly
11. Encourages language and/or action by approving that behavior in others

What Clinician Does to Enhance Children's Attending

12. Shows natural enthusiasm through speech and action
13. Creates a feeling of anticipation
14. Plans activities and materials that stimulate and hold children's attention
15. Encourages children to pay attention

What Clinician Does to Enhance Children's Imitating

16. Has children rehearse language and/or action

What Clinician Does to Enhance Children's Cooperating

17. Discourages misbehavior through logical consequences: withholding, firmness, etc.

What Clinician Does to Enhance Children's Caring, Helping, Sharing

18. Demonstrates caring toward children: listens to, directs comments to, gently touches, smiles, shows concern for children's interests
19. Encourages children to look out for the interests of others, to show concern for others' well being
20. Encourages children to help others to participate
21. Plans situation that provides for children to give to and receive from others help, information, and materials
22. Encourages children to give to and receive from others help, information, and materials

What Clinician Does to Enhance Children's Self-Initiating

23. Plans situation that provides for children to act or speak spontaneously
24. Plans situation that provides natural consequences for spontaneous language and/or action

What Clinician Does to Enhance Children's Trying to Cause

25. Plans situation that provides for children to communicate powerfully in a way to make something happen
26. Encourages children to communicate powerfully in a way to make something happen

What Clinician Does to Enhance Children's Leading

27. Structures situation to provide for children to take the lead in activities

CHAPTER 9 Auditory Considerations in Treatment

Articulation errors cannot be treated easily by a single approach. Generally, the developers of treatment methods for articulation disorders do not intend their methods to apply to all circumstances. Rather, a treatment approach is recommended for application to a restricted set of conditions, because articulatory acquisition involves several different albeit interrelated processes.

The recognition that several process levels are relevant was reflected in Van Riper's (1939) insightful and comprehensive presentation on articulation disorders. As described in chapter 5 of this text, Van Riper outlined three primary process levels in articulation learning: (a) auditory practice, (b) articulatory production, and (c) carryover.

Van Riper held that the first step in articulation treatment should involve extensive auditory experience with the sound the child is to acquire. Not all clinicians endorse the principle that auditory experience is to be emphasized in articulation training. However, there has been reconsideration of the usefulness of auditory experience with the increased use of phonological theory in descriptions of articulation disorders. A phonological approach is particularly useful because it provides a method for describing systematically patterns of

Harris Winitz, Ph.D., is a professor of speech science and psychology at the University of Missouri–Kansas City.

articulation errors. Treatment methods based on phonological theory are discussed in chapters 7, 12, and 14. In this chapter the role of auditory considerations in relation to these and other approaches will be the focal point of discussion.

LEVELS OF ARTICULATION BREAKDOWN

Until about 1970, functional articulation disorders were generally thought to be caused by an inability to execute the motor movements of speech even when no evidence of an underlying organic pathology existed (Winitz, 1969). Several factors were implicated as potential causes of functional articulation disorders, such as poor auditory memory span, malocclusion, and structural deficiencies of the articulators. It can be said with some degree of confidence that these factors and a host of others have not provided evidence for the identification of deficiencies or causes that underlie functional articulation disorders.

In recent years, the emphasis has largely shifted from specific causes to defects in the systems that underlie articulation performance. In addition to the motor execution system, the perceptual system, the phonological system, the phonetic system, and the articulation motor control system are now regarded as important areas of study in that each is believed to contribute to the development of articulation errors in children. The most active area of study involves the phonological system, but it is generally recognized that a breakdown in each of these five systems can result in articulation deviations.

Often investigators, in their discussion of these systems, group them into the perceptual, the phonological, and the motor systems. Some investigators use the term *phonological disorders* as a cover term for articulation disorders that can be caused by a breakdown in each of these several systems. Additionally, some investigators implicate one or more of these systems to explain deviations in another system. For example, because of the influence of the writing of Stampe (1969) and subsequent research in phonological processes, there is renewed interest in the motor basis of articulation errors. Stampe expressed the position that there are universal linguistic processes present in the human that must be suppressed for a particular language to be learned. These processes, presumably, have a basis in articulation and perception. For example, the process of reducing all consonant clusters to single sounds, as in the reduction of /sl/ and /str/ to /s/ would be an example of a universal process. Suppression is necessary, according to this theory, if consonant clusters are to be acquired in languages in which they occur. Accordingly, the use of phonologically immature forms is the result of unconstrained universal phonological processes that operate on the developing phonological system.

The term *phonological process* refers to a systematic set of articulation "errors," resulting from a failure to suppress underlying universal phonological constraints, usually interpreted to be motor. Cluster reduction and the stopping of fricatives— that is, the conversion of all fricatives into stops —are systematic "errors" or systematically deviant articulation performance because they are instances of phonetic classes, in this case the frica-

tives and phoneme cluster units. The presence of these processes is frequent in the normally developing child. However, when they persist beyond the age level when they no longer appear in the speech of the normally developing child they are regarded, according to the theory posited by Stampe, as instances of failure of suppression of universal phonological forces.

Clinicians who apply the theoretical tenets of the phonological process approach often view articulation treatment to involve the suppression of phonological processes, that is, suppression of their underlying motor correlates (Hodson & Paden, 1983; Tyler, Edwards, & Saxman, 1987) largely through production practice. Emphasis on suppression of underlying processes is only one aspect of this method, as discussed in chapter 7, but because motor suppression is a primary consideration, many of the training procedures involve production practice. Procedures such as stimulus-response imitation and the elicitation of sounds through visual and auditory cues are generally associated with methods that emphasize motor production training (Hodson & Paden, 1983; Tyler, Edwards, & Saxman, 1987).

Other interpretations may be made of children's use of systematic errors, and these interpretations will be discussed relative to the auditory component, the primary emphasis of this chapter. It will present the viewpoint that the auditory component is a theoretical system underlying articulation performance and that treating articulation disorders involves auditory considerations, but not without taking into consideration that the auditory system is interactive with the phonological and motor systems.

Auditory System

In the writings on auditory discrimination and its relation to articulation disorders, two general premises have been advanced. The first pertains to the discrimination of acoustic features and the second to the influence of the child's phonological system on perception.

Acoustic Features and Perception. Failure to discriminate between sounds or to identify sounds correctly may be the result of an inability to distinguish between the essential acoustic characteristics of sounds (Dalston, 1975) or the inability to focus on the relevant acoustic cues (Winitz, 1975). Stated somewhat differently, children may not hear the difference between two acoustic features such as between the two fricatives [s] and [ʃ], whose spectra of energy across frequency range is somewhat similar, or they may hear the difference but not focus on the relevant acoustic cues.

The first of the two acoustic-feature hypotheses, the inability to distinguish between essential acoustic cues of sounds, requires consideration of the individual variability of children's articulation errors (Dinnsen & Elbert, 1984; Tyler, Edwards, & Saxman, 1987). The acoustic-feature hypothesis would seem to require that there is a broad range of highly specific auditory dysfunctions in children with articulation errors. One child, for example, might not discriminate between [w] and [r], and another child might not discriminate between [r] and [l]. A third child might have perceptual difficulty with both contrasts and several others. A fourth child might have difficulty with a particular feature, frication, for example, that affects all fricative-stop distinctions. When the variability of children's phonological processes is considered, the number of specific auditory dysfunctions possible is almost unlimited in number. To justify this hypothesis, it would be necessary for the hearing mechanism to exhibit highly specialized speech sound dysfunctions, of which more than one dysfunction may be present, and that one dysfunction does not necessarily imply the presence of another dysfunction. This consideration is unlikely, as we would need to postulate feature detectors for each specific acoustic-phonetic relationship and assume that each can become defective independent of all others. Additionally, this theory would need to show why these auditory dysfunctions are so easily altered with auditory discrimination training (Winitz & Bellerose, 1967) or minimal pair training (Tyler, Edwards, & Saxman, 1987).

Research on acoustic-feature dysfunctions has largely been limited to language-disordered children, perhaps with the exception of an early study by Sommers, Meyer, and Furlong (1969), who used the Seashore pitch test to investigate the perceptual ability of children with articulation errors. By using this measure, they assessed the acoustic property of frequency independent of speech and demonstrated that children with moderate articulation errors performed poorer on pitch perception than children with mild articulation errors. More recently, Tallal and Piercy (1975) utilized rapidly changing acoustic spectra to examine the discrimination ability of dysphasic children. The children experienced difficulty distinguishing between units, such as /ba/ and /da/, which involve acoustic transitions that are brief and whose frequencies show rapid changes. These investigators demonstrated that by slowing the rate of these temporally varying transitions the children's discrimination improved. Despite this interesting finding, Rees (1981) has pointed out that a correlation between the children's articulation and perception has not been adequately demonstrated. Often the stops, such as /b/ and /d/, are correctly articulated by children who exhibit a severe delay in language development. Stark and Tallal (1979) found that dysphasic children's stop consonants are about 13% in error, mostly because of voicing errors (/p/ for /b/, for example) and in a few instances because of place of articulation errors (/p/ for /d/, for example). Of course, these children exhibit consonant errors, such as fricatives, that do not reflect rapidly changing speech segments. This particular point can be applied to the Sommers et al. (1969) investigation also. Their investigation used a single measure, pitch perception, independent of the children's particular class of sound errors. Meaningful interpretations might be forthcoming from this direction of research if the acoustic cues and articulatory performance of the children are correspondingly considered.

The second acoustic-feature hypothesis pertains to incorrect focusing or utilization of the acoustic cues during the period in which the phonological system is developing. Children may be endowed with certain perceptual skills in infancy enabling them to discriminate between certain sounds, as investigators have observed (Eilers, 1980). Additionally, however, investigators have noted that there are developmental trends with regard to perception and production. Zlatin and Koenigsknecht (1975, 1976) observed with regard to the acoustic measurement of voicing, or voice onset time, in the stop contrasts /p–b/, /t–d/, and /k–g/, that perception and production show changes from 2 years of age to adulthood, although by 6 years of age children's performance on this phonetic measure closely resembles adult performance. In all three age groups (2 years, 6 years, and adulthood), Zlatin observed that perception and production showed increased correspondence. This finding, as well as others, leads us to the conclusion that the perception and production of speech sounds continue to be refined throughout childhood (see chapter 3). Some children may experience difficulty in the perception of certain acoustic features during this developmental period. One possibility is that the acoustic characteristics, especially those that are relatively similar, in some instances may not be identified or discriminated by children during the years when speech sound development is taking place.

Difficulty in perception may persist for only a relatively short period of time, but sufficiently long to affect articulatory performance. Menyuk and Anderson (1969) examined the perception of young children on /r–w/, /l–w/, and /l–r/. In their group of children of about 4½ years of age, they found that perception was generally more accurate than production. Of interest is that in their sample of subjects were four children who did not produce the /l/ and the /r/ sounds. In the perception test, which involved the identification of a range of synthetic stimuli for each of these three sounds, two children had difficulty with the /l–w/ synthetic contrasts and three with the /l–r/ contrasts. Is it possible that children who evidence this type of perception-production behavior may retain their articulation errors despite the fact that the devel-

opment of correct speech perception occurs at a later time? We wonder whether this situation may be analogous to adults who acquire a foreign language, and whose perception of sounds is excellent, but who retain speech sound deviations regarded as nonnative. Along these lines of thinking, Winitz and Bellerose (1963) set up a situation in which children would make speech sound generalization errors of /ʃ/ for /s/. This generalization was accomplished by having children listen to and repeat a nonsense word beginning with /ʃ/ for 10 trials and then inserting on the 11th trial /s/ for /ʃ/. Most children produced the /ʃ/, indicating that generalization had taken place. Then half of the children were rewarded for continuing to make /ʃ/ for /ʃ/, and half were rewarded only if they did not say /ʃ/. The first group, by and large, continued to produce the /ʃ/ sound for /s/, but the second group changed their response to /s/. Therefore, possibly some children retain speech deviations that have developed early, through inappropriate generalization, despite further growth in speech perception. Gierut, Elbert, & Dinnsen (1987) refer to these forms as fossilized forms; that is, misarticulations in certain morphemes are not representative of a child's phonological system, suggesting they were acquired early and stabilized.

Phonological Systems and Speech Perception. Speech perception has been the subject of intensive investigation by speech scientists and psychologists. A particularly important finding regarding the way in which sounds, especially consonants, are perceived was discovered by Liberman, Harris, Hoffman, and Griffith in 1957. The type or form of perception that was observed was called categorical perception to reflect the noncontinuous form of the perception. As will be illustrated, in noncontinuous perception, generally referred to as categorical perception, each acoustic stimulus is designated by the listener as belonging to a category.

In the investigation of speech perception, synthetic speech stimuli were used, but here categorical perception will be explained with letters. For this demonstration, assume you are asked to label the stimuli in row 1 of Figure 9.1 as letters E and F. You would complete this exercise by designat-

FIGURE 9.1
Example of labeling
letters as E or F.

E   F   F   E   F   E

E   F   F   E   F   E

ing each letter as E or F by printing the appropriate letter below each item, as in row 2. In row 3 the letters are rearranged to show at what point the determination of the letters changed from E to F.

Suppose you participated in a second experiment involving discrimination of letters rather than the labeling of letters. Each letter is paired with each other letter, as in Figure 9.2, and the assignment is to indicate whether the letters are the same or different. Your responses are indicated in row 2. Note that same pairs are pairs composed of letters labeled as both E or both F, and different pairs are pairs composed of letters in which one is labeled E and one F.

Both the labeling experiment, which involved designating a letter as E or F, and the discrimination experiment, which involved classifying a pair of letters as same or different, resulted in similar findings. These findings are: (a) letters are categorized as either E or F; (b) letters are regarded as the same when they have been labeled as belonging to the same letter category; (c) letters are regarded as different when they are categorized as belonging to different letter categories; and (d) discrimination between E and F was as good between the items that straddle the two letter categories (items 3 and 4 in row 3 of Figure 9.1) as those from the different letter categories that are more distant from each other (for example, items 1 and 5 in row 3 of Figure 9.1). This type of perception, in which there is an abrupt shift from one category to another category (in our example from E to F) is called categorical perception.

Categorical perception, it is believed, is the result of phonological experience. Having acquired a language, the language learner will know the phonetic distinctions that are required by the language. Two perceptual processes may be involved. Acquired distinctiveness of cues refers to the formation of boundaries between phonemes because of a heightening in distinction between the relevant phonetic elements through experience with the language. There is another possibility. The phoneme boundaries are innate distinctions that remain intact if the language in question demands these distinctions. If the phonological distinctions are not demanded by the language, then the perceptual distinctions atrophy. This perceptual process is called acquired similarity of cues.

When individuals know two languages, the appropriate perceptual distinctions are different, a consideration taken into account by the speaker. In a recent investigation, Flege and Eefting (1987) reported that distinctions between /d/ and /t/ for voice onset time were different for the same speakers depending upon whether they were examined in a way that made them believe the sounds were Dutch or English. As the same acoustic cues were present in both experimental assessments, the individuals' perception of the task to involve Dutch or English sounds accounted for the difference. Perceptual bias, then, can be strong in the perception of sounds. Possibly, then, children whose phonological systems are nonstandard—that is, they evidence one or more phonological processes—may not show accurate speech sound identi-

FIGURE 9.2
Example of discrimination
between E and F.

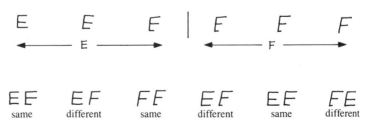

247

fication and discrimination because their phonological system biases them to perceive sounds differently. Their perception reflects the particular phonological system that they invoke.

In summary, when children with articulation disorders are unable to discriminate between speech sounds, it may be the result of two factors: an inability during the developmental period to discriminate appropriately between certain acoustic properties of sounds and a phonological system different from the adult system that biases the speech perceptual system to ignore relevant phonological distinctions.

Phonological System

A second type of breakdown in articulation acquisition can take place, regardless of the quality of the auditory input, at the phonological level (Compton, 1970; Haas, 1963; Ingram, 1976; Winitz, 1969). Auditory factors may contribute to this impairment, but there is the possibility that an impairment in reasoning, memory, or motivation may be responsible for the delay in phonological development. It is also possible that individual children, as they are acquiring language, may minimize their attention to the phonological system in order to concentrate on other language components, such as syntax or semantics (Edwards & Shriberg, 1983; Panagos, 1982).

Currently there are conflicting interpretations of the phonological basis for children's articulation errors. Some investigators (Shriberg & Kwiatkowski, 1980; Stampe, 1969) posit that children's phonological systems are the same as the community language. According to this position, the children know the correct phonological forms, but, as already discussed, constraints operate on the articulatory system to prevent use of the phonological knowledge in expression. Sometimes the term "output constraint" is used to describe this phenomenon. Constraints reflect organizational properties in that a particular phonological feature may be altered for a group of sounds; e.g., all fricatives

become stops. This is the reason for the adoption of the linguistic term *phonological process.*

A second point of view, expressed by Dinnsen and Elbert (1984), is that the underlying phonological knowledge may be absent. Some children with articulation errors, in fact, may not have the same underlying phonological representations as adult speakers of their language community. This premise rests largely on a different model. Here it is assumed that children are active involvers in the construction of their phonological system within the constraints of universal restrictions on the type of phonological systems humans can acquire.

Because of cognitive constraints or restricted environmental experiences children may construct underlying representations that are incorrect. In the case of the phonological process stopping of fricatives, children who show this phonological behavior may represent words in their mental lexicon as having stops for fricatives. Their phonetic performance, of course, may be similar to a child who also shows this same behavior of stopping because of a constraint on motor output or perception. Dinnsen and his colleagues have executed a number of investigations, using generalization procedures, to assess the validity of this particular premise (Dinnsen & Elbert, 1984; Gierut, Elbert, & Dinnsen, 1987; McReynolds & Elbert, 1981). The procedures are somewhat indirect and the results are difficult to interpret.

Their primary criterion for establishing psychological validity for underlying phonological knowledge is generalization of this knowledge from a sound that has undergone articulation training to sounds that have not received training and that represent similar levels of phonological knowledge. The procedure they employ works as follows. A phonological assessment is made and an inference about a child's phonological representations is made. Consider two children who delete final consonants and produce utterances such as [dɑ] for *dog,* and [i] for *eat.* However, child A says [dɑgi] and [itin] for *doggie* and *eating,* respectively. Child B says these words by adding a second syllable of one vowel: [dɑ·i] and [ii]. Based on this evidence, it may be inferred that child A's underlying phonological representations include consonants in word final position and that child B does not have underlying knowledge of medial and final stops. Although the phonological process *final consonant deletion* describes the articulation behavior of both children, the mental representations of these two children may be different.

Subsequent to the phonological analysis, child A and child B would be trained to acquire one or more final consonants. If child A acquired the sounds faster and generalized them to final consonants more than child B, it might be inferred that child A's underlying phonological knowledge represents consonants in word final position. A variant of this procedure is to establish levels of knowledge ranging from most to least phonological knowledge for a particular subject for a range of sounds, and then to assess generalization across knowledge levels (Gierut, Elbert, & Dinnsen, 1987). However, this indirect method of using generalization to validate information that was obtained from the phonological analysis has some shortcomings. Only with the top category, most phonological knowledge, that of never producing the target sound incorrectly in all contexts, can we be certain that perception, phonological representation, and motor skill are appropriately acquired. At other levels, it is difficult to discern whether there is an impairment at one or more of the three system levels. In some cases, good guesses may be made as to whether the motor, the perceptual, or the phonological system is implicated, but for a high degree of certainty additional investigation is required. For example, child A would appear to have phonological representation and would fall into level 2 knowledge. However, it is possible that child A does not have phonological knowledge of final consonants. If this child, for example, is unable to discriminate between the presence or absence of final consonants or unable to identify final contrasts correctly, there would be some support for this conclusion. In these studies the training procedures preceding the tests of generalization seem to confound the interpretations, because they involve a mixture of motor and phonological training, in that production training and minimal pair contrasting were used.

Although not well developed at this time, procedures are available that appear to be more direct than the generalization procedures that have been employed. For example, Locke and Kutz (1975) studied the serial memory of children with /w/ for /r/ substitutions for the word *ring*. They report that the children showed accurate discrimination between *wing* and *ring* yet performed poorly, relative to children who did not have this articulation error, on the serial memory task. The memory task involved the presentation of three words orally (e.g., *wing, shack, ring*) followed by presentation of a four-picture set. The subject's task was to point to each of three pictures in the order in which the words were presented. Although the children were able to discriminate between the words *ring* and *wing,* the presentation of the /w/ for /r/ substitution affected their performance. This finding seems to suggest that the children's underlying phonological representations for /r/ were not adult-like.

In a series of investigations with very young children whose vocabulary generally contained fewer than 100 words, Leonard and his colleagues (Leonard, Fey, & Newhoff, 1981; Schwartz, Leonard, Loeb, & Swanson, 1987) found that children were more likely to acquire newly taught words as expressive units when the words represented phonological elements that were present in their spontaneous speech patterns. The new words were systematically taught to the children through the use of concepts represented by objects that were unfamiliar to the children. The procedures might be adapted for assessing underlying phonological representation. Lexical learning involves phonological coding of words in memory. It would be ideal to determine whether differences in receptive vocabulary might be obtained with children with articulation errors. Although comprehension was not a consistent factor in the studies conducted by Leonard and his colleagues, it may operate for older children for whom the phonological analysis suggests that the phonological representation is not correct.

It is of interest to speculate that auditory discrimination may reflect underlying phonological representation, but it may also, in the case of some children, be independent of it. That is, we might reason that children who fail an auditory discrimination test of phonological contrasts do not have appropriate phonological representation of the sounds in question. On the other hand, performing appropriately on a speech sound discrimination test does not ensure phonological knowledge, judging from the results of Locke's investigation on serial memory. The tentative conclusion is that the phonological system can be independent of the perceptual system for children with articulation errors, an issue that will be reconsidered along with articulation treatment.

Phonetic System, Motor Control System, and Motor Execution System

The third, fourth, and fifth sites of breakdown will only be briefly discussed because they do not reflect the primary content area of this chapter.

The third site of breakdown is the link between the phonological system and the articulatory system (Macken, 1980; Smith, 1973), originally defined by Chomsky and Halle (1968) as the systematic phonetic level. In contrast to the phonological component, which contains abstract phonological units, the systematic phonetic level contains the phonetic specifications, somewhat abstract in form, of the sounds of a language. For example, at this level are represented the many phonetic forms of the English /t/ phoneme and the contexts in which they appear. As described in chapter 2, the abstract phonological units are the underlying representation, and the phonetic specifications determine the surface representation. In English the /t/ may have one or more phonetic features such as dentalization, aspiration, and rounding.

Conceivably, a child could acquire correct phonological forms, but be unable to learn the corresponding systematic phonetic units. An example might be a child who produces fricatives appropriately, but systematically alters place of articulation so that the fricatives are distorted. Speakers of a foreign language sometimes show distortion of phonetic units, even though they have acquired

complete knowledge of the underlying phonological system. Perhaps one way to identify children with a deficit at the systematic phonetic level would be to devise discrimination tests that evaluate both phonetic and phonemic differences. An investigation of this type was conducted by Hoffman, Stager, and Daniloff (1983), and their results seem to provide evidence that some children with errors of /r/ do not have auditory knowledge of the phonetic parameters of /r/, although they have acquired auditory distinctions that indicate that /r/ has been acquired as a phonological unit, i.e., they can distinguish among /r/, /l/, and /w/.

A fourth possible type of breakdown is at the system level that involves the planning of articulatory acts. In this case, the phonetic instructions to the articulatory system may be correct, but there may be difficulty in establishing articulatory programs or schemata. A motor scheme starts with knowledge of articulatory targets and the context in which these targets occur. From this information, an articulatory plan is formulated that serves as the input to the speech motor system. It is possible that some children have difficulty in formulating articulation programs. This difficulty is called *apraxia* (to be considered in chapter 10).

The fifth and final source of difficulty is the inability to execute an intended motor schema. Here sensory, tactile, and auditory systems are involved. The breakdown may occur because damage to the central or peripheral nervous system impairs the initiation of speech motor movements or causes feedback systems, which provide information after an articulatory movement has been initiated, to operate poorly. This type of breakdown may result in *dysarthria* (see chapter 10). When neurological tests do not confirm the presence of apraxia or dysarthria, a breakdown at the fourth and fifth levels cannot be confirmed by using traditional tests of the speech peripheral mechanism (Williams, Ingham, & Rosenthal, 1981; Winitz, 1975). As pointed out by Kent and Lybolt (1982), levels four and five are inextricably woven together in that the formation of articulatory plans rests, in part, on the development and use of feedback systems that are involved in the execution of speech motor movements.

TABLE 9.1
Five System Levels for Potential Breakdown in Articulatory Acquisition

1. Level of auditory input—Child may not discriminate among sounds.
2. Level of phonological system—Child may fail to learn the rules of the system.
3. Level of systematic phonetics—Child may be unable to link the phonological system to the phonetic specifications.
4. Level of articulatory planning—Child may be unable to plan the motor acts to produce sounds or sound sequences.
5. Level of articulatory production—Child may be unable to execute the motor movements to produce sounds or sound sequences.

Table 9.1 summarizes the five system levels of articulatory breakdown. Although the levels were presented as a "top" to "bottom" system, it should not be assumed that, in development and in usage, the process of articulation is one that begins at the top with auditory discrimination and proceeds through each step until the bottom is reached. The levels interact with each other in complex but as yet unknown ways as children acquire and use the phonological and articulatory patterns of their language. In addition, current diagnostic procedures do not reliably distinguish among these five potential levels of breakdown in articulation acquisition. Nevertheless, it is possible that a particular child may have more difficulty at one level of articulatory functioning than at another level.

The focus of this chapter is on the auditory component as it contributes to each of these five potential areas of breakdown in the acquisition of articulation. Auditory processing will be discussed with regard to the discrimination, production, and carryover of speech sounds, often regarded as three fundamental phases of articulation acquisition, and the relationships of each to the five areas of potential breakdown.

TESTING AUDITORY DISCRIMINATION

In its most narrow sense, *auditory discrimination* involves distinctions between sounds. This definition does not restrict the process to phonological distinctions, although it is often used in this specific way. A phonological distinction or phonological contrast refers to differences between the sounds of a language that signal semantic intent. For example, in English the /p/ and /b/ distinguish between the words *pat* and *bat*. A third word, namely *sat,* is indicated by placing /s/ within this same context. These words are called *minimal pairs* because the distinction among these three words in each case is due to a difference of one sound. The difference between the words *pat* and *bad,* however, is not a minimal-pair distinction because the word difference is signaled by the contrast between /p/ and /b/ in the initial word position and /t/ and /d/ in the final word position.

In standardized tests of auditory discrimination, phonological distinctions generally are tested. However, when children produce nonstandard errors or distortions it is often useful to determine their ability to distinguish between each nonstandard error and the corresponding target sound, as, for example, when a child produces an /r/ sound whose production is intermediate between /r/ and /w/.

A common procedure in discrimination testing is to ask the child to indicate whether two sounds are the same or different. For example, the traditional format for testing the distinction between /r/ and /w/ is illustrated as follows:

Clinician: Tell me whether these two sounds are the same or different: /ru/ /wu/.
Child: Responds by saying either "same" or "different."

Clinician: /ri/ /wi/.

Child: Responds by saying either "same" or "different."

There are other approaches (Locke, 1980a, 1980b) that can be used to assess auditory discrimination, but it is not presently clear that these alternate methods assess different processes or produce different results in testing (Winitz, 1984).

The overriding question that usually surfaces when the auditory discrimination of children with articulation errors is considered is: Does the performance of articulatory-defective children on auditory discrimination tests differ from that of normal-speaking children? The answer to this question has been mixed. Some investigators have concluded from their research that children with articulation errors are not different from normal-speaking children on tests of auditory discrimination (Locke, 1980a, 1980b; McReynolds, Kohn, & Williams, 1975). Other investigators take the opposite position by citing evidence that indicates a positive relationship between articulation performance and auditory discrimination. In 1967, Weiner provided a comprehensive summary of the major research efforts to that date, and concluded that a strong relationship exists between auditory discrimination skills and articulation performance when certain testing constraints, to be described, are met. Subsequent investigations, as reviewed by Winitz (1969, 1975, 1981, 1984), have supported Weiner's position.

Selection of Contrastive Items

Two testing constraints Weiner and others have discussed pertain to the composition of the test items. First, the auditory discrimination items should be relevant; that is, they should involve the specific sounds that each child misarticulates. Second, the paired items of the auditory discrimination tests should contain the child's specific error response. For example, consider a child who misarticulates /r/ with a [w] substitution. Relevant discrimination items are those that examine the auditory discrimination of /r/ in contexts in which it is misarticulated, such as a particular word position, blend, or the preceding or following vowel. Paired items that contain /w/ to form contrasts, such as /rɑ/–/wɑ/ and /drim/–/dwim/, utilize the specific error response of the child. Similarly, when a child substitutes [θ] for /s/, the /s/ should be examined in the contexts in which it is misarticulated. Furthermore, /θ/, not other typically observed errors, such as /t/, a lateralized /s/ or an omission of /s/, is regarded as the appropriate contrast for /s/ in the paired items of the auditory discrimination test.

Several writers (Locke, 1980a; Weiner, 1967; Winitz, 1969, 1975, 1981, 1984) have commented that most auditory discrimination tests are designed to measure general sound-discrimination ability. These tests, of which the Wepman (1960) test is the most widely used, are called *general auditory discrimination tests* (Monnin, 1984; Winitz, 1969, 1981, 1984). The paired items of a general discrimination test contain a wide range of paired sound contrasts, such as /s/–/θ/, /r/–/l/, and /p/–/b/; however, only one example of each type is generally included. The reason this test format is used is that auditory discrimination is considered to be a general underlying ability that is assessed by administering to each child a large number of auditory contrasts. This procedure, however, does not take into account the sounds that each child misarticulates or the type of errors that he makes.

A *specific auditory discrimination test* is a test that is individualized for each child. There are no standardized specific discrimination tests. The clinician selects items that are relevant and contain the appropriate error response, taking into account the contexts in which each sound is misarticulated.

Context is important in the design of specific discrimination tests. Often children are able to distinguish between two sounds in one context and not in another, or in one word and not in another (Spriestersbach & Curtis, 1951). Examples of four contexts for a /θ/ substitution are (a) vowel contexts (/θi/–/si/ and /θɑ/–/sɑ/), (b) word position *(think–sink, pathway–passway,* and *bath–bass),* (c) consonantal context *(tenth–tense* and *frothed–frost),* and (d) morphological environment *(eighths-eights).* Additionally, there is a degree of variability or test error that cannot be avoided when testing individuals, especially children. For this reason a large number of contexts should be included for each target sound that is misarticulated.

When auditory discrimination tests containing a limited number of contexts and few item-pairs for each sound have been used to assess the auditory discrimination of articulatory-defective children, a small or nonexistent relationship is found between auditory discrimination and articulation (Locke, 1980b; McReynolds, Kohn, & Williams, 1975). However, in investigations in which the test protocols contained a sufficient number of relevant contrasts in which each child's errors were reflected in the paired items in a number of contexts, a strong relationship was found between articulation performance and auditory discrimination (Broen, Strange, Doyle, & Heller, 1983; Monnin & Huntington, 1974; Strange & Broen, 1981; Weiner, 1967; Winitz, 1969).

Weiner (1967) made another interesting observation regarding the use of general discrimination tests. He commented that children with few articulation errors are unlikely to show a deficit in auditory discrimination when general discrimination tests are used. However, he noted that the auditory discrimination performance of children with moderate and severe articulation disorders on general discrimination tests often is below that of children who do not have articulation errors. Weiner recognized that when children have a large number of articulation errors, the chances are increased that at least some of the items of the discrimination test are relevant to the sounds that they misarticulate, their specific errors, and the contexts in which the errors occur. For this reason, a positive relationship between articulation and discrimination often is found for children with multiple articulation errors when general discrimination tests are used.

Developmental Considerations

Another important consideration in the testing of auditory discrimination involves the complex relationship between the development of auditory discrimination and the development of articulation. Recent investigations indicate that the development of auditory discrimination precedes the acquisition of articulation (Edwards, 1974; Eilers & Oller, 1976; Winitz, Sanders, & Kort, 1981). An interpretation of this finding is that the process of learning how to articulate the sounds of a given language involves learning the correspondence between auditory input and the mechanisms involved in the production of speech sounds. It is believed that children first acquire an auditory concept of a speech sound. This concept then provides the perceptual framework for the formation of the phonological and articulatory systems. As we know, however, there are many dimensions to each of these processes. Therefore, although auditory learning may precede a particular aspect of speech-sound learning, it is not implied that all phases of auditory learning must precede each developmental step in phonology and articulation (see chapter 3).

Partial and interactive learning is exemplified by instances in which children have been found to produce error sounds that are variations or distortions of standard sounds (Kornfield, 1971). For example, a child may substitute a sound for /r/ that is intermediate between /r/ and /w/. The production of intermediate or distorted sounds may be the result of articulation acquisition that takes place without full development of each auditory contrast (Greenlee, 1980; Hoffman, Stager, & Daniloff, 1983).

Although it is recognized that auditory input is the primary source through which information about the phonological system and its phonetic properties is acquired, there are, no doubt, complex interactions among auditory perception, phonology, and articulation, such that the development of each influences the development of the other. For example, articulation learning may provide certain sources of feedback to the auditory system to cause it to attend in a certain way to incoming signals. Similarly, one's implicit knowledge about the phonological system and other dimensions of language no doubt influences the perception of the speech signal. These considerations notwithstanding, the developmental constraint of discrimination first, articulation second must be taken into account when analyzing the results of studies on the relationship between auditory discrimination and articulation.

This developmental process may be identified as having three acquisitional stages:

1. Neither auditory discrimination nor articulation has developed.
2. Auditory discrimination has developed, but articulation has not developed.
3. Both auditory discrimination and articulation have developed.

When articulatory-defective children are selected as subjects, they may fall into either Category 1 or Category 2 as some investigators have observed (Broen, Strange, Doyle, & Heller, 1983; Eilers & Oller, 1976; Winitz, Sanders, & Kort, 1981). If an overwhelming number of subjects in a given study fall into Category 2, no difference in auditory discrimination between the articulatory-defective and the normal-speaking children will be found. The conclusion that there is no relationship between articulation performance and auditory discrimination is correct when the majority of articulatory-defective children fall into Category 2. However, it does not necessarily follow that auditory discrimination is unimportant in the development of articulation. In those investigations in which no relationship was found, this particular developmental constraint may have been a consideration.

In summary, we have identified three conditions that may be responsible for the observation that in some investigations a positive correlation between articulation performance and auditory dis-

crimination was not found. These conditions are inadequate sampling of the relevant auditory contrasts, paired contrasts that do not take into account the type of articulation error the individual child makes, and developmental constraints. When these considerations are taken into account, the experimental evidence indicates that a certain proportion of children with functional articulation errors show a deficit in auditory discrimination. Furthermore, it is recognized that the auditory discrimination deficit is restricted to the individual articulation errors of each child. There is no evidence to indicate that the auditory discrimination deficit is caused by an underlying auditory disability of general origin. We conclude from these findings that auditory discrimination training is an important component in the rehabilitation of children with misarticulations.

TEACHING AUDITORY DISCRIMINATION

The procedures of training that are described in this section place almost exclusive emphasis on an extended period of auditory discrimination training prior to productive practice. As indicated earlier, this approach does not ignore the relationship that may exist between the perceptual system and other systems of articulation development. It does, however, consider auditory input to be a fundamental skill in that its development, for the most part, precedes that of other systems that contribute to the development of articulation.

A number of procedures can be used to teach children to attend to the relevant phonetic cues of sounds that they misarticulate after it has been determined that they do not discriminate between a target sound and its respective error sound. Discrimination testing should be thorough. It should involve a variety of phonetic and linguistic contexts, and, if possible, the target sounds and the child's substitutions should be tested in full sentences as well as in single words. For example, the difference between the syllables /sɑ/ and /θɑ/ can be assessed in short sentences, as in *He put the* /sɑ/

meaningful units, as in the following pair of sentences: *The artist sketched the mouth with a pen –The artist sketched the mouse with a pen.* Children are to indicate whether the sentences are the same or different. Sentences should be said at a moderately fast pace to determine whether or not accurate discriminations can be made when the test items approximate normal conversational speech rate. It is well known that some speech sounds are reduced or altered in significant ways in the normal flow of speech. If a child discriminates well when the test items involve isolated words, but does poorly when the test items are sentences, there is a strong possibility that accurate discriminations are not being made in conversational speech.

Formal Approach

When children do not discriminate well in isolated word contexts and/or in sentence contexts, the primary goal is to teach them to hear the relevant differences. Both a formal approach and an informal approach can be used. In the *formal approach* the child is drilled on sound pairs. The training method is essentially the same as the testing format just described. The training should be fairly extensive and should include sentence contexts that are said at a rapid rate. Production practice is not introduced at this point.

Informal Approach

Informal practice involves training in communicative contexts. Goal-oriented activities, tasks, and situations that involve completion of an activity or the accomplishment of a goal are used by the clinician to provide meaningful and realistic listening situations. Activities such as arts and crafts, games, and minor work situations are used to focus the child's attention on speech for communicative purposes. The clinician selects objects and activities in which the target sound will appear often. Through these activities the child is motivated to

request items, ask questions, and listen attentively so as to be able to participate.

When listening skills are trained through informal practice, the communicative activities serve as the focus of training. Children are never directly aware that listening is being trained because formal exercises are not used. Nor are they directly aware that their performance is being evaluated because all evaluations are part of the communicative process. For example, the paired contrast between /r/ and /w/ can be presented by devising a game about "witch people" and "rich people." The clinician can say, "Pick up the witch people and we will play that game." If the child responds inappropriately by picking up the objects that go with the rich people, the clinician might say, "No, I said the witch people. These are the witch people and these are the rich people. Let's play the witch game." At another training session the clinician might ask, "Which game would you like to play?" If the child responds "witch people" the clinician would pick up the objects for the "witch people" game. The child might respond, "No, I meant the witch people," and then immediately point to the "rich people." The clinician may respond, "These are the rich people, and these are the witch people," in order to emphasize again the contrast. Although in this latter example the child is engaged in conversation, the purpose of the activity is to teach auditory discrimination in meaningful contexts.

It is particularly difficult to find /r/–/w/ minimal pairs for the frequently misarticulated /r/ because /w/ and /r/ show few contrasts for the same part of speech. For example, *wag* is a verb, and *rag* is a noun. Also, *red* is an adjective and *wed* is a verb. Additionally, there are many other /r/ words for which there is no /r/–/w/ contrast, such as *rabbit, road,* and *reach,* or the contrast is an infrequent word. For /r/, artificial minimal-pair contrasts need to be devised within the context of activities and games. One activity is to line pictures whose labels or names are in minimal contrast up against a wall and place an object in front of each picture. Then ask the child to find the object in front of a particular picture, and to place it somewhere else to win the game (e.g., ''Put the pencil in front of the *wag* (or *rag*) on the table.'') In this way, minimal contrasts can be utilized in a context that is meaningful for children. Pictures that represent words might be used, such as *wag* (a dog wagging his tail) and *rag, run* and *one,* and *rent* and *went.* Other suggestions regarding the use of minimal pairs can be found in chapters 7 and 14.

The informal approach has two primary objectives. One is to provide meaningful input in which the target sound and the respective error sound are in contrast frequently. A second objective is to use the communicative process to indicate to the child in an indirect way that a correct discrimination is important for effective communication. As a consequence, it is expected that a substantial amount of phonological restructuring will take place.

Informal teaching is preferred for reasons described in chapter 8. Nevertheless, there are instances in which formal instruction seems appropriate. Usually formal instruction is provided when discrimination training must be direct and highly focused. It is used as a last resort when informal training has failed to teach auditory discrimination.

Amount and Timing of Auditory Discrimination Training

Whether a formal approach or an informal approach is used, two frequent questions that surface pertain to the amount of time to be spent on auditory training, and whether the auditory training is to precede or coincide with articulation training. Some clinicians take the position that no direct training in auditory discrimination should be provided prior to articulation training. Others take intermediate positions.

The approach we recommend is that auditory discrimination training should be *intensive* and should precede all levels of articulation production training. It should extend over several weeks and perhaps months of training. No production should

be insisted upon during this period, although in an informal training situation children will make spontaneous attempts to produce the target sound because communicative, goal-oriented activities most generally stimulate children to talk. There is no easy solution as to when to begin articulation production practice. This decision is largely subjective. However, regardless of the position one holds, the child should not be asked to produce sounds at each succeeding production level (e.g., sound, syllable, sentence, and conversational utterance) until it has been determined that the appropriate speech sound discrimination for that level can be made easily and rapidly.

CONSIDERATIONS REGARDING LEVEL OF BREAKDOWN

Thus far, this chapter has considered primarily Level 1 of the five levels of potential breakdown (Table 9.1). One goal of auditory training is to alter a child's underlying phonological system in the direction of the adult phonological code. Discrimination training is a necessary first step. However, improving auditory discrimination will not necessarily cause a child's underlying system of phonemes to change; conceivably, children may be able to hear phonetic distinctions, but be unable to apply this knowledge at the phonological level (Level 2). It is also possible that the underlying phonological system can be correct, but for some reason, this information is not provided to or cannot be utilized at the phonetic and articulatory levels (Levels 3, 4, and 5). Each of these possible sources of breakdown will be discussed.

Correct Sound Discrimination with Incorrect Underlying Phonological System: Level 2 Breakdown

Some children with misarticulations have normal auditory discrimination. The source of their difficulty apparently lies along other dimensions. One area of difficulty may be in the organizational processes that are involved in learning complex rule systems like phonology. However, the source of this difficulty cannot be easily explained. Generally, children who are unable to learn concepts are thought to show a retardation in intellectual ability. However, intelligence is not related to articulation performance for children whose IQs are above 70 (Winitz, 1964). Children with IQs below 70 will often show a greater number of articulation errors than normally intelligent children, but this observation does not explain phonological retardation for normally intelligent children. Possibly, some children acquire phonological concepts slowly because of specific language deficits, or because their language experience or language acquisitional strategies have in some way inhibited the development of phonological competence.

One procedure for determining whether the breakdown occurs at the phonological level involves the use of context-free sentences in which both the target sound and the respective error sound are appropriate. According to a procedure we have developed recently, children hear three sentences, all of which contain the target sound or the error sound. After hearing these three sentences, the children signify their understanding by selecting the appropriate picture from a set of two pictures. For example, a child listens to three context-free sentences in which the same /w/ or /r/ word is used in all three sentences, and then is immediately asked to point to one of two pictures, choosing the one that represents the meaning of the three sentences. Two sets of three sentences are as follows:

A. 1. I was to wake it up.
   2. I didn't want to wake it up.
   3. Finally I was told to wake it up.
B. 1. I was to rake it up.
   2. I didn't want to rake it up.
   3. Finally I was told to rake it up.

After the three sentences from set A or B are presented, the child is shown the two pictures in Figure 9.3 and is asked to point to the picture that correctly describes the sentences.

This procedure, termed the *phonological performance test,* is currently being tested with children who substitute /w/ for /r/. We are interested in determining whether children who are able to discriminate between /w/ and /r/ in single words and sentences perform poorly on the test. If they do, a reasonable interpretation is that they can *hear* the difference between /w/ and /r/, but they do not *utilize* this distinction in their phonological system when words occur in context.

A second procedure is to determine whether the children can detect mispronounced words (Cole, 1981). For example, a story is read and some of the words beginning with /r/ and /w/ are purposely mispronounced. The substitution of [w] for /r/ and [r] for /w/ provides a way to determine whether children who can discriminate between /w/ and /r/ readily detect mispronunciations of these sounds. If they fail to detect these mispronunciations, we may infer that the /r/–/w/ distinction is not part of their phonological system because the mispronunciations of /r/ and /w/ are considered to be correct. It should be noted, however, that this is a metalinguistic task in that the child is asked to make a judgment about the phonological system. It may thus be influenced by metalinguistic as well as discrimination abilities.

The focus of treatment for children who *can* discriminate between the target sound and the error sound, but who do not *utilize* this distinction in their phonological system, centers on instructing the child to make changes in his or her underlying phonological system. The same goal-oriented communicative activities that are used to teach speech discrimination can be applied here without the need to focus exclusively on the teaching of minimal-pair distinctions.

Informal Training in Phonological Restructuring. Training in phonological restructuring is regarded as somewhat different from training in speech sound discrimination. In auditory discrimination training there is concentration on teaching the paired difference between two contrasting

FIGURE 9.3

Example of picture test items used to assess phonological performance. One of the following two sets is read to the child prior to the simultaneous presentation of these two pictures:

I was to rake it up.
I didn't want to rake it up.
Finally I was told to rake it up.

I was to wake it up.
I didn't want to wake it up.
Finally I was told to wake it up.

sounds. In phonological training all error sounds that are presumed to be governed by a particular phonological rule are treated simultaneously. Children are taught to alter the underlying phonological rules that govern their sound errors without at first being required to produce the target sound.

Of primary importance is the way the clinician responds to the child's verbal and nonverbal remarks. When a child does not respond appropriately, either through nonverbal expression or through verbal expression, the clinician should not show understanding of the child's communicative intent. For example, when a child substitutes a [w] for /r/ in conversation or selects a /w/ item when the clinician says an /r/ item, the clinician should respond only to what the child says or does.

If the child requests a toy by saying, ''I want the 'wabbit,' '' the clinician may respond, ''I don't know what you mean. There is a rock, radio, ring, and rabbit on the shelf. Which one do you want?'' At this point the child may signify through gestures that the intended word is *rabbit*. The clinician may respond by saying, ''Oh you mean the rabbit, the

toy rabbit. At first I didn't understand you.'' In this instance the error sound does not produce a linguistic contrast; therefore, it is not recommended that the clinician say, ''Oh you meant the rabbit, but you said the wabbit.'' Possibly, in communicative situations, the use of the error sound may reinforce its incorrect pronunciation. In formal auditory discrimination training the error sound is often presented as a nonlinguistic contrast, but here the child is advised that one production is correct and the other is incorrect, and usually nonsense items are used so that words are not mispronounced.

An important aspect of informal training in phonological restructuring is to teach children with articulation errors to realize that errors often cause the clinician, and, by generalization, peers, teachers, and parents, to misunderstand them. As a result children may attend carefully to the communicative process and may modify their articulatory errors without conscious attention to their speech. The purpose of the informal approach, then, is to convey to the child, in an indirect way, that com-

258

municative responses must be accurate if appropriate communication is to take place.

Formal Methods in Phonological Restructuring.

When informal procedures do not work well, formal methods may be used. A number of formal procedures have been used to teach children to change the underlying set of phonological rules that govern their misarticulations. Although these procedures vary in approach, they all include production practice. One approach is to present the error sound and the target sound to the child and ask him to imitate both (Ingram, 1976). A second approach (Weiner, 1981) is to point to objects or pictures that the child names. If the names of these items are in minimal contrast, and the child uses the same sound in both words of a minimal pair (e.g., [wæg] for *rag* and *wag*), the clinician will point to the incorrect picture or object when the target sound is misarticulated. This procedure will indicate to the child that his articulation errors contribute to a failure to convey the correct meaning. As a consequence, the child may be motivated to correct articulation errors by paying close attention to phonological distinctions that are important for communication (see chapters 7 and 14 for further discussion). These two approaches are not always successful because, although children may understand the purpose of each of the two training procedures, they may require initially standard procedures of auditory training and articulation correction in order for them to learn the production of the target sound so that they can participate effectively (Shelton, 1982).

A third approach to altering underlying phonological structure is to use standard procedures of articulation correction (Compton, 1970). Investigators who stress articulation procedures as a means of changing underlying phonological structure assume that production practice is an essential component in the restructuring process. However, the use of articulation practice *only* is somewhat problematic in that it does not necessarily follow that correct understanding of a phonological pattern results from practice in correct articulation.

We recommend another strategy to begin the teaching of phonological restructuring. In this ap-

proach, children are taught to identify categories of sounds prior to and independently of articulation practice, adapting a procedure used with adults (LaRiviere, Winitz, Reeds, & Herriman, 1974). The target sound and the error sound are presented in groups. For example, consider the pattern of stopping. In this case the clinician would tell the child to listen to a series of sounds and to notice that each sound in the series is similar. The child hears the first series (the target sounds, or in this illustration fricatives) followed by a pause, and then hears the second series of sounds (the error sounds, or stops). The child is then told that each series is to be identified by a number and to try to learn that number. The clinician then presents in random order each group of sounds followed by the number 1 or 2, e.g., all the fricatives followed by the number 1, and all the stops followed by the number 2. After several trials, the clinician no longer says the numbers. At this point the child is to say the correct number after the clinician says the sounds of each group and the clinician immediately tells the child whether the number was correct or incorrect. The objective here is to teach the child that stops and fricatives are categories of sounds and that stopping is an inappropriate category for fricatives.

Correct Underlying Phonological System with Incorrect Underlying Phonetic System: Level 3 Breakdown

Currently, precise diagnostic procedures do not exist that distinguish between errors of underlying phonology and underlying phonetics. Auditory discrimination tests might be used for this purpose if the error sound is a nonstandard sound. For example, if children distinguish well between contrasts of English, and also do well on the phonological performance test, but have difficulty distinguishing between a target sound and its corresponding nonstandard error sound, there is the possibility that the error sound has been internalized as an underlying phonetic unit. On the other hand, if auditory discrimination is normal, the problem may lie at the articulatory level.

If the formation of underlying phonetic units is incorrect, our recommendation is to postpone production practice until an individual child can discriminate reliably between the target sound and the corresponding nonstandard error sound. Previous research has indicated that intensive auditory discrimination training is a satisfactory method for achieving this objective (Winitz & Bellerose, 1967).

Correct Underlying Systems with Incorrect Articulatory Programming/Execution: Level 4/5 Breakdown

When no apparent difficulty exists at the auditory, phonological, or phonetic level, training in articulation production should be started immediately. Perhaps one final check of auditory coding should be made. Before production practice is begun, we should be confident that the level of breakdown resides with production. For example, it would be useful to know whether discrimination can be made between sequences of phonemes such as *tan −nat* and *books−boosk*. It is possible that some children with functional articulation errors perceive strings of sounds incorrectly. A disorder of this type may be evident from their performance on specific discrimination tests. If this disorder is present, auditory discrimination training should be evaluated and, if necessary, given careful attention prior to training in articulation production.

MOTIVATIONAL CONSIDERATIONS

Some children may have the capability for learning all of the component levels of articulation that have been discussed, but fail to want to alter their articulatory patterns beyond a certain point. In second-language learning, stabilizing grammatical usage at a certain point in the acquisition of a foreign language prior to full mastery is called *fossilization* (Selinker & Lamendella, 1978). Fossilization in second-language learning and in native-language learning is not well explained at this time. Social factors, especially the motivation to talk and communicate, are important considerations in the treatment process, as has been indicated. Children who discriminate between sounds well and who imitate the target sound correctly on stimulation, or who show in other ways by their ''inconsistent'' production of sounds or features that they can articulate the sounds they misarticulate, should receive training that is geared to motivate them to listen and to communicate.

One question that often arises when the intervention strategies of communication and intensive listening are recommended is: Why do these procedures, administered by a professional in a professional setting, provide greater motivation than the everyday communicative experiences of children, as they seem to resemble the kinds of communicative and listening experiences that children receive in the classroom or in the home, where apparently they have failed to be effective? The answer to this question lies in how the communicative listening experiences provided in the speech and language clinic differ from those already taking place in the natural environment of the child. First, the clinic experiences are focused to provide practice with specific sounds and speech contexts. Second, the communicative contexts that are set up to make the child a better listener involve strategies of responding that indicate directly or indirectly to the child that correct articulation usage leads to clarity and understanding in communication. Third, the clinician responds within the communicative context, but does not cause children to have anxiety about their speech difficulty. Children with few articulation errors will benefit especially from planned communicative experiences because they are usually intelligible, and therefore often communicate well with their peers, teachers, and parents. Planned communication experiences will place them in a setting in which their articulatory errors will be the focal point of the communicative process.

AUDITORY DISCRIMINATION
TRAINING AND ARTICULATION
TRAINING

CHAPTER 9
Auditory Considerations in Treatment

261

Auditory training should not be limited to pretraining phases of articulation training. There are three reasons for continuing auditory discrimination training during articulation production training. The first pertains to the degree of auditory perception that is required to achieve the standard articulatory productions of the community language. The second pertains to the type of monitoring that may be necessary in order to learn new articulatory productions. The third concerns the number of different phonetic and speech contexts that must be taken into account when learning speech sounds.

Degree of Auditory Perception

Speech sounds contrast on a number of phonetic dimensions, and usually not all of these are critical in learning to hear differences between sounds. For example, English /l/ and /r/ can be distinguished on the basis of the lateral or nonlateral place feature. No other differences need to be considered when making a discrimination between them. Yet this limited information about the differences between these two sounds will *not* enable one to articulate these sounds correctly. Learning to articulate correctly often requires a greater degree of discrimination training than is involved in learning to hear differences between two sounds.

It may be that full attention is not given to the auditory cues that mark a speech sound unless an imitative response is required. For this reason, partial learning of auditory contrasts may represent a legitimate stage in the perceptual development of sounds. As children acquire the sounds of their language, they continue to refine their auditory discrimination as they improve their articulation. This reciprocal relationship between articulation and discrimination in the normally developing child may come about because children attend to phonetic cues closely when they are required to imitate them correctly. Children with articulation errors who also show a deficit in auditory discrimination initially may show little progress in the development of articulation unless auditory discrimination training is given special emphasis in articulation training. Not only may such children require special attention before articulation practice is begun, but this special attention may need to be carried out throughout all stages of articulation training.

Monitoring

The acquisition of articulatory responses requires continuous monitoring on the part of the child. In most training procedures the auditory channel is used by the child to evaluate the accuracy of a newly learned articulatory production. A typical articulation training paradigm begins with the clinician's production, followed almost immediately by the child's production, and concluded by an evaluation of performance that the clinician conveys to the child. In effect, the child's articulatory productions are monitored with reference to the clinician's productions in that judgments of self-performance involve a comparison between self-produced responses and those of the clinician.

Later, when the production of a sound is acquired, children judge auditory output with reference to an abstract, internally derived conceptualization of the sound. Similarly, adult listeners judge a sound as right or wrong by comparing it with an internally generated concept of the sound held in memory. In this regard, successful learning in articulation training relies heavily on the auditory channel to monitor the acquisition of articulation productions. As more is learned about how auditory feedback is used as a monitor in articulation learning and usage, clinicians will be better able to use auditory feedback in treatment.

Phonetic and Speech Contexts

Articulation training, as practiced by most speech-language pathologists, usually involves the training of sounds in isolation or in syllable contexts.

As the sound is acquired, the complexity of the context is increased. However, auditory training is usually ignored when the shift is made from isolation and syllables to words, and finally to sentences. Earlier, intensive discrimination training prior to articulation training was recommended. As training in articulation production is implemented, continuing discrimination training is needed so as to provide auditory experience for the target sounds in contexts that closely approximate those of conversational speech.

Carryover

Clinicians often report that carryover is the most difficult area of articulation treatment. A number of procedures are often used to provide for effective carryover in settings outside the clinical environment. All of these approaches have one common purpose in mind: to "remind" the child to continue to use the newly acquired sounds in conversational contexts when not in the clinic.

My recommendation is not to begin carryover training until children can detect errors in the speech of others and in their own speech. Detection of errors of other speakers can be trained effectively by reading children stories in which some of the words are purposely mispronounced when uttered at a conversational rate. Children can learn to monitor their own speech errors by reading a story and reporting after each sentence whether any words were said incorrectly. These procedures do not assure that children will consistently monitor their speech in settings outside the clinic, but they do provide a beginning in this direction.

SUMMARY

Intensive auditory training prior to articulation production practice is regarded as an important component in articulation treatment along several dimensions. Auditory discrimination training directed to the differences between the target sound and the error sound provides the special kind of listening that children with articulation disorders need in order to acquire phonological distinctions. It was recommended that children with articulation disorders be given auditory discrimination training in communicative situations in order to utilize newly acquired phonetic distinctions as part of their developing phonological system. It was also recommended that auditory training be continued throughout all later stages of articulation treatment to provide the kinds of experiences that are essential in learning to monitor speech and in the acquisition of carryover.

REFERENCES

Broen, P. A., Strange, W., Doyle, S. S., & Heller, J. H. (1983). Perception and production of approximant consonants by normal and articulation-delayed preschool children. *Journal of Speech and Hearing Disorders, 26,* 601–608.

Chomsky, N., & Halle, M. (1968). *The sound pattern of English.* New York: Harper and Row.

Cole, R. A. (1981). Perception of fluent speech by children and adults. In H. Winitz (Ed.), *Native language and foreign language acquisition, Annals of the New York Academy of Sciences, 379,* 92–109.

Compton, A. J. (1970). Generative studies of children's phonological disorders. *Journal of Speech and Hearing Disorders, 35,* 315–339.

Dalston, R. M. (1975). Acoustic characteristics of English /w, r, l/ spoken correctly by young children and adults. *Journal of the Acoustical Society of America, 57,* 462–469.

Dinnsen, D. A., & Elbert, M. (1984). On the relationship between phonology and learning. In M. Elbert, D. Dinnsen, & G. Weismer (Eds.), *Phonological theory and the misarticulating child* (pp.

59–68). Rockville, MD: American Speech-Language-Hearing Association.

Edwards, M. L., (1974). Perception and production in child phonology: The testing of four hypotheses. *Journal of Child Language, 1,* 205–220.

Edwards, M. L., & Shriberg, L. D. (1983). *Phonology: Applications in communicative disorders.* San Diego: College Hill Press.

Eilers, R. (1980). Infant speech perception: History and Mystery. In G. Yeni-Komishian, J. Kavanagh, and C. Ferguson (Eds.), *Child phonology: Vol. II. Perception.* New York: Academic Press.

Eilers, R. E., & Oller, D. K. (1976). The role of speech discrimination in developmental sound substitutions. *Journal of Child Language, 3,* 319–329.

Flege, J. E. & Eefting, W. (1987). Cross-language switching in stop consonant perception and production by Dutch speakers of English. *Speech Communication, 6,* 185–202.

Gierut, J. A., Elbert, M., & Dinnsen, D. A. (1987). A functional analysis of phonological knowledge and generalization learning in misarticulating children. *Journal of Speech and Hearing Research, 30,* 462–479.

Greenlee, M. (1980). Learning the phonetic cues to the voiced-voiceless distinction: A comparison of child and adult speech perception. *Journal of Child Language, 7,* 459–468.

Hass, W. (1963). Phonological analysis of a case of dyslalia. *Journal of Speech and Hearing Disorders, 28,* 239–246.

Hodson, B. W., & Paden, E. P. (1983). *Targeting intelligible speech.* San Diego: College Hill Press.

Hoffman, P. R., Stager, S., & Daniloff, R. G. (1983). Perception and production of misarticulated /r/. *Journal of Speech and Hearing Disorders, 48,* 210–215.

Ingram, D. (1976). *Phonological disability in children.* New York: American Elsevier.

Kent, R.D., & Lybolt, J. T. (1982). Techniques of therapy based on motor learning theory. In W. H. Perkins (Ed.), *Current therapy of communication disorders: General principles of therapy.* New York: Thieme-Stratton.

Kornfield, J. (1971). What initial clusters tell us about a child's speech code. Massachusetts Institute of Technology Research Laboratory of Electronics. *Quarterly Progress Report,* 218–221.

LaRiviere, C., Winitz, H., Reeds, J., & Herriman, E. (1974). The conceptual reality of selected distinctive features. *Journal of Speech and Hearing Research, 17,* 122–133.

Leonard, L. B., Fey, M. E., & Newhoff, M. (1981). Phonological considerations in children's early imitative and spontaneous speech. *Journal of Psycholinguistic Research, 10,* 123–134.

Liberman, A. M., Harris, K. S., Hoffman, H. S., & Griffith, B. C. (1957). The discrimination of speech sounds within and across phoneme boundaries. *Journal of Experimental Psychology, 54,* 358–368.

Locke, J. L. (1980a). The inference of speech perception in the phonologically disordered child: Part I. A rationale, some criteria, the conventional tests. *Journal of Speech and Hearing Disorders, 45,* 431–444.

Locke, J. L. (1980b). The inference of speech perception in the phonologically disordered child: Part II. Some clinically novel procedures, their use, some findings. *Journal of Speech and Hearing Disorders, 45,* 445–468.

Locke, J. L. & Kutz, K. J. (1975). Memory for speech and speech for memory. *Journal of Speech and Hearing Research, 18,* 176–191.

Macken, M. A. (1980). The child's lexical representation: The "puzzle-puddle-pickle" evidence. *Journal of Linguistics, 16,* 1–17.

McReynolds, L., & Elbert, M. F. (1981). Generalization of correct articulation in clusters. *Applied Psycholinguistics, 2,* 119–132.

McReynolds, L. V., Kohn, J., & Williams, G. C. (1975). Articulatory-defective children's discrimination of their production errors. *Journal of Speech and Hearing Disorders, 40,* 327–338.

Menyuk, P., & Anderson, S. (1969). Children's identification and reproduction of /w/, /r/, and /l/. *Journal of Speech and Hearing Research, 12,* 39–52.

Monnin, L. M. (1984). Speech sound discrimination testing and training: Why? Why not? In H. Winitz (Ed.), *Treating articulation disorders: For clinicians by clinicians.* Baltimore: University Park Press.

Monnin, L. M., & Huntington, D. A. (1974). Relationship of articulatory defects to speech-sound identification. *Journal of Speech and Hearing Research, 17,* 352–366.

Panagos, J. M. (1982). The case against the autonomy of phonological disorders in children. *Seminars in Speech, Language and Hearing, 3,* 172–181.

Rees, N. (1981). Saying more than we know: Is auditory processing disorder a meaningful concept? In R. W. Keith (Ed.), *Central auditory and language disorders in children.* San Diego: College Hill Press.

Schwartz, R. G., Leonard, L. B., Loeb, D. M. F., & Swanson, L. A. (1987). Attempted sounds are sometimes not: An expanded view of phonological selection and avoidance. *Journal of Child Language, 14,* 411–418.

Selinker, L., & Lamendella, J. T. (1978). Fossilization in interlanguage learning. In C. E. Blatchford & J. Schacter (Eds.), *On TESOL '78, EFL policies, programs, practices.* Washington, DC: Teachers of English to Speakers of Other Languages.

Shelton, R. (1982). Response to Weiner. *Journal of Speech and Hearing Disorders, 47,* 336.

Shriberg, L. D., & Kwiatkowski, J. (1980). *Natural process analysis (NPA): A procedure for phonological analysis of continuous speech samples.* New York: Wiley.

Smith, N. V. (1973). *The acquisition of phonology: A case study.* London: Cambridge University Press.

Sommers, R. K., Meyer, W. J., & Furlong, A. K. (1969). Pitch discrimination and speech sound discrimination in articulatory defective and normal speaking children. *Journal of Auditory Research, 9,* 45–50.

Spriestersbach, D. C., & Curtis, J. F. (1951). Misarticulation and discrimination of speech sounds. *Quarterly Journal of Speech, 37,* 483–491.

Stampe, D. (1969). *A dissertation on natural phonology.* New York: Garland.

Stark, R. E., & Tallal, P. (1979). Analysis of stop consonant production errors in developmentally dysphasic children. *Journal of the Acoustical Society of America, 66,* 1703–1721.

Strange, W., & Broen, P. A. (1981). The relationship between perception and production of /w/, /r/, and /l/ by three-year-old children. *Journal of Experimental Child Psychology, 31,* 81–102.

Tallal, P., & Piercy, M. (1975). Developmental aphasia: The perception of brief vowels and extended stop consonants. *Neuropsychologia, 13,* 69–74.

Tyler, A. A., Edwards, M. L., & Saxman, J. H. (1987). Clinical application of two phonologically based treatment procedures. *Journal of Speech and Hearing Disorders, 52,* 393–409.

Van Riper, C. (1939). *Speech correction, principles and methods.* New York: Prentice-Hall.

Weiner, F. (1981). Treatment of phonological disability using the method of meaningful minimal contrast: Two case studies. *Journal of Speech and Hearing Disorders, 45,* 97–103.

Weiner, P. S. (1967). Auditory discrimination and articulation. *Journal of Speech and Hearing Disorders, 32,* 19–28.

Wepman, J. M. (1960). Auditory discrimination, speech, and reading. *Elementary School Journal, 58,* 259–268.

Williams, R., Ingham, R. J., & Rosenthal, J. (1981). A further analysis for developmental apraxia of speech in children with defective articulation. *Journal of Speech and Hearing Research, 24,* 496–505.

Winitz, H. (1964). Research in articulation and intelligence. *Child Development, 35,* 287–297.

Winitz, H. (1969). *Articulatory acquisition and behavior.* New York: Appleton-Century-Crofts.

Winitz, H. (1975). *From syllable to conversation.* Baltimore: University Park Press.

Winitz, H. (1981). Considerations in the treatment of articulation disorders. In R. Rieber (Ed.), *Communication disorders.* New York: Plenum Press.

Winitz, H. (1984). Auditory considerations in articulation training. In H. Winitz (Ed.), *Treating articulation disorders: For clinicians by clinicians.* Baltimore: University Park Press.

Winitz, H., & Bellerose, B. (1963). Phoneme-sound generalization as a function of phoneme similarity and verbal unit of test and training stimuli. *Journal of Speech and Hearing Research, 6,* 379–392.

Winitz, H., & Bellerose, B. (1967). Relation between sound discrimination and sound learning. *Journal of Communication Disorders, 1,* 215–235.

Winitz, H., Sanders, R., & Kort, J. (1981). Comprehension and production of the /-əz/ plural allomorph. *Journal of Psycholinguistic Research, 10,* 259–271.

Zlatin, M. A., & Koenigsknecht, R. A. (1975). Development of the voicing contrast: Perception of stop consonants. *Journal of Speech and Hearing Research, 18,* 541–553.

Zlatin, M. A., & Koenigsknecht, R. A. (1976). Development of the voicing contrast: A comparison of voice onset time in stop perception and production. *Journal of Speech and Hearing Research, 19,* 93–111.

CHAPTER 10 Considerations for Organic Disorders

Thus far, the focus of this book has been on functional articulation problems, i.e., those problems for which no organic cause has been determined. However, there are certain disorders of articulation that are quite different in nature from functional articulation problems, although they often share similar perceptual characteristics. This group of disorders is referred to as *organic articulation disorders*.

Organic articulation disorders can be defined as those disorders that arise from physical anomalies affecting structure or function of the mechanisms of speech. The damage may be to the structures of the oral mechanism as well as to the central and/or peripheral nervous systems.

The etiological or causal differences between organic and functional articulation disorders lead to a number of points of special consideration. First of all, the umbrella term *organic disorders* should not be interpreted as meaning a single disorder. Within the category of organic disorders are a number of types of disorders, each with its own

Dorothy H. Air, Ph.D., is the associate director of audiology and speech pathology at the University of Cincinnati Medical Center. **Ann Stace Wood,** Ph.D., is a clinical speech and language pathologist in private practice in Cincinnati and an adjunct faculty member at the University of Cincinnati. **Jean R. Neils,** Ph.D., is an assistant professor at the University of Cincinnati.

specific causes, speech and language characteristics, and associated problems. This, of course, has implications for diagnostic procedures, treatment, and prognosis.

Treatment for organic problems tends to be multidisciplinary, because rarely is speech the only affected area. For example, in cerebral palsy, the same motor dysfunction that affects speech affects more generalized motor function as well. Therefore, both evaluation and treatment will involve several disciplines working together. Another example of a multidisciplinary problem is cleft palate, where the total treatment program may require the efforts of the surgeon, orthodontist, prosthodontist (the specialist who provides artificial oral devices), speech pathologist, and audiologist, to name but a few. Although in some cases a team approach may be necessary in the treatment of a functional articulation problem, frequently the speech pathologist is the only professional involved due to the more narrow scope of the problem.

Another major difference between organic disorders and functional disorders is that of prognosis. Prognosis has a direct relationship to the degree of organicity. Therefore, the success that can ultimately be achieved is related to the degree of physical damage. This has important ramifications for goals, treatment planning, and counseling.

Because of these physiologic limitations, success for the organic problem may be defined differently than for the functional problem. Rather than in maximum potential for *speech,* success in treating the organic problem lies in maximum potential for *communication.* In some cases, it may be possible to achieve normal, or at least a useful, articulation level. This may be done by using standard approaches to articulation therapy to improve articulatory accuracy, or it may involve teaching compensatory methods to more closely approximate normal articulation. In severe disorders, such as degenerative neurological disease or severely involved static neurological problems, prognosis for oral communication may be quite poor. For individuals with these disorders, nonoral communication strategies may be necessary either as an augmentative measure or as a total approach.

Working with severely involved organic disorders requires that the speech pathologist be knowledgeable enough to plan realistic goals. While it may seem obvious that an individual cannot progress beyond her physiologic limits, the speech pathologist must be able to recognize those limits and respond accordingly. It has not been unheard of to find patients who have spent years in speech therapy working on very limited goals and making minimal progress, when some of that energy might have been more productively directed toward nonoral communication. On the other side of the coin, all clinicians have seen patients who were never referred because the referral source felt there was no potential for improvement. When, in fact, these patients finally did make their way to the clinic, there was indeed some potential present. If a realistic appraisal is made, the most effective management can follow.

Counseling for organic communication disorders may be a difficult task, as many sensitive issues must be considered. Issues such as changing roles, acceptance of limited skills, deteriorating conditions, etc., are critical issues to patients. How they ultimately handle these crises affects the course of therapy. Counseling should always be honest, yet maintain a balance between the positive and the negative factors. For the individual with a poor prognosis, consideration of negative factors alone may destroy motivation and limit progress beyond the physiologic constraints. Emphasizing positive factors alone is misleading and may result in the patient setting very unrealistic goals for herself. One must always remember that recognizing the potential of the individual and communicating information to the family and patient in an honest and realistic way are as essential to the treatment process as are the specific treatment techniques used.

One final reminder should be mentioned concerning articulation problems. The population with organic disorders may also have functional problems; it cannot be assumed that all symptoms reflect organicity. Those who have organic disorders are subject to maturational lags and environmental influences just as everyone else is.

As has been mentioned, a number of types of organic disorders can affect articulation. Each of these will be considered in some detail.

APRAXIA OF SPEECH

Apraxia of speech is a term used to describe a motor disorder of speech programming that occurs in adulthood or in childhood. Although both the adult form and the child form share similar articulatory characteristics, the two forms have important differences. The adult form of apraxia of speech occurs long after completion of normal speech and language development. In childhood, apraxic speech errors become evident as the child's language develops. Furthermore, adult apraxia of speech occurs as a result of structural brain damage, whereas a neurological basis for childhood apraxia of speech has not been specified. The following sections deal with, first, apraxia of speech in adulthood and, secondly, developmental apraxia of speech.

Apraxia of Speech in Adulthood

Historically, much controversy has surrounded the adult form of apraxia of speech. There are some who insist that the articulatory manifestations labeled apraxia should be considered a linguistic impairment (Martin, 1974) and others who maintain that an isolated apraxia of speech almost never exists (Geschwind, 1975). However, Darley, Aronson, and Brown (1975) note that for 100 years observers of the speech and language of the left-brain-damaged person have identified the same characteristics over and over again, although each observer gave the symptom complex a different name—*expressive aphasia, aphemia,* and *cortical dysarthria,* to name a few. Darley et al. (1975) maintain that the term *apraxia of speech* is an all-inclusive label for the motor speech disorder that often accompanies aphasia.

We believe that there is an apraxia of speech and that it can be differentiated from other types of speech sound disorders. Clinical experience shows that it can be resolved via a method of treatment that does not produce results with other speech or language problems.

Definition. Apraxia of speech is defined as a sensorimotor speech disorder. It is manifested as an impairment of the central motor programming for the voluntary production of phonemes and the sequencing of muscle movements for the production of words (Darley et al., 1975; Wertz, 1978). In simpler terms, it might be said that the person cannot call up the commands for the motor programming necessary to produce individual or sequenced speech sounds. In the last chapter, Winitz outlined five levels of articulatory breakdown. Apraxia of speech results from breakdown at the fourth level, which is the level of articulatory planning. The most salient characteristics are errors in articulation of consonants and changes in the normal patterns of prosody. The articulatory programming problem, apraxia of speech, may appear alone in a left-brain-damaged person. However, the symptoms are most commonly seen in conjunction with aphasia, which refers to language disorders resulting from brain injury, and sometimes with dysarthria, the other motor speech disorder to be described later in this chapter. The point to be remembered is that aphasia and dysarthria are not the causes of apraxia; they are coexisting disorders.

Etiologies. Apraxia of speech is caused by the same insults to the brain that cause aphasia, namely, stroke, trauma, tumors, and infection. The probable site of lesion is the third frontal convolution of the left hemisphere, which is also called Broca's area. There is controversy regarding the exact site of damage causing apraxia; however, it is important to remember that a lesion causing apraxia of speech is not discrete. It nearly always results in the coexistence of aphasia and apraxia.

Speech Characteristics. Darley, Aronson, and Brown, in the classic book *Motor Speech Disorders* (1975), provide a detailed description of the characteristics of apraxia of speech. The following is a summary of their findings.

Apraxia of speech is most easily identified by difficulties in articulation. However, inability to coordinate phonation, rate, and/or stress may be observed. The manifestations of articulatory involvement are as follows:

1. Articulatory struggle occurs, during which the patient many times shows awareness of her difficulty. Some patients will get disgusted and give up with a gesture of "forget it."
2. Errors increase as the length of the word increases.
3. The articulation errors are inconsistent and vary among substitutions, repetitions, prolongations, and additions.
4. Sometimes the error will be perseverative with rearticulation of an already completed phoneme (*bottle-bobble*). Other times, the error seems to be anticipatory (*hospital-hostital*).

5. Consonants are more difficult than vowels.
6. Initial consonants are more troublesome than final consonants.
7. Articulation errors increase as the complexity of the motor pattern increases. Therefore, vowels are easier than single consonants, and single consonants are easier than consonant clusters. Of single consonants, fricative and affricate phonemes evoke the most errors.
8. To confound the clinician, the patient, and the patient's family, there are often islands of perfectly articulated speech, particularly when these are automatic or highly practiced utterances (Hi! How are you? Fine. What's going on? Where have you been?).
9. Patients articulate more easily when they can watch a highly visible word being pronounced by a clinician.

More recently, Canter, Trost, and Burns (1985) found that errors of *transition* were common for individuals with apraxia of speech. These are errors where the normal flow of articulation from sound to sound and syllable to syllable is disturbed. More specifically, this included errors such as stə rit/strit, f:laʊr/flaʊr and silent periods between the productions of phonemes in a word.

Associated Problems. Other impairments may or may not appear with apraxia of speech. Some patients present an oral apraxia, which is the inability to perform oral vegetative movements such as blowing, chewing, protruding the tongue, or licking the lips voluntarily upon request. Other apraxic patients may present an oral-sensory perceptual deficit (Rosenbek, Wertz, & Darley, 1973), such as the inability to recognize the form of an object placed in the mouth.

A great number of apraxic patients also manifest an accompanying aphasia, an inability to understand and use symbolic aspects of communication. They may have problems with auditory memory, sequencing, and discrimination. They

may have difficulty with reading and reading comprehension. Writing and speaking may be marked with reduction of available language and difficulty in sentence formulation, use of correct syntax, and organization of material.

Furthermore, all of the physical, social, and emotional problems associated with brain damage are likely to be present. The physical problems may include hemiplegia, or weakness of the arm or leg, on the right side of the body. Patients with these symptoms are easily fatigued and sometimes unable to withstand frustration. When their frustration tolerance has been exceeded, they may experience such physical symptoms as hyperventilation, fainting, and rapid heartbeat. Apraxic patients may experience reduced sensation in the mouth and extremities and visual problems such as hemianopsia (loss of vision in one half of the visual field) and diplopia (double vision).

Emotional problems may include emotional lability, which is defined as inappropriate laughing and crying. Depression may set in earlier with apraxic patients than with aphasic patients, because apraxic patients are usually more aware of the loss of their speech ability than are aphasics. When it can be demonstrated to a patient that relearning can take place, the depression begins to lift. Anger and low self-esteem are often present due to the patient's loss of abilities and changes in relationships at home and at work.

The apraxic patient sometimes has even greater problems with adjustment to the condition than do the aphasics. Because the individual with apraxia of speech can self-monitor production so well, and because there is more language available, frustration with the inadequate production, the inconsistency of production, and the necessary slowness is at a high level.

Assessment. Although oral assessment has been covered in chapter 4, the following additional measures are especially important.

Because there is a high probability of the presence of both apraxia and aphasia in the same left-hemisphere-damaged patient, test batteries used for aphasia are appropriate for helping the clinician to ascertain the presence of apraxia. In addition, there are informal methods of assessing the motor and sensory involvement of the articulators in both vegetative and verbal performance. These informal measures are often among the first tasks the clinician requests of the patient. By knowing the extent of the motor programming deficit, the clinician can better judge the oral language responses.

Assessing oral apraxia can be accomplished by making the following requests (La Pointe & Wertz, 1974):

Lip function

1. Show me how you blow.
2. Show me how you kiss.
3. Show me your teeth.

Jaw function

4. Show me how you chew.
5. Show me how to bite.
6. Show me how your teeth chatter.

Tongue function

7. Stick out your tongue.
8. Put your tongue on your teeth.
9. Lick your lips.

Observation of verbal apraxia can be facilitated by remembering the characteristics of the disorder and requesting tasks to elicit the presence or absence of the characteristics. The following checklist is adapted from Wertz (1978):

1. Vowel production is least likely to be affected. Ask the patient to produce all vowels in isolation.
2. Consonant blends, affricates, or fricatives are likely to be most difficult. Ask the patient to repeat words beginning and ending with /f, s, ʃ, tʃ, dʒ, z/. Also ask for production of a representative sample of blends of /l, r, s/.
3. Because no sequencing is involved, sometimes the repetition of single phonemes will be intact. Ask the patient to repeat single consonant phonemes, such as /b, p, t, d, g, k/ with a neutral vowel /ʌ/.
4. Repetition of multisyllable sequences should show error. Ask the patient to say [pʌ–tʌ–kʌ]. Ask the patient to produce

multisyllabic words (*snowflake, considerable, synchronization*). Ask the patient to produce words of increasing length (*funny, funnier, funniest, seem, seeming, seemingly*).

5. Words with the same initial and final phoneme should show a greater number of errors in the initial position (*cake, tot, church, judge, fife, peep,* etc.).
6. Repetition of sentences and descriptions of action pictures will be very difficult. Sometimes the patient will refuse the task.

Additional oral evaluative instruments are oral sensory measures, such as those used by Rosenbek, Wertz, & Darley (1973), and the articulation tests listed in Appendix 4.1 at the end of chapter 4. The oral sensory measures aid in determining the severity of the inability to recognize forms in the mouth, and the articulation test provides data on the hierarchy of difficulty of speech sounds and selected clusters.

One of the most common clinical questions and one of the most difficult to answer unequivocally is how to differentiate paraphasia from apraxia-of-speech errors, because speech resulting from either condition may sound the same to the inexperienced clinician. Paraphasic errors are articulatory errors resulting from difficulty with grammatical and phonological rules, whereas apraxia results from difficulty in motor programming of the articulators. Some attempts to document the differences between apraxia and paraphasia have been made. Trost and Canter (1974) suggested that apraxic patients are phonetically logical in their errors. For example, they may substitute p/f, w/r, d/dʒ and often show only one-feature errors. Canter et al. (1985) found that errors of transition differentiated apraxic errors from paraphasias. Clinically, we have observed that apraxic errors tend to occur within the framework of a speech struggle, whereas paraphasic errors occur in a run of fluently articulated and prosodically normal speech. Unless the patient is mute, performance will improve vastly if there is instruction to watch the mouth of the clinician. Patients making paraphasic errors do not benefit from visual cues or repetition; in fact, they seem to get more confused. Often, apraxic patients are very aware of their errors. On the other hand, patients exhibiting paraphasic errors usually go blithely on, making no effort to self-correct, although there are exceptions to this in mild cases. Vowels tend to be involved in paraphasic errors, whereas in apraxia of speech, the vowel is sometimes involved, but the distortion of it seems to be related to the consonant struggle before it.

One of the classic examples of a paraphasic error occurred when a patient was ordering a steak. He first told the waitress he wanted it "medium rear," then he changed to "medium roar," and finally settled on "medium rare." In contrast, the apraxic patient might have said, "bedium mare, no—medium mare, no—redium rare, no—porget it."

Prognosis. Because the lesion that produces apraxia is the same one that produces aphasia, the prognostic variables relevant to aphasia—such as type and interaction of the size and location of the lesion—are also applicable to apraxia. In addition, there are some other behavioral characteristics associated with apraxia of speech that are prognostic. A coexisting oral apraxia is a negative prognostic indicator for recovery from verbal apraxia (Rosenbek, Wertz, & Darley, 1973; Vignolo, 1964). The more severe the accompanying aphasia, the poorer the prognosis. When a patient with a moderate to mild apraxia demonstrates awareness of the errors and attempts self-correction, the prognosis can be considered more positive (Wepman, 1958). Other factors, such as age, physical health, family environment, motivation, and early therapeutic intervention affect recovery from apraxia, as they do recovery from aphasia.

Therefore, a young, motivated, healthy patient with a supportive family, who has only a verbal apraxia resulting from trauma, will recover better than the older, depressed, physically debilitated patient, with an accompanying oral apraxia from vascular etiology (stroke), who lives alone.

Remediation. Depending on the severity of the oral and/or verbal apraxia and the presence or absence of an accompanying aphasia, therapy will vary. Many times, the first move is to help the speechless patient work through the accompanying oral apraxia. Often in a moderate to severe apraxia (with relatively good auditory comprehension), the motor speech problem will need to be improved first. After some improvement is observed, expressive language tasks can be incorporated into the apraxia drill. Sometimes very mild verbal apraxics learn quite soon that if they slow their rate of presentation, they experience fewer difficulties.

Severe apraxics may have no speech in the early days of their recovery. However, they should not be confused with severe aphasics, who are also often speechless, but in addition, have a severe auditory comprehension deficit, which the apraxic patient does not. It is frustrating to the patient and the therapist to begin only apraxia therapy with a severe aphasic. The key to differentiation between the two, which must be accomplished in order to plan the appropriate therapeutic task, is the degree of auditory comprehension difficulty.

When the diagnosis of apraxia of speech has been made, there are several possible avenues of therapeutic intervention. However, they all include the concepts of imitation, auditory-visual stimulation, motor repetition, and phonetic placement. Darley et al. (1975) state that the goal of apraxia therapy is to regain voluntary control over articulation, and that the articulation therapy should therefore be direct. There will be no need to work on auditory discrimination, respiration, phonation, or resonation. The essentials of their therapeutic approach are as follows:

1. Choose a phoneme that is typically easy for the patient and one that is easily visible (/w, m, b, f/). Phonemes worked on in succession should be as dissimilar as possible so that the patient is not confused.
2. Begin with phonemes in isolation and then move to consonant-vowel combinations.

The instructions might be, "You watch my mouth, and say what I say. We will say each sound three times together. Let's say *buh*. Ready—buh, buh, buh. Good. Now let's try *bah*. Bah, bah, bah. Good."

3. Then add consonant-vowel-consonant combinations to be repeated three times (*bab, bub, beeb*, etc.).
4. Then string these syllables together (*bab-bub-beeb, bab-bub-beeb*).
5. Next work on words with the phoneme in initial, then medial, then final position (*bat, rubber, cob*).
6. Provide repetition of two-word phrases using the phoneme (*big boy, Bob bites babies*).
7. Then ask questions and provide sentence frames that require answers using the practice words the patient has learned (*What do you do to the candles on your cake? What color is the sky on a sunny day? The day you were born is called your _____. The opposite of white is _____.*)

The patient should watch the clinician's mouth during production. Some patients are also helped by using a mirror, but this must be an individual decision. Some patients are upset by the change in their appearance since the onset of the illness and find the mirror distracting. Other patients will need phonetic placement instructions and sometimes actual manipulation of the articulators.

Rosenbek, Lemme, Ahern, Harris, and Wertz (1973) have developed an eight-step program that emphasizes the transfer from imitative to volitional purposive utterances. This program also incorporates other language modalities. A summary of this technique follows.

1. The clinician encourages the patient to watch and listen while they make the utterance together.
2. The patient imitates the clinician after a slight delay. At this point, the auditory cue is faded and the visual cue remains.
3. The patient is asked to repeat after the clinician in the absence of any cues.

4. The patient is asked to repeat after the clinician several times without any intervening visual or auditory cues.
5. The clinician presents a written stimulus and the patient reads it aloud.
6. The written stimulus is shown and then removed so that the patient gives a delayed response.
7. The imitative model is replaced with experiences that provide the opportunity for spontaneous and meaningful utterances. The appropriate utterance is elicited by asking a question.
8. Appropriate spontaneous responses are stimulated through role playing.

A third variant of therapy for apraxia of speech is melodic intonation therapy (MIT) described by Sparks, Helm, and Albert (1974) and Sparks and Holland (1976). These authors have used some of the results of current research concerning the roles of the right and left hemispheres in language to create a therapy model. Although the final integration of language function occurs in the dominant left hemisphere, the right hemisphere possesses an auditory vocabulary and seems to be the area in which the suprasegmental aspects of language (stress and intonational contours) are processed. Because the right hemisphere is also dominant for music, Sparks et al. (1974) theorize that by combining basic language with musical form, they can facilitate cooperation between the two hemispheres and tap the latent language abilities of the right hemisphere. The entire method must be learned under supervision. However, a summary of the philosophy and the techniques are provided here.

Melodic intonation therapy should be used on patients with relatively good auditory comprehension, but severely restricted verbal output. Essentially, the patient is asked to "intone" or sing phrases in a very restricted melodic pattern that resembles the true pitch varieties of speech. It is not true singing, and overlearned and popular melodies must be avoided because the patient will often sing the words to the popular song rather than the language being practiced.

Melodic intonation therapy consists of several levels, each of which has several substeps. Progression through the levels occurs only after the patient has had 10 successful therapy sessions at the previous level. The four steps of the first level are as follows.

1. The clinician intones a phrase such as *salt and pepper* or *apple pie* and helps the patient to tap her hand to the rhythm and stress of the sentence. Hand tapping accompanies all four steps of the first level.
2. The patient is asked to join the clinician in intoning the sentence.
3. This step is like step 2, except that the clinician begins to fade her participation so that the patient continues independently.
4. The clinician intones a sentence and the patient repeats it solo.

If the patient progresses to the second level, there are five steps. The goal of this level is to move the patient from the intoning of phrases to speaking of phrases. Patient selection, criteria for moving from one step to another, scoring of responses, and what to do if a patient fails are all incorporated into the program (Sparks et al., 1974; Sparks & Holland, 1976).

There is some evidence that gestural language can be offered as a facilitating, supplementary, and/or alternative form of communication for some severely apraxic patients. The gestural program presented by Skelly, Schinsky, Smith, and Fust (1974) used an adaptation of Amerind, American Indian Sign Language, as a facilitator of speech. Gestural communication is not a language in that it has no grammatical structure and uses a logical associative order. Although gestural communication has limitations, it is in daily use by most people. Putting the finger to the lips means "be quiet," and crooking the finger means "come here." Any gesture or group of gestures that adequately conveys the idea is acceptable. Skelly et

al. reported improved and expanded oral communication after the improvement of manual gesturing. As they suggest, more systematic clinical research is required. Indeed, this is an avenue of communication that must not be underestimated. This approach is further supported by Kimura (1976), who presented material indicating that speaking and manual activities are closely associated in the left hemisphere.

While the patient is working to develop usable speech, writing, gestures, and augmentative communication aids may be considered, if the patient is an appropriate candidate and desires this kind of intervention.

Conclusion. Apraxia of speech is a disturbance of the volitional motor programming of the articulators. Although it coexists with both aphasia and dysarthria, it must not be confused with them. Its correct diagnosis terminates in a unique type of therapy that is based on imitation, auditory-visual stimulation, oral motor repetition, and phonetic placement. This therapeutic approach is not effective with any other expressive disorder.

Developmental Apraxia of Speech

When apraxia of speech occurs in childhood in the course of speech and language development, it is referred to as developmental apraxia of speech or developmental verbal apraxia. The diagnosis of developmental apraxia of speech is not universally accepted, however. Guyette and Diedrich (1981), for example, state that "developmental apraxia of speech is a label in search of a population" (p. 34).

Speech-language pathologists with a strong linguistics orientation might refer to such children as having a severe phonological disorder. Because children with apraxia of speech are relatively rare or may have coexisting problems that obscure a pure form of apraxia of speech, few definitive research studies have been conducted. The work of Aram and Glasson (1979), Yoss and Darley (1974a), Rosenbek and Wertz (1972), and Chappell (1973) has helped to begin to clarify this diagnostic category and to separate developmental

Three characteristics found in all
the studies were (a) a high incidence of an accompanying oral apraxia; (b) efforts at imitation
marked by struggle and groping responses from the
articulators; (c) unusual substitutions and distortions, which indicated confusion of features and/or
two- and three-features errors, such as m/s or t/f;
and (d) much more difficulty in producing multisyllabic words than monosyllabic words.

Crary (1984) proposed a general error hierarchy: clusters > fricatives > affricates > stops >
nasals. According to Crary, this hierarchy is modified by the environment the sounds are produced
in or the syllable configurations required for word
production.

Children diagnosed as presenting apraxia of
speech often demonstrate other associated problems. They may display a number of "soft" neurological signs, such as difficulty in fine motor
skills and/or difficulty in coordination of the extremities, particularly in alternating movements
(Haynes, 1978; Yoss and Darley, 1974a). Despite
behavioral symptoms of neurological dysfunction,
these children do not show localized cortical pathology on CT scan studies (Aram and Glasson,
1979). Oral sensory deficits may be observed in
some children when they are tested on oral form
identification and two-point discrimination
(Haynes, 1978).

To further complicate diagnosis (just as in
adults), these children often present a concomitant
language problem. Generally, their receptive skills
are normal and/or may appear quite accelerated in
relation to their speech. When the apraxia has begun to clear, some children will clearly demonstrate an expressive language problem. Aram and
Glasson (1979) suggested, in contrast to other investigators, that the articulatory disorder and the
syntactic language disorder do not simply coexist
but that both stem from a common breakdown in
the selection and sequencing of both language and
articulatory elements. Some children with a developmental apraxia of speech do not demonstrate
language problems until they reach the third or
fourth grade, where they begin to manifest difficulty in the higher language processes such as cat-

egorizing, organizing, and abstracting. Yoss and
Darley (1974a) reported that some of the children
in their study were classed as learning disabled.

Assessment. Diagnosing developmental apraxia of
speech should begin with a thorough articulation
test. Some apraxic children do fairly well in a
single-word articulation test. However, in connected conversation, they become completely unintelligible, with numerous inconsistent substitutions, distortions, and omissions that were not
present at the one-word level. Therefore, it is imperative to engage the child in conversation and
picture-description activities also.

Yoss and Darley (1974a), Rosenbek and Wertz
(1972), and Chappell (1973) all noted the high
incidence of an accompanying oral apraxia. Consequently, testing for this condition is diagnosti-
cally significant. Yoss and Darley (1974a) noted
that some children produce isolated oral movements quite well. (The movements requested are
the same as those requested of adults.) However,
when the children were asked to sequence oral
movements—coughing, sticking out the tongue,
and showing how they kiss, for example—they
were unable to perform. This difficulty in sequencing can be demonstrated by asking the child to do
the following:

1. As quickly as you can, say puh-puh-puh.
2. As quickly as you can, say tuh-tuh-tuh.
3. As quickly as you can, say kuh-kuh-kuh.
4. As quickly as you can, say puh-tuh-kuh.

The child will probably be unable to perform
puh-tuh-kuh correctly if developmental apraxia of
speech is present. In addition to testing oral motor
function, the clinician should examine oral sensory
function. Ringel, House, Burk, and Dolinsky
(1970) constructed a test of oral form discrimination for children. The results of their testing indicated that the more severe the articulation problem, the poorer the performance will be on tasks of
oral discrimination.

Because developmental apraxia of speech often appears in concert with expressive and sometimes receptive language disorders, no diagnostic evaluation is complete without in-depth testing of language abilities.

Remediation. Little information is currently available from which to draw therapy approaches. Children with apraxia of speech vary in their articulation, language, and cognitive abilities; therefore, no one therapy approach is likely to be beneficial for all children considered to be apraxic.

Therapy for developmental apraxia of speech follows the same principles of visual cuing and motor repetition used for adult apraxic patients (Darley et al., 1975; Haynes, 1978; Rosenbek, Hensen, Baughman, & Lemme, 1974; Rosenbek, Lemme et al., 1973; Yoss & Darley, 1974b). Variations for children may include extensive work on vowels and introduction of age-appropriate syntactic and semantic rules. Children with developmental apraxia must always be cautioned to slow their speech. Carryover to conversational skills is based on their being able to produce the phonemes they have learned at a slower rate than is usual in conversation. Yoss and Darley (1974b) made further suggestions for the treatment of developmental apraxia of speech. Because some degree of oral apraxia is present, oral imitation and sequencing tasks of the tongue, lips, and jaw can be initiated early. In addition to having the child imitate sustained vowels and visible consonants, the clinician can help the child imitate CVC syllables (just as in adult therapy) by using some type of body movement, such as arm swinging, to accent stress patterns. The children should be taught self-monitoring skills early in therapy. Some children will spontaneously begin to produce phonemes that have not been directly practiced in therapy. However, even if this does happen, apraxia therapy for children is a long process, because usually each phoneme and consonant blend must be taught individually. Nightly parental drill with the child is a necessity.

In some children with severe developmental apraxia of speech, sign language may be used to augment communication. The use of signs will allow the child to interact with his environment until verbal abilities further develop. In our experience, the use of sign language requires that the child's cognitive and language comprehension abilities are better than her verbal skills. In addition, the child's parents must be willing to use signs with the child outside of the therapy setting. The introduction of signs should not preclude continued work with oral-motor skills and articulation.

Because language and learning problems may be associated with developmental apraxia of speech, it is wise to carefully evaluate these children, as well as children with other speech sound disorders, as they enter school. They should be evaluated for reading competence in the first and second grades and then evaluated for higher language functions upon entering the fourth grade. By monitoring and ultimately treating the possible associated problems, the speech pathologist can contribute significantly to the child's successful education.

Conclusion. Developmental apraxia of speech is a sensorimotor speech disorder that interferes with the voluntary motor programming of the articulators. In children, this disorder is often accompanied by an oral apraxia (the inability to perform oral vegetative movements upon request), articulatory struggle, and unusual substitutions and distortions that involve confusion of features and/or two- and three-feature errors. Careful testing by the speech-language pathologist, who recognizes that disordered communication can take place at the sensorimotor level as well as the symbolic level, will lead to the appropriate therapeutic strategies.

DYSARTHRIA

The subject of dysarthria is a complex one. Dysarthria most commonly occurs in adulthood as a result of a neurological impairment caused by a stroke, head trauma, or progressive disease, to name a few of the causes. In childhood, dysarthria is most often associated with cerebral palsy. Only recently have standardized dysarthria tests been developed, and treatment approaches are still evolving.

The course of treatment undertaken will be greatly affected by the cause of the dysarthria, the severity of the problem, and the stage of the disease process. Etiological factors weigh heavily in determining realistic achievement. The speech pathologist must decide whether the best communicative success will be accomplished through increased speech skills, maximized speech skills accompanied by augmentative measures, or augmentative measures alone.

Definition

Dworkin (1984), drawing on the work of Darley, defines *dysarthria* as "disorders of phonation, articulation, resonation, and prosody which occur either singly or in combination as a result of weakness, paresis, incoordination, and/or abnormalities in the tone of the muscles of the speech mechanism . . . and are due to impairment of the central nervous system, peripheral nervous system or both . . ." (p. 264). In contrast to apraxia, which results from difficulty in programming speech sounds, dysarthria results from difficulty in the actual production of them. This is a disorder at the fifth level of articulatory breakdown discussed in chapter 9.

As indicated by the definition, dysarthria cannot be strictly equated with faulty articulation, because articulation represents only one of the processes of speech. The muscles of respiration, phonation, and resonation may also be involved and therefore their function affected as well.

It has been established that dysarthria is not a single entity, but a group of related problems. The specific symptoms depend on the cause and location of the damage within the nervous system. The most detailed and classic contribution on the classification of dysarthria comes from Darley et al. (1975). They described the motor system as being organized into six hierarchical levels of function,

and they identified clusters of symptoms that are related to different levels of nervous system impairment.

Speech Characteristics

Typical speech characteristics of dysarthria fall into the areas of phonation, resonation, respiration, articulation, and prosody. A summary of the types of symptoms that might occur are found in Table 10.1 The specific symptoms that appear depend on the level of motor system impairment. Darley et al. (1975) describe six types of dysarthria in terms of the following primary characteristics.

Flaccid Dysarthria. The two major characteristics of this type of dysarthria are weakness and lack of muscle tone. Enervation of the muscles of all of the speech processes can be affected. The speech characteristics most often associated with flaccid dysarthria are hypernasality, imprecise consonants, monopitch, nasal emission, breathiness, and audible inspiration.

Spastic Dysarthria. The four major problems of this type are spasticity, weakness, limited range of movement, and reduced diadochokinetic rate. The most typical speech characteristics include imprecise articulation, reduced rate, low pitch, harsh voice and strained-strangled phonation. Prosody may also be affected, in the form of reduced stress, limited pitch, and loudness changes.

Ataxic Dysarthria. Patients with this type of involvement experience movements that are slow, inaccurate, and irregular. There is reduced muscle tone and tremor. The speech characteristics, as described by Yorkston and Beukelman (1981b) in concurrence with Darley et al. (1975), include imprecise articulation, often with irregular articulatory breakdowns, prosodic abnormality with slow rate, excess and equal stress, monoloudness, monopitch, and prolonged syllables.

TABLE 10.1
Dimensions of Dysarthria

I. *Phonation*
- A. Pitch
  1. Pitch level
  2. Pitch breaks
  3. Monopitch
  4. Voice tremor
- B. Intensity
  1. Monoloudness
  2. Excess loudness variation
  3. Loudness decay
  4. Alternating loudness
  5. Loudness (overall)
- C. Quality
  1. Harsh voice
  2. Hoarse (wet) voice
  3. Breathy voice (continuous)
  4. Breathy voice (transient)
  5. Strained/strangled voice
  6. Voice stoppages

II. *Resonation*
- A. Hypernasality
- B. Hyponasality
- C. Nasal emission

III. *Respiration*
- A. Forced inspiration/expiration
- B. Audible inspiration
- C. Grunt at end of expiration

IV. *Articulation*
- A. Imprecise consonants
- B. Phonemes prolonged
- C. Irregular articulatory breakdown
- D. Phonemes repeated
- E. Vowels distorted
- F. Intelligibility
- G. Bizarreness

V. *Prosody*
- A. Rate
- B. Phrases short
- C. Increase of rate in segments
- D. Increase in rate overall
- E. Reduced stress
- F. Variable rate
- G. Intervals prolonged
- H. Inappropriate silences
- I. Short rushes of speech
- J. Excess and equal stress

VI. *Other*

Note. The specific characteristics (e.g., pitch level, pitch breaks, monoloudness) are from *Motor Speech Disorders* by F. Darley, A. Aronson, and J. Brown, Philadelphia: W. B. Saunders & Co., 1975.

Hypokinetic Dysarthria. In hypokinesia, muscle functions for speech and other motor movements are generally slow and limited in range and mobility. Speech is characterized by monotone and monoloudness, reduced stress, and imprecise articulation. Rapid, short bursts of speech, inappropriate silences, and a tendency to "trail off" and run speech together are other typical characteristics.

Hyperkinetic Dysarthria. Within this category two distinct types can be identified. In the quick form, movements are quick, random, and include involuntary movements. The speech pattern includes imprecise consonants, prolonged intervals, voice stoppages, limited pitch variation, harshness, vowel distortion, and hypernasality.

In the slow form, movements are slow and sustained. By contrast to the quick form, characteristics include harsh voice, strained-strangled voice, monopitch, monoloudness, and unplanned variations in loudness.

Mixed Dysarthria. The dysarthrias already discussed occur when only one part of the motor system is involved. However, frequently more than one part of the motor system is impaired, and when this occurs a combination of problems occurs.

276

Associated Problems

The type of motor system impairment that affects speech affects other motor function in a similar manner. Depending upon the level of motor impairment, patients might experience difficulty with gait, balance, fine motor coordination, and gross motor coordination.

Etiologies

Numerous problems can affect the central or peripheral nervous system and result in dysarthria. Among the causes that have been identified are cerebrovascular insult (stroke), head trauma, degenerative diseases, and tumors. Cerebral infections and toxic conditions are also potential threats to speech integrity. Specific incidence figures for dysarthria are difficult to find because dysarthria is associated with so many different causes. However, the highest incidence results from stroke and certain degenerative neurological diseases. Studies indicate that the occurrence of some neurological and congenital problems is influenced by geographic, racial, and age factors, so incidence figures may also vary according to the population being studied (Rosenbek & LaPointe, 1981).

Assessment

Although this chapter focuses on evaluation of the speech processes, a complete diagnosis of dysarthria is based not only on speech involvement but also on other motor involvement. The evaluation process, therefore, involves an interdisciplinary approach.

Numerous assessment approaches are described in the literature, each having its own philosophical basis. Peterson and Marquardt (1981), however, state that a complete evaluation should include the structural and functional integrity of the five processes of speech (i.e., respiration, phonation, articulation, resonation, and prosody). *Structural integrity* refers to the size, shape, and relationship of

the speech structures to each other. *Functional integrity* refers to the adequacy of these structures to perform speech movements.

Assessment of structural and functional integrity can be accomplished through the use of instrumentation, such as biofeedback equipment, manometers to measure airflow, cinefluorography to observe structure and function through X-ray photography, and others, as well as through a perceptual approach. Instrumentation will not be considered in this chapter. Instrumentation can produce information that might be considered more scientific and exact, but it can be very costly and is not accessible to all speech pathologists. Even when instrumentation is possible, it must be used in combination with other traditional evaluative procedures.

Although specific evaluative procedures may vary from patient to patient, a general evaluation procedure would include an orofacial examination and evaluation of function for nonspeech movements and speech movements.

Orofacial Examination. Examination of the structures involved in articulation is described in some detail in chapter 4. Of specific interest to the dysarthria evaluation are the following:

1. Symmetry of the articulatory structures: One should observe whether the structures are equal in appearance and movement on both sides of the midline.
2. Other neurological symptoms: The examiner should note any evidence of tremor, signs of atrophy (wasting away of tissue structure) or ridging of the tongue, weakness, and the occurrence of involuntary contractions. Drooling or the presence of food in the oral cavity after a meal should also be noted.

Gross Motor Function. The procedures described in chapter 4 for evaluation and function of the mandible, lips, velum, pharynx, and tongue are appropriate for the evaluation of dysarthria. Specific observations of function should include the following:

1. Smoothness: Movement should be smooth and even, without groping, tremor, or jerkiness.
2. Range: Movement should have full excursion and be equal on both sides of the midline.
3. Strength and duration: Position should be maintained against mild resistance, and movements should be sustained over time with no evidence of deterioration.
4. Rate: Diadochokinetic rates should fall into normal range.
5. Coordination: Alternating sequential movements should be accurately produced.

The focus of this book is on articulation, and the evaluation procedures discussed so far have been limited specifically to articulation. However, in dysarthria, the other processes of speech (respiration, phonation, resonation, and prosody) are also often significantly altered and have an influence on articulation. Although evaluation of these processes will not be detailed in this chapter, the following basic observations should be included in the complete evaluation:

1. Respiration: adequate breath support and coordination of respiration with speech. Adequate loudness should be demonstrated.
2. Resonation: evidence of hypernasality, nasal emission, or hyponasality.
3. Phonation: evidence of abnormalities of pitch or voice quality, such as high pitch, monopitch, uncontrolled pitch fluctuations, pitch breaks, voice tremor, breathiness, hoarseness, and strained-strangled quality.
4. Prosody: abnormalities of timing, melody pattern, and stress.

Speech Function. Evaluation of nonspeech performance is only one level of function. Adequate performance at this level does not mean that function will be adequate for the more complex demands of speech. Therefore, standardized articulation tests as well as a speech sample should be included in the evaluation of all dysarthric patients unless the patient is so impaired that this is impossible. Deep testing of articulation is more useful than testing individual phonemes or testing phonemes in a limited context, because errors may vary according to different coarticulatory combinations. It is important that a speech sample be long enough to determine the individual's consistency over time. In some types of problems the patient may do well initially but break down when performance must be maintained for a period of time. Error patterns are as important as specific phoneme errors, and stimulability for improved production should also be tested.

According to Yorkston and Beukelman (1981a), measures of general intelligibility in relation to rate are as important as assessing specific articulation performance. These authors state that, although symptoms vary, intelligibility is a constant factor. It can also serve as a measure of severity and provide an understandable scale to patients and families. In many cases normal articulation will not be achievable; improved intelligibility may be a more practical and realistic goal.

Prognosis and Remediation

There are special considerations for dysarthric patients not only in the assessment process but in the treatment process as well. As mentioned earlier, the emphasis of treatment will be on *communication,* which may mean speech, augmented speech, or alternative communication methods.

Determining realistic goals is critical to the success of the treatment program. The speech pathologist does not want to set the patient up for failure or lead her to expect unrealistic levels of accomplishment. Unlike most functional problems, the ultimate goal for the dysarthric patient is generally compensated rather than normal speech (Rosenbek & LaPointe, 1979). One must also recognize that goals may fluctuate and have to be revised downward, depending on the course of the disease. When a patient's condition is a deteriorating one, goal planning must consider this, and utilize approaches and augmentative or alternative systems that are flexible enough to accommodate changing status. One would not want to recommend an expensive augmentative communication system that seemed practical now but would not be usable by the patient later when the disease process is more advanced.

Improving communication skills may require interdisciplinary cooperation. For example, a given case may require the expertise of a physical therapist for positioning the patient for better muscle tone during speech activities or providing girdling for support when significant muscle weakness is present; a physician for supervising girdling recommendations or for administering medication; and a prosthodontist for assistive devices.

With these preliminary considerations in mind, we can discuss more specific aspects of treatment.

General Principles of Therapy. According to Darley et al. (1975), five principles form the foundation of dysarthria therapy: (a) compensation, (b) purposeful activity, (c) monitoring, (d) an early start, and (e) motivation.

No one knows how actual improvement of function occurs; however, it is suggested that the system compensates for impaired areas and develops the ability to make maximum use of the potential that remains. Speech, once an automatic process, must be brought under intentional control. This involves developing an awareness of the activity of the articulators and producing these activities in a deliberate manner. Self-monitoring is, with dysarthria as with all other disorders, an important element. If the patient is unable to identify errors, she cannot make the necessary adjustments and corrections for improvement. Therapy should begin early, before faulty speech patterns have had an opportunity to become too firmly established. If the disease process is progressive, patients may be able to learn in the early stages to conserve or maximize skills they presently have. The importance of motivation in any disorder cannot be overemphasized. There are no passive exercises to which a patient can be subjected. Improvement relies heavily on active participation of the patient. Only a motivated patient will be vigilant in the monitoring and practicing that is so necessary.

Goals and Techniques of Therapy. The importance of establishing realistic goals for ultimate level of accomplishment has already been mentioned. Now let us consider more specific goals. Rosenbek and LaPointe (1979), recognizing the many differences among dysarthric patients, suggest eight treatment goals as a model for therapy. These include

1. assisting the patient to develop a productive attitude, i.e., a willingness to cooperate with the therapeutic process and to assume an active role
2. increasing physiological support for speech by modifying abnormalities of posture, tone, and strength
3. modifying the five processes of speech production, i.e., respiration, phonation, resonation, articulation, and prosody, for improved function
4. assisting in the use of augmentative communication when functional speech is limited

Therapy for dysarthria is very structured and very repetitive. Building muscle strength, increasing rate of movement, increasing range of movement, and improving muscle tone for speech are like building any other muscle functions. They require appropriate techniques to stimulate development and they require practice. The improvement that occurs will probably be in the form of progressive approximation. When adequate return does not result, therapy may turn to initiating compensatory strategies.

Articulation is affected by an interaction of all of the processes of speech, and improvement in articulation may occur in conjunction with improvement in other areas. Accordingly, LaPointe (1982) states that "lately there seems to be less primary emphasis on treating articulation in motor speech disorders. In both apraxia of speech and the dysarthrias, attention to the interaction of rate, stress and durational factors in the accuracy of speech sound production is gaining favor" (p. 395).

To elaborate on this point, articulation can often be improved through indirect approaches or through methods that have generalizing effects on articulation. For example, slowing rate has been shown to have a significant effect on intelligibility (Yorkston & Beukelman, 1981b). This can be accomplished by tapping out rhythms or using a metronome. The Delayed Auditory Feedback Unit has been suggested as a possible technique to slow rate and increase loudness (Hanson & Metter, 1980). Exaggeration of consonant production can increase accuracy and slow rate.

Articulation therapy may involve techniques similar to those used for other types of articulation problems when working on specific articulation goals (see chapter 5). However, because in dysarthria the speech pathologist is dealing with an impaired motor system, therapy must be directed to those specific problems as well. Proper positioning is important so that the patient's energy can be directed toward speech goals rather than trying to maintain head or trunk control. Poor positioning may create negative force on muscles and make speech postures more difficult to achieve. Exercises designed to extend range of movement, to increase strength and speed, and to improve coordination of movements may be necessary preliminary steps before specific articulation therapy can begin. Examples of such exercises might be:

□ Range of movement: After stabilizing the mandible, have the patient elevate the tongue tip to the alveolar ridge. Patient may accomplish this in gradual stages.
□ Increase strength: Protrude tongue and see if the patient can maintain position against resistance applied by tongue depressor.

□ Increase speed: Have the patient perform alternating movement such as lateral tongue movement or protrusion/retraction at gradually increasing speeds.
□ Coordination: Produce alternating movement patterns in controlled fashion. Examiner may have patient perform movement according to a pattern tapped out or spoken by therapist. Exercises with increasing difficulty levels for alternating or sequential movements can also be used.

When the patient can perform these types of exercises on gross motor movement tasks, she can move on to incorporating phoneme production into the exercises. Following that, syllable, word, and sentence production may be undertaken, assuming that each of these stages is potentially feasible. In addition to traditional articulation approaches, electrical stimulation techniques, described by Netsell and Cleeland (1973), have been used. Biofeedback techniques have been applied to assist the patient in monitoring movement and accuracy.

When the process just described is not feasible, alternative goals must be established. According to Logemann (1984), these alternative goals fall into three areas:

1. compensatory speech production (e.g., substituting a perceptually similar phoneme for a phoneme that cannot be produced normally)
2. surgical compensation (such as Teflon injection or pharyngeal flap when velar movement is inadequate)
3. prosthetic devices (such as palatal lift for reduced velar function)

The speech pathologist should be familiar with all of the compensating strategies and be able to recognize when such measures are appropriate.

Again, the importance of the other speech processes to articulation and intelligibility cannot be ignored. Although discussion has been limited to direct and indirect articulation strategies, when problems of respiration, phonation, resonation, and prosody exist, these must also be addressed in therapy. In some cases, treatment in these areas may precede articulation goals and at other times occur concomitantly.

Conclusion

The study of dysarthria is still in an early stage. Dysarthria affects all speech processes, and specific symptoms vary according to the level of neurological involvement. It is generally agreed that many patients can benefit from direct therapy even though they will not achieve normal speech. When prognosis is poor, the emphasis of therapy must be upon facilitation of communication rather than speech.

CEREBRAL PALSY

Cerebral palsy is a developmental disability often accompanied by speech and/or language disorders. It is not a diagnostic label for a unique speech or language disorder. In fact, the most common motor speech disorder in children who are diagnosed as having cerebral palsy is dysarthria.

Why, then, is cerebral palsy singled out for individual discussion if the speech manifestations are not unique? Cerebral palsy must be studied separately because diagnosis and treatment begin much earlier than in discrete speech and language problems in children. Furthermore, cerebral palsy must be differentiated from pure articulation disorders because, as a developmental disorder, it encompasses so many other problems that the speech pathologist cannot treat the individual without being a member of a ''cerebral palsy team'' that includes the physical therapist, the occupational therapist, the physiatrist, the psychologist, the social worker, and the teacher. In cerebral palsy the articulation disorder can be best understood by understanding the entire disability.

Definition

Cerebral palsy is a developmental disability in which the main clinical feature is a lack of motor control presented most commonly as spasticity or increased muscular tone. Less often the motor control problem may be involuntary movements or incoordination (Paneth, 1986). The individual's

ability to walk is always affected. The term *cerebral palsy* does not refer to one disorder but to a collection of nonprogressive neuromotor disorders that appear early in life. The insult causing the symptom complex of cerebral palsy must occur in utero, at birth, or early in life. Early in life means up to the age of 2 years (Mysak, 1980) for some authors, and up to the age of 6 for others (Boone, 1972).

Proponents of neuro-developmental treatment (NDT) have put forth another definition of *cerebral palsy*. NDT, which was developed by Berta Bobath (1967), involves early team intervention for the treatment of cerebral palsy. In this approach all types of cerebral palsy are seen as a problem of abnormal coordination of muscle action rather than paralysis or weakness of muscles. The brain lesion interferes with normal maturation of the brain, which then interferes with normal motor development. Adherents of the neuro-developmental approach consider the accompanying intellectual, cognitive, sensory, and perceptual deficits secondary to the cerebral palsy. In other words, the primary inability to coordinate muscle movement has deprived the child of the ability to explore the environment and develop other abilities. The Bobaths consider ''movement'' to be the foundation of learning.

According to neuro-developmental treatment theory, cerebral palsy caused postnatally, after a certain degree of motor development has already occurred, will require different assessment procedures and treatment planning.

Etiology

Cerebral palsy is caused by damage to, or malformations of, the brain. Many factors can contribute to these brain anomalies. The causes of cerebral palsy are often classified according to three vulnerable periods in the life of the fetus-infant-child: prenatal, perinatal, and postnatal or early infancy.

Some prenatal factors (those that occur during pregnancy) include infection, RH factor, hemorrhage, and anoxia (lack of oxygen to the fetal brain), which is the most common.

Perinatal factors, or those that occur from the onset of labor until the baby is visible, include anoxia as the main contributor, and trauma as the second most common.

Postnatal factors account for only 10% to 15% of the cases of cerebral palsy. Some of these factors are traumatic injury such as auto accident, falls, and blows to the head; and infectious diseases such as meningitis and encephalitis.

In a recent study by Nelson and Ellenberg (1986) of 189 children with cerebral palsy, the authors concluded that the cause or causes of most cerebral palsy is still a mystery and that factors of labor and delivery play a relatively small role in accounting for cerebral palsy.

Associated Problems

Cerebral palsy presents itself in many forms. There are so many variations of these forms that problems other than the actual neuromotor handicap may cause more difficulty than the condition itself. Newton (1977) mentions that the degree to which the child's disability handicaps her increases proportionately to the number and severity of related problems. Therefore, it is necessary to attend to the problems related to cerebral palsy in order to understand their nature and effects. The three major categories of problems that must be conquered by the cerebral palsy child and, of course, the family, are physical problems, psychological problems, and learning difficulties.

The physical problems of children with cerebral palsy include difficulty in ambulation and learning self-care activities. Cerebral-palsied children also have impaired ability in chewing, sucking, and swallowing, which interferes with one of the most important early relationships of the child—feeding. Between 35% and 60% of cerebral-palsied children will have a seizure in their life (Perlstein, Gibbs, & Gibbs, 1947). Although anticonvulsive

drugs, such as Dilantin, control seizures, they have side effects that impair attention and learning. Visual defects are found in 50% of cerebral-palsied children (Pearlstone, 1969) and about 20% have hearing loss (Nober, 1976). Dental problems may also result from the oral motor difficulties of cerebral palsy.

Emotional disorders experienced by those with cerebral palsy are not necessarily typical of the cerebral palsy population, but are the kinds of problems that are common to people in trouble. It is easy to understand why low self-esteem, immaturity, and dependency are fostered in the child with cerebral palsy.

Mental retardation is estimated to affect 50% to 75% of the cerebral-palsied population (Cruickshank, 1976). Thus, educational problems are common in this group, yet they vary with the abilities of each individual child. Perceptual problems are not as obvious as physical disabilities, but nevertheless are a significant contributor to learning disabilities and educational failure. Some of the children are hyperactive and/or easily distracted, which adds to the burden of learning.

About 68% of cerebral-palsied children have speech and/or language disorders (Cruickshank, 1976). The diversity of these problems is wide. The disorders include all varieties of dysarthrias, articulation problems, and language disorders, such as difficulty in abstracting, organizing, and drawing conclusions.

The remainder of this section will be devoted to the articulation problems of the cerebral-palsied child and will address the characteristics, assessment, and remediation of these problems.

Speech Characteristics

The articulation problems in the cerebral-palsied child are usually the most obvious component of the speech problem. These disorders are often referred to as *developmental dysarthria*. However, the articulation of a cerebral-palsied child cannot be separated from the other motor processes of speech, which include respiration, phonation, and resonation. These processes need to operate at fundamental levels before useful articulation patterns can be taught. In addition, the posture of a cerebral-palsied child needs to be considered. If it is inadequate, then it should be improved before working with the speech. Some of the articulation problems in children with cerebral palsy are caused by persistence of feeding reflexes, such as rooting, lip-mouth opening, and sucking. Another cause of articulation problems is paralytic involvement of some of the articulators. Articulation of the cerebral-palsied child can also be hampered by involuntary movements or by inconsistency or limitations in the range, strength, and direction of movements. Apraxia may also be present in cerebral-palsied children, creating difficulty in making voluntary movements. In general, there is no typical articulation pattern for the cerebral-palsied child.

Assessment

Twenty-five years ago, this section on assessment would have begun directly with the traditional methods of evaluating the oral musculature as described in chapter 4. However, the concept of early intervention in the treatment of cerebral palsy has significantly changed the content of the speech assessment of cerebral-palsied children. What was thought to be early intervention at ages 3 and 4 is now not considered early. Early intervention in the comprehensive treatment of cerebral palsy is some time before the end of the first year, and the earlier the better.

In 1966, Kong reported the results of an early intervention program based on the neuro-developmental approach developed by the Bobaths (1972). The rationale was that early intervention in cerebral palsy could improve the long-term prognosis of the children. The program initiated intervention in the first 6 months of the infant's life. The goals were inhibition of the abnormal movements and reflexes and facilitation of normal automatic movements, so that more normal sensorimotor patterns of development could be acquired. The program provided for active participation of the parents, so that the program's goals were in-

corporated into the child's routine of handling by the mother. At the end of 4 years, 75% of the 69 children who remained in the program demonstrated a normal gait. It was also observed that there were fewer mentally retarded children in the group than would be expected. Kong's impression was that early normal motor experience had given these children a chance to develop their normal potential.

Because of this study, and others by Denhoff and Holden (1954) and Jones, Barrett, Olonoff, and Anderson (1969), as well as much work by Bobath (1967) and Finnie (1975), the concept of neuro-developmental treatment and early intervention has received much support from professionals and the United Cerebral Palsy Association. The basic tenet of this approach seems to be that physical competence is the most important factor relating to later success, including the development of normal speech. Normal speech is dependent on the successful acquisition of feeding and prespeech skills, and the evaluation of these skills can, and must, be done early in life.

Several *nonspeech aspects* of normal development involve physiological structures needed for articulation development:

1. head control with stability of the neck and shoulder girdle, because stability provides for later mobility of the oral structure
2. a coordinated pattern of respiration and phonation, which is related to development of abdominal muscles
3. a variety of feeding experiences with foods of different textures, temperatures, and tastes, in order to provide normal development of feeding patterns
4. babbling practice

When evaluating oral motor function, it is necessary to note the presence or absence of these sensorimotor prerequisites. In addition, oral motor function must be assessed in relation to whole body movements, and in a variety of body positions. For example, a child may find sitting to be such an effort that there can be no control over the oral mechanism, whereas the same child, placed in a different position, will have more control. At this point, it is important to mention again the concept of a neuro-developmental treatment *team*. The speech pathologist can receive invaluable assistance from physical and occupational therapists in the evaluation and treatment of speech-related areas, such as head control and breathing.

The Pre-Speech Assessment Scale (Morris, 1975a) assists the speech pathologist on the team to evaluate systematically the areas of prespeech behavior in which cerebral-palsied children deviate from normal. The scale examines areas such as postural tone and movement, response to sensory stimuli, and the prespeech behaviors of (a) feeding, (b) biting and chewing, (c) sucking, (d) swallowing, (e) respiration and phonation, and (f) sound play.

In the Pre-Speech Assessment Scale, Morris suggests that the following observations be made regarding postural tone and movement patterns:

1. Observe the general postural tone in terms of hypertonicity (excessive muscle tone) or hypotonicity (insufficient muscle tone), normalcy or fluctuation of tone. These observations should be made when the child is at rest, in various positions, and when the child tries to communicate or talk to someone. Typical patterns of tone and movement should be noted.
2. Head and trunk control should be evaluated in terms of symmetry, positions that enhance control, and responses of head and trunk when the child rolls, sits, or talks.
3. Responses to sensory stimulation should also be assessed. Auditory, visual, vestibular, and tactile modes should be questioned. The tactile mode is of special interest around the mouth. The clinician needs to know what responses the child has to sensory stimulation around the mouth, because many children are hypersensitive and must have a therapeutic approach to feeding and speech that incorporates a series of graded stimuli.

The prespeech skills section of the Pre-Speech Assessment Scale examines 12 components of prespeech behavior:

1. The clinician and team should note the influence of abnormal body tone and movements on the speech mechanism. Are there certain tensions and movement patterns in the jaw, lips, tongue, etc., that are related to the gross movement abnormalities?
2. Structural deviations and deformities of the speech mechanism, as well as of other parts of the body, should be noted.
3. Facial expressions are very much a part of communication. Some cerebral-palsied children do not possess a repertoire of facial expressions because of poor muscle tone. The clinician needs to watch for variety and symmetry in facial expression and, especially, to see if the face is used communicatively.
4. General feeding behavior is often abnormal in cerebral-palsied children. They do not suck well from the beginning, are slow, and do not tolerate new foods. Normal sucking activities, as well as normally coordinated actions of the tongue, lips, and mandible in chewing and swallowing prepare the child for the more precise oral movements necessary for articulation. Here again, the cerebral-palsied child is doubly penalized. The child was born with abnormal enervation and control to use the oral structure, and, because it cannot be used maximally, the child cannot profit from the developmental experiences that it provides. Therefore, the clinician needs to observe length of time, and amount and types of foods needed by the child. Positioning and behavioral problems related to mealtime are also of interest.

5. Sucking behavior should be observed in terms of jaw, lip, and tongue involvement and control. What is sucking like when taking pureed foods from a spoon? Does a tongue thrust or bite reflex interfere with these activities?

6. Swallowing is reflex behavior in the normal infant. In the cerebral-palsied infant, it is often marked with coughing, choking, and leakage from the corners of the mouth. Some foods are easier to swallow than others. Drooling sometimes accompanies fine motor and speech activities because a voluntary swallow has not yet been accomplished.

7. The acts of biting and chewing are composed of a number of subskills and sometimes interfered with by reflexes, such as the bite reflex and a jaw thrust. The observer needs to see what kinds of food the child will chew or bite, and if there are overflow movements into the body while biting and chewing. Are the tongue, lips, and jaw active and efficient in chewing?

8. The clinician should observe what kinds of imitative control over the oral mechanism the child can demonstrate. Is there imitative behavior of basic oral movements such as puckering lips and protruding the tongue? In addition, the child needs to have some imitative responses for vowels, consonants, and syllables.

9. Two manners of breathing are recognized. Vegetative breathing, or silent involuntary breathing, is characterized by an almost even inspiratory and expiratory cycle through the nose. Breathing rates of children under 2 are also usually quite variable and may range from 20 to 40 breaths per minute. As the child matures, the rate decreases. In contrast to vegetative breathing is speech breathing, which is characterized by a quick inspiratory phase and a long expiratory phase, accomplished through the mouth. Productive speech breathing should be stabilized at the rate of about 20 breaths per minute. Breathing difficulties are reported to be seen in 40% to 80% of children with cerebral palsy. The problems include shallow breathing; incoordination of the thorax and abdomen, which produces simultaneous inspiratory and expiratory movements, or "oppositional breathing"; and a high rate of breaths per minute (over 30) (Crickmay, 1966). An additional difficulty may be the delay in changing from the state of vegetative breathing to the state of speech breathing. Some children cannot make the change at all. Morris (1975a) suggests that while looking at the child's breathing one should keep in mind tone of the musculature, depth and regularity of breathing, rib-flaring effects of other body movements, and use of the nose or mouth for breathing.

10. Control over breathing is essential to control over phonation, although there are abnormalities of phonation that may be present in spite of adequate breathing patterns. There may be poor control over the opening and closing of the vocal folds and/or velopharyngeal port. There may be weakness and/or incoordination in the intrinsic and/or extrinsic muscles of the larynx. Among the things the clinician wants to note about the child's phonation patterns are the ease and variability of phonation. Are respiration and phonation well coordinated, or is there a voice quality problem of hoarseness or harshness? Does the child have appropriate stress patterns and does she use these as phonation patterns to communicate?

11. In addition to assessing articulation in the usual way, the clinician on a neuro-developmental treatment team must also look for earlier articulatory gestures. Babbling and the variability, spontaneity, and speed of the articulators should be noted.

12. Assessment for augmentative communication skills is also a necessity. Are the child's cognitive and linguistic abilities now more advanced than her speaking abilities? Can she use her eyes to indicate direction, or can she fingerpoint?

The prespeech assessment scale is a vital component in assessing the communication disorders of cerebral-palsied children. It should be used by a speech pathologist who is knowledgeable about normal oral motor development, because sometimes even subtle deficits in three or four areas of prespeech development can combine to produce a very complex clinical picture.

For several reasons, the evaluation of isolated articulation patterns can be done only after the clinician has evaluated the prespeech behaviors. One reason is that the isolated articulation evaluation should be done in terms of how prespeech behaviors have affected articulation. Secondly, because of the age at which the prespeech evaluation is done, an actual articulation evaluation is not appropriate until later. However, when the speech pathologist facilitates and stimulates normal bodily movements and prespeech behaviors, neuro-developmental theory postulates that articulation will begin more normally because other interfering variables have been eliminated and new patterns have been taught upon which articulation patterns can be based.

When a traditional articulation evaluation can be done, the methods suggested in chapter 4 are applicable. However, phonation, respiration, and resonation must also be assessed in the context of articulation, as suggested in the dysarthria section of this chapter.

Remediation

Speech pathologists who are interested in serving the cerebral-palsied population must be prepared to be members of a team that will begin to deal with these children in infancy. The speech pathologist does not have to wait until speech fails to develop; the role is expanded to one of a prespeech-language therapist. Therapies can be initiated in infancy, so that early interactions with the mother are productive for language learning and speech development. Early intervention by the speech pathologist can prevent, or lessen, the effects of poor head control, abnormal patterns of respiration and phonation, and feeding difficulties.

Neuro-developmental treatment (Bobath & Bobath, 1972) stresses that therapeutic physical handling by all professionals (as well as parents) will inhibit the abnormal and primitive reflexes, while providing stimulation for the development of more normal postural adjustments and coordinated movements. For example, a spastic child will experience extensor spasticity in the legs when she is carried. However, this pattern can be broken, and more normal patterns stimulated, if the mother will open the child's legs and carry her on her hip. This type of action also stimulates head control and balance reactions in the trunk. In other ways of physical handling, the child's breathing and oral activities can be stimulated into more normal patterns while the abnormal movements are extinguished.

In the prespeech and language treatment of the cerebral-palsied infant, the speech pathologist has three priorities: (a) parent education, (b) communication and language stimulation, and (c) facilitation of prespeech skills.

A team approach involving an occupational therapist, physical therapist, speech pathologist, and an educational specialist is especially beneficial for the preschool child with cerebral palsy. Multidisciplinary classes are structured to include play that elicits cognitive, physical, and language goals. Parents also have an opportunity to discuss problems with other parents and the team. A snack time allows the speech pathologist and the occupational therapist to observe and modify oral motor skills.

Parent education is an integral part of treatment. The parent can observe strategies that various specialists employ. Early language stimulation is natural to most parents; the parents of cerebral-palsied children, however, are under special stresses, and they will need special help.

Because cerebral-palsied children do not have normally integrated sensory systems, early initiation of graded sensory stimulation may be needed to facilitate development toward normal sensory experiences, which are important for language development. The therapist should verbalize the principle being demonstrated after the parents have observed it in action. Then the parent should be asked to practice the principle while being observed. Suggestions for placing the child so that she can obtain abundant visual stimulation are also helpful to language development. Facilitation of body positions should be of prime concern so that the child will be free of abnormal postures when directing attention to verbal and visual material.

A priority in prespeech therapy is facilitation of nonspeech skills related to articulation development. This includes work on the four sensorimotor prerequisites, which are head control, coordinated respiration and phonation, normal development of feeding skills, and babbling practice. The speech pathologist must consult with the physical therapist in order to learn how to facilitate the development of normal head control. For example, if there is an excess of movement, the speech pathologist must discuss with the physical therapist methods for stabilizing the trunk and extremities. The effectiveness of the entire prespeech program will often depend on the speech pathologist's ability to deal with abnormalities of postural tone, movement patterns, and reflex activities. Consequently, it is necessary for the clinician to maintain a good working relationship with the physical and occupational therapists.

Coordinated respiration and phonation, again, depend on the functioning of other larger muscles, particularly some abdominal muscles. Examples of some of the problems that the speech pathologist addresses are (a) lack of coordinated voicing and breathing and (b) inadequate duration of phonation to sustain babbling. Lack of coordinated voicing and breathing can be remediated by stimulating laughing or crying, and then using light vibration on the sternum during exhalation. This vibration then becomes associated with phonation on exhalation and can be used to initiate voice as control progresses. Increasing the duration of phonation

can be aided by placing the child in a position that is conducive to phonation and babbling. This might be on the stomach (prone) or on the side. Another maneuver might be to use slow physical movement, such as lap jiggling or light rapid vibration of the therapist's hands over the chest and shoulders during exhalation.

A variety of feeding experiences are structured to assure normal development as well as to inhibit abnormal reflexes and improve coordination of the jaw, lips, tongue, and soft palate in sucking, swallowing, biting, and chewing. Morris (1975b) presents the following principles:

1. Carefully analyze the task. For example, in chewing, there must be control of the jaw, lateral movement of the tongue, and inhibition from sucking and inward pressure of the cheeks. In what aspects is the child unable to succeed?
2. Observe what is happening in the rest of the body and use the positions that will facilitate or elicit the desired oral movements.
3. Because many cerebral-palsied children are hypersensitive to facial or oral stimulation, controlled stimulation must be used in the orofacial area to reduce hypersensitivity and build more normal oral sensory perception.
4. All types of food and liquids should be used. However, careful attention must be paid to grading of stimulation and variations of taste, texture, and temperature.
5. The mother should be an active participant in therapy. When she is skilled and confident, she can begin to incorporate the new routines in the home.
6. Successful experience of more normal feeding patterns will produce oral movements that can be modified for use in babbling and speech.

Because of the large amount of very specific information on therapeutic feeding, only the principles have been mentioned. More information on specific techniques can be found in Morris (1975b), Connor, Williamson, and Siepp (1978), and Finnie (1975).

Another sensorimotor prespeech skill is babbling practice. The child should be placed in a position that has been found to stimulate vocal play. Some techniques that have been used are facilitation of a sustained sound by using vibration, or by actually manipulating the jaw and lips to produce a variety of sounds. A wider variety of sound play may be stimulated by encouraging the child to voice while chewing. The therapist should praise jargon behaviors and set up little conversations by responding to jargoning with such statements as, ''Oh, tell me more about that'' or ''Oh, that is very interesting.'' Imitating the child's babbling may also be helpful.

The therapeutic principles that have been discussed are taken from the philosophy of neurodevelopmental treatment and are intended to apply to the very young child. However, some speech pathologists will be involved with cerebral-palsied children who are older and/or who have not had the benefit of early treatment. In addition to the articulatory remediation practices utilized with functional disorders, the following treatment strategies are applicable to these children.

Speech therapy for the older child without a language problem follows procedures similar to those discussed earlier in the treatment of dysarthria. However, there are modifications due to the nature of cerebral palsy as a developmental disorder.

A basic part of treatment is facilitating the desired movements while inhibiting the abnormal reflex patterns. Before the speech pathologist can address the problems of respiration, phonation, and articulation, the child must be able to assume and maintain some reflex-inhibiting postures that the physical therapist recommends. Articulation develops in the normal child when primitive reflexes have disappeared and coordination of respiration and phonation are established. A cerebral-

palsied child who has been in a neurodevelopmental treatment center since infancy will have experienced much therapy for inhibiting abnormal reflexes and stimulating normal movements before articulation develops. When this therapy is successful, articulation should begin and develop fairly normally. If there are errors, they can be treated in the same manner as articulation errors in a non-cerebral-palsied child would be treated (Newton, 1977). However, if the cerebral-palsied child is severely involved or has not had the advantage of neuro-developmental treatment, special procedures must be applied. Some children may still need therapeutic feeding and desensitization of the oral area before articulation therapy can be initiated.

The goals of articulation therapy are to increase the speed, range, and accuracy of the tongue, lips, and jaw movements. The goals are pursued in concert with the maintenance of body and head tones as well as respiration, phonation, and resonation normalcy (Mysak, 1980). Mysak divides therapy for articulation into three processes: (a) differentiation, or ability to move articulators in isolation from other body parts, (b) praxis, or the ability to make specific movements, and (c) diadochokinesia, or speeding up the movements.

In the differentiation phase, the child is stabilized and then asked to move her tongue or lips. If the child cannot do it, the clinician assists in this endeavor, but also should investigate why the child cannot make these movements. Is the difficulty related to body positioning, inability to perform some oral movement in feeding, or inability to inhibit abnormal reflex patterns? If these kinds of questions are not asked, treatment may be focusing on a symptom and not the cause. The sequence includes being able to independently move the mandible from the head, the tongue from the mandible, and the lips from the mandible. The final movements are when the child is able to move the mandible, lips, and tongue independently of the head and each other, as in normally articulated speech.

After independent movement is established, specific articulatory movements are introduced, such as lingua-alveolar, linguavelar, and linguadental. Movements should be carried out in conjunction with appropriate audiovisual stimulation by the clinician.

Speeding up the movements can be done by serial production of voiced and voiceless, or nasal and nonnasal sounds. Using phonemes that she can produce, the child can practice two-, three-, and four-syllable sets to increase speed. An example might be /nɑ–tɑ/, /nɑ–dɑ/, /nɑ–nɑ/, /nɑ–kɑ/, /nɑ–gɑ/. Three- and four-syllable combinations can be used and eventually two-word combinations can be introduced.

Although prognosis for a cerebral-palsied child is almost impossible to ascertain early in the treatment, all children will develop some kind of communicative skill, be it speech or not. In some children, speech may be severely impaired and alternative means of communicating must be explored. The generic term *communication augmentation* refers to any approach designed to support, enhance, or augment the communication of individuals who are not independent, verbal communicators in all situations (Beukelman, Yorkston & Dowden, 1985). Augmentative communication may involve gestural communication, pointers, boards containing words and pictures, or electronic devices. For the individual who has a severe motor impairment, these devices may provide the only means for unlocking language and intellectual potential.

Conclusion

No specific articulation therapy program is available for the cerebral-palsied child. This child needs to begin at a much more basic level than most children with articulation disorders and needs to have articulation interrelated with all the other processes of bodily development and speech.

Neuro-developmental treatment is a philosophy of treatment that is based on early intervention. The basic tenets of this approach are to inhibit abnormal and primitive reflexes while stimulating the development of normal postural adjustments and the acquisition of coordinated movements. NDT appears to offer a new perspective on an old and yet-unsolved problem.

Augmentative communication should be attempted with cerebral-palsied children who are not reaching their fullest potential due to a severe motor impairment restricting speech.

CLEFT PALATE

Cleft palate is a problem quite different from apraxia and dysarthria, but one that can have considerable effect upon speech. Speech problems result from inadequate structures, poor muscle function, compensatory strategies, and/or functional causes.

Treating the problems of cleft palate involves closing the actual defect as well as improving function of the structures for speech. Recently, many exciting medical/surgical and technological advancements have occurred that reduce or eliminate the devastating effects of cleft palate that once existed. However, the role of speech pathology in the management of cleft palate remains an important one.

Definition

Cleft palate is a structural anomaly that can affect the tissues, muscles, and bony processes of lip, alveolar process, hard palate, soft palate, and uvula (see Figure 10.1). A cleft of these structures occurs during embryonic development, when there is a failure of structures to unite. Nonunion most typically occurs between the median and lateral frontonasal processes that normally form the primary palate, including the lip, alveolar process, and incisive foramen; or at the midline between the palatal plates that form the secondary palate, including the hard and soft palates (Morley, 1970). This development takes place during the first trimester of pregnancy.

Clefts of the lip and palate together affect boys more frequently than girls (2:1), whereas cleft pal-

FIGURE 10.1
Normal palate.

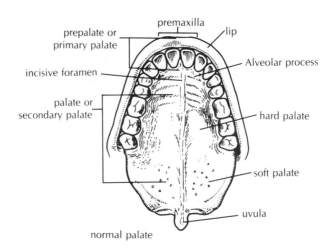

ate only affects girls more frequently (2:1) (Koepp-Baker, 1971).

Numerous classification systems exist. In an attempt to establish common terminology and an acceptable conceptual framework, a classification system was established by the American Cleft Palate Association (Harkins, Berlin, Harding, Longacre, & Snodgrass, 1962). It is based on embryological development and defines structures involved, location, size of cleft, and type of distortions present. The system includes submucous clefts, i.e., clefts that affect the underlying muscle and bony structures but leave the membrane covering intact. It also includes palatal shortness, a frequently neglected problem in classification systems. This classification system is found in Table 10.2.

Etiology

Numerous causal factors have been associated with cleft palate, although no single explanatory factor has emerged (Koepp-Baker, 1971). Possible environmental causes cited by Morley (1970) include trauma, malnutrition, drugs, rubella, and viral disease during the first trimester of pregnancy. Interference from other embryonic structures such as the hands, feet, cord, or tongue which prevent the

structures from uniting have also been cited as possible causes.

Genetic transmission is suggested by observation of a familial tendency, although the mode of transmission is not known (Longacre, 1970; Woolf, Woolf, & Broadbent, 1963). According to current literature, there may be a genetic predisposition which, when coupled with certain environmental factors, can result in a cleft (Koepp-Baker, 1971; McWilliams, 1982).

Speech Characteristics

Typical speech characteristics associated with cleft palate fall into the areas of resonation, articulation, and phonation. A brief summary of all three areas is included because all three have an impact on overall intelligibility; they also have an interactive effect upon one another.

Resonance. The most typical resonance characteristic associated with cleft palate is hypernasality. This results from inability of the velum to close off the nasal cavity in order to maintain a balance between oral and nasal resonance. Too much air is allowed to enter the nasal cavity. The cause may be structural, as in a short palate, submucous cleft, or an opening in the palate; or it may be functional,

TABLE 10.2
American Cleft Palate Association Classification System

*Clefts of Prepalate**	*Cleft of Prepalate*
Cleft lip	Any combination of foregoing types
Unilateral	Prepalate protrusion
Right, left	Prepalate rotation
Extent in thirds ($\frac{1}{3}$, $\frac{2}{3}$, $\frac{3}{3}$)	Prepalate arrest (median cleft)
Bilateral	
Right, left	*Clefts of Palate***
Extent in thirds	Clefts of soft palate
Median	Extent
Extent in thirds	Posteroanterior in thirds
Prolabium	Width (maximum in mm)
Small, medium, large	Palatal shortness
Cogenital scar	None, slight, moderate, marked
Right, left, median	Submucous cleft
Extent in thirds	Extent in thirds
	Cleft hard palate
Cleft of Alveolar Process	Extent
Unilateral	Posteroanterior in thirds
Right, left	Width (maximum in mm)
Extent in thirds	Vomer attachment
Bilateral	Right, left, absent
Right, left	Submucous cleft
Extent in thirds	Extent in thirds
Median	Cleft of soft and hard palate
Extent in thirds	
Submucous	*Clefts of Prepalate and Palate*
Right, left, median	Any combination of clefts described under Clefts of Prepalate and Clefts of Palate

*Prepalate or primary palate includes the lip, alveolar ridge, and triangular area of the palate just behind the alveolar ridge but anterior to the incisive foramen.
**Palate or secondary palate refers to the remaining portion of the palate lying posterior to the incisive foramen, i.e., hard palate and soft palate.

Source: "Classification of Cleft Lip and Palate" by A. J. Berlin. In *Cleft Lip and Palate: Surgical, Dental and Speech Aspects,* W. C. Grabb, S. W. Rosenstein, & K. Bzoch (Eds.), 1971, Boston: Little Brown & Co. Copyright 1971 by Little Brown & Co. Reprinted by permission.

as in a repaired cleft with poor or uncoordinated velar mobility or poor tongue positioning. A symptom of hypernasality is nasal emission, which is a sound that results from airflow going through the nasal cavity. It is perceived as an audible nasal escape of air, especially on plosive, affricative, and fricative phonemes.

Much less frequently found are problems of hyponasality and cul-de-sac resonation. Hyponasality is most often caused by an obstruction or a pha-

ryngeal flap (a type of surgical repair) that provides too much occlusion. Cul-de-sac resonance is a combination of hypernasality and hyponasality. This type of resonance could result from a blockage in the nasal passages.

Articulation. The severity of the articulation deficit was found to be related to the severity of clefting (Riski & DeLong, 1984). In this study, children with cleft lip only had normal articulation.

Articulation ability decreased in the following order: 1) cleft lip and alveolar ridge, (2) cleft palate
only, and (3) cleft lip and palate. The specific phonemic errors may vary according to cause as discussed in the following sections.

Decreased Intraoral Pressure. Hypernasality results in a decrease in intraoral pressure and hence
affects articulation. Stops (/p, b, t, d, k, g/), fricatives (/s, z, ʃ, ʒ/), and affricatives (/tʃ, dʒ/) are
all affected because these phonemes require intraoral pressure for accurate production.

When intraoral pressure is limited, several effects might be anticipated. The consonant produced might be weak or distorted. If intraoral airflow is increased, nasal emission results. Although
the patient is often capable of normal articulatory
placement, she may develop compensatory patterns in an attempt to prevent nasal emission.

In most instances where compensatory articulations are substituted for target phonemes, the correct *manner* of articulation is preserved while correct *place* of articulation is sacrificed (Trost,
1981). Generally, the place of articulation is
moved posteriorly or perhaps, as Estrem & Broen
(in press) suggest, away from the center of the oral
tract to the periphery of the oral tract. According to
Trost (1981), frequently observed compensatory
substitutions are the glottal stop, pharyngeal fricative, velar fricative, pharyngeal stop, mid-dorsum
palatal stop, and posterior nasal fricative. In all but
the glottal stop (voiced) and the posterior nasal
fricative (unvoiced), the compensatory articulation
may be voiced or unvoiced.

1. A *glottal stop* is an attempt to implode
   before the air reaches the oral cavity, especially on stop consonants, by creating a
   valve at the level of the glottis.
2. The *pharyngeal fricative* results from an
   attempt to shift the valve to the pharynx to
   compensate for inadequate intraoral breath
   pressure on fricatives and affricates.

3. The *velar fricative* is a lingua-alveolar articulation made in the approximate place
   of /k/ and /g/.
4. The *pharyngeal stop* is produced as a /k/
   or /g/ with the tongue positioned posterior
   and inferior to its normal target place. The
   place of articulation varies from near the
   level of velopharyngeal closure to a lower
   position closer to the glottis.
5. The *mid-dorsum palatal stop* is a stop consonant made in the approximate place of
   the glide /j/. This substitution is used to
   replace /t/, /d/, /k/, or /g/.
6. The *posterior nasal fricative* occurs when
   there is an airway constriction as the velum approximates the pharyngeal wall, but
   there is no velopharyngeal seal, and the air
   is released nasally. The speech
   consequence is an audible friction with
   associated nasal air emission. Posterior
   nasal fricatives are typically accompanied
   by nasal emission but are distinguishable
   from nasal emission alone.

Posterior nasal fricatives, pharyngeal fricatives,
and glottal stops may be produced simultaneously
with a more anterior place of articulation, such as
bilabial or lingua-alveolar articulation produced in
the same manner.

Dental and Occlusal Abnormalities. Although the
specific effects of dental and occlusal anomalies
remain unclear, both may interfere with normal
articulation. Any deviations that produce a class III
malocclusion, or open bite, may have an effect on
consonant production, especially the sibilant
sounds (Starr, 1979). Any other dental abnormality that restricts tongue movement may likewise
affect articulation. When there is a disproportion-
ate relationship between the mandible (lower jaw)
and maxilla (upper dental arch), bilabials, the fricatives /f/ and /v/, and lingual-alveolar consonants
may also be affected. These kinds of problems
may result in the development of compensatory
movements and/or phoneme distortions or approximations. According to Starr, the conditions most
likely to result in an articulation problem are open

bite, missing central incisors, or any anomaly affecting the relationship between the tongue and the lower incisors. However, although articulation problems may result from these problems, many individuals are able to compensate for dental and occlusal problems and have normal speech.

Hearing Loss. Cleft-palate children have a higher incidence of conductive hearing loss than the normal population (McWilliams, 1982).

The prevalence of fluctuating hearing loss during the language-learning period has been commonly cited as a potential cause of articulation problems. The research to support this, however, has been poorly controlled (Ventry, 1980). This remains a viable possibility but needs further documentation to establish a cause/effect relationship.

Other Causes. Finally, one must consider the possibility of functional articulation problems in the cleft-palate population. These are problems that are not caused by the organic deficit of cleft palate, and which the normal population is subject to as well.

Phonation. Although problems of phonation are sometimes overlooked (Edwards, 1980), such problems as decreased loudness, which is used as a means of decreasing nasal resonance, often occur. This results in a weak and breathy voice. Individuals who have difficulty maintaining loudness levels may increase efforts to speak louder. This additional effort may produce hoarseness (Ross & Johnson,1972). Vocal abuse, especially frequent glottal stops, may also contribute to phonatory problems, as seen by the increased incidence of vocal nodules in the cleft-palate population.

Associated Problems. Numerous other problems are associated with cleft palate. The most frequently cited problems include hearing loss (Bennett, 1972; Bluestone, 1978; Chaudhuri & Bowen-Jones, 1978; Yules, 1970; Walton, 1973), impaired intelligence (Estes & Morris, 1973; Lencione, 1980; Phillips & Harrison, 1969; Ruess, 1965), psychological problems (Clifford, 1979; Ruess, 1965; Watson, 1964; Wirls & Plotkin,

1971), emotional problems of patient and family, medical complications, and feeding problems.

Assessment

The cleft-palate child can have numerous interrelated problems. Dealing with the deformity alone may require the skills of an oral surgeon, plastic surgeon, orthodontist, and prosthodontist. When associated problems are present, additional specialists may be needed, such as a speech pathologist, audiologist, otologist, psychologist, cardiologist, radiologist, etc. Because of the numerous professionals who might be required, assessment and treatment are best carried out within the structural framework of a cleft-palate team, where an exchange of information and coordinated planning can occur. As with other types of articulation disorders, the assessment includes orofacial examination and evaluation of function of nonspeech and speech tasks.

Orofacial Examination. In performing the examination of the oral structures described in chapter 4, there are considerations specific to cleft palate. At this point, the reader might want to review the orofacial examination procedures in chapter 4. In regard to cleft palate, the examiner should especially note the following:

Lips. It has been found that the lips do not contribute significantly to articulation problems found in cleft-palate speech, although gross deviations of the lips might affect production of bilabial phonemes. The examiner should look for evidence of a cleft, location of the cleft, evidence of surgical repair, general appearance and symmetry of lips, tightness or mobility of the lips, and diadochokinetic rate of movement.

Occlusion and Dentition. Although dental abnormalities can have an effect on articulation (especially the sibilant and fricative sounds), occlusion abnormalities have a greater effect. The examiner should observe the general condition of the teeth (healthy versus carious), number of teeth, alignment of teeth, and occlusion pattern. When examining the occlusion pattern, one should particularly watch for anterior crossbite or class III (open bite) malocclusion.

Alveolar Ridge. Alveolar lingual phonemes such as /t, d, n, l/ are most notably related to the condition of the alveolus. Observations include: evidence of a cleft, location of the cleft, evidence of surgical repair, and use of an orthopedic appliance.

Palate. Defects of the velum have a primary effect on resonance patterns. Articulation is also affected by the inability to implode adequate air pressure and by the consequent development of compensatory movements. As discussed in chapter 4, the velopharyngeal sphincter cannot be viewed via intraoral inspection. However, a certain amount of information can be obtained by observation of the visible structures. The hard palate should be examined for height and shape of the palatal arch, size and location of fistulas, evidence of a repair, and evidence of a submucous cleft.

The soft palate should be examined for height and shape of the arch, especially during phonation; extent and location of the cleft, if still unrepaired; evidence of submucous cleft, such as velar dimple or transparent appearance of membrane covering; bifid uvula; and length and mobility of velum. In most cases, the soft palate will have been repaired, because this is usally done early.

Pharynx. The examiner should look for evidence of posterior and lateral pharyngeal wall movement. Other observations should include evidence of an abnormally deep pharyngeal area, previous surgical repair such as pharyngeal flap, and possible upper airway obstructions. Abnormalities should be noted but, because the velopharyngeal valve cannot be fully observed, normal appearance does not necessarily mean normal function.

Tonsils. The examiner should observe whether tonsils are present or absent and, if present, size of the tonsils.

Tongue. The positioning of the tongue in the mouth may have an influence on resonance. Observations of the tongue should include size of the tongue, ability to perform gross motor movements described in chapter 4, and position of the tongue at rest.

Speech Evaluation. In the speech evaluation the following areas are especially important.

Resonance. Both objective and subjective measures of resonance should be obtained. Objective measures include airflow studies, direct observation via nasopharyngoscopy, and X-ray studies such as videofluoroscopy and cineradiography. These measures can be employed to evaluate the balance between oral and nasal resonance and to determine the factors creating the resonance problem.

Additional testing for resonance is done in conjunction with articulation testing. Vowels, as well as the consonants described previously, are especially affected by hypernasality. Having the patient produce vowels and CV combinations with the nares occluded and unoccluded is a method of testing for hypernasality. The hypernasality will diminish when the nares are occluded. Hypernasality should also be evaluated at the single-word and sentence level. Some individuals are able to achieve proper balance for limited segments but cannot maintain it in ongoing speech.

Evidence of nasal emission, nasal snort, facial grimacing, nasal flaring, and compensatory productions such as glottal stops and pharyngeal fricatives should be noted.

Articulation. The articulation evaluation is performed not only to determine specific deviant phonemes but, more importantly, to determine error patterns or deviations in the phonological system. The patient is routinely administered an articulation test. Tests that are frequently used include the McDonald Deep Test (McDonald, 1964), Iowa Pressure Test (Morris, Spriestersbach, & Darley,

1961), C-PAC (Secord, 1981), or Bzoch Error Pattern Diagnostic Articulation Test (described in Bzoch, 1971). Typical substitutions, distortions, and omissions are noted as in any articulation evaluation. However, the examiner is particularly interested in types of errors and compensatory production.

Edwards (1980) points to a number of phonological differences that have been observed in the literature. Most of these are similar to those observed in children with functional articulation problems. Some cleft-palate children have been found to demonstrate final consonant omission, deletion of unstressed syllables, and cluster reduction. They also have difficulty in making binary contrasts such as oral versus nasal, stop versus continuant, and voice versus voiceless.

In cleft-palate speech, the resonance problem may be difficult to separate from the articulation problem. One of the most common problems when inadequate intraoral air pressure is present is a weakness of consonants, despite normal placement. The examiner should attempt to determine the influence of resonance problems on articulation problems.

There are individuals who can produce isolated phonemes or even individual words due to the fact that the speech mechanism is able to function more efficiently at a slower rate. Therefore, analyzing spontaneous speech is as important as doing formal articulation testing. In addition, since cleft-palate children are subject to the typical delays of other children, the examiner should determine which problems are related to the cleft palate and which problems are due to other causes.

Phonation. Breathiness is frequently found in cleft-palate individuals as they attempt to reduce pressure and use a soft attack. The examiner should look for signs of vocal abuse such as hard glottal attacks, abnormal head and neck postures, and excessive tension (Edwards, 1980). Hoarseness may be present if vocal nodules have developed. If phonatory problems are present, evaluation of the voice problem is indicated following typical voice evaluation procedures.

Other Evaluation Considerations. All cleft-palate children should be suspected of having potential for language delay and hearing loss. Hearing testing and screening for both receptive and expressive language problems should be included in every evaluation.

Remediation and Prognosis

The earliest concerns for the cleft-palate child relate to surgical and/or prosthetic management. Cleft of the lip is generally repaired during the first few months of life. Repair of the alveolar ridge may be done at the same time or may be delayed. In severe defects, orthodontic intervention may precede surgery to bring structures into better alignment for surgery.

Surgical procedures to improve velopharyngeal function are frequently recommended for speakers with cleft palates. Such secondary surgeries are usually performed between 4 and 8 years of age. Surgical management often improves speech production in children with cleft palates and velopharyngeal incompetence, but surgical procedures do not guarantee normal articulation. Letcher, Broen, and Moller (1986) found that children's articulation gradually improves over a period of several months following surgery.

All cleft-palate children should be considered at risk for speech and language problems. Therefore, the most effective approach is of a preventive nature in order to minimize the risk of speech problems. This approach differs significantly from that for functional problems in that, with functional problems, it is assumed that speech will develop normally, and so intervention does not occur until after symptoms begin to appear. For cleft-palate children, early speech and language stimulation is important. Philips (1979) feels that a stimulation program should begin as early as 18 to 24 months. Stimulation should be geared toward vocabulary, syntax, and phonological development.

When problems of resonance, articulation, and phonation occur, direct intervention is needed. Let us consider each of these areas.

Resonance. Therapy will not improve resonance defects that are the result of an inadequate structure. When structures are deficient, surgical and/or prosthetic intervention should precede speech therapy. In unclear cases, a trial period of therapy can be attempted. If no improvement has occurred within 3 months, the child should be referred for reevaluation to determine the need for secondary surgery or prosthetic alternatives.

Muscle-training techniques have been used by some to increase velopharyngeal function. According to Cole (1979), there are three approaches to muscle training for resonance problems: (a) indirect, as in articulation therapy; (b) semidirect, as in blowing and sucking exercises; and (c) direct, as in direct muscle stimulation designed to bring involuntary and reflexive muscle action under voluntary control. These approaches have had varying degrees of success.

Articulation therapy designed to improve resonance problems has not proven to be an effective approach for improving velopharyngeal closure. Sucking, and especially blowing exercises, have been used to redirect airflow into the oral cavity as well as to increase velopharyngeal closure. The efficacy of blowing techniques has been questioned on the basis that the closure pattern for blowing is different from that for speech (Edwards, 1980). The success of direct muscle-training techniques has been variable, and patient selection must be done carefully. Additional research into this area is needed to determine its value (Cole, 1979). Various biofeedback techniques have been used to offer visual and auditory feedback to develop kinesthetic and auditory awareness for reduced nasality. Therapy should also focus on eliminating extraneous movements such as facial grimacing when such behaviors exist.

Articulation. Riski and Millard (1979) suggest that articulation therapy should precede therapy for resonance disorders. The rationale for this is that, with improved articulatory postures, hypernasality will often decrease as well, thereby saving unnecessary efforts in that area later on.

Many articulation defects relating to cleft palate are difficult to separate from resonance problems. However, the relationship between the two should be determined before establishing therapy goals. Although improved articulatory postures may decrease hypernasality, if there is a significant impairment of structure and/or function that causes hypernasality, articulatory postures will be unable to compensate totally. In planning therapy goals one must consider whether surgery or prosthodontia should precede extensive articulation therapy in order to achieve success.

Typical articulation and phonological procedures applicable to other types of articulation disorders are appropriate for therapy with cleft-palate individuals. Articulatory placement is important and should receive early emphasis. Auditory, visual, tactile, and kinesthetic cues can all be used to develop normal production. If structural distortions are present that obviate normal production, compensatory productions can be taught so that production may at least be improved.

Phonation. Because there is a high incidence of vocal nodules due to abusive vocal behaviors, potentially abusive behaviors such as yelling and screaming should be identified and eliminated. Since many of the vocally abusive behaviors are associated with abnormal compensatory articulation productions and difficulty achieving intraoral pressure, phonation therapy may sometimes be used simultaneouly with resonance and articulation therapy. At other times, specific voice therapy techniques such as those used for decreasing breathiness or reduction of tension in the laryngeal area may be employed.

With appropriate intervention, prognosis for articulation outcome is quite good (Bzoch, 1979). Karnell and Van Denmark (1986) reported the articulation performance of three groups of children

FIGURE 10.2

Mean percentage correct on the Iowa Pressure Articulation Test for each group and age. Templin-Darley normative data are included at ages 4, 6, and 8 for reference. (*Source:* "Longitudinal Speech Performance in Patients with Cleft Palate: Comparisons Based on Secondary Management," by M. P. Karnell and D. R. Van Denmark, 1986. *Cleft Palate Journal, 23,* p. 281.) Copyright 1986 by American Cleft Palate Association. Adapted by permission.

with cleft palates tested at 2-year intervals from age 4 through age 16: Group A children with low Iowa Pressure Articulation Test performance who received secondary surgery by age 8; Group B children with low Iowa Pressure Articulation performance who *did not* receive secondary surgery; Group C children with *relatively high* Iowa Pressure Articulation Test performance who did not receive secondary surgery. As seen in Figure 10.2,

all three groups displayed a dramatic improvement by 8 years of age. Some children, perhaps those who had poor articulation performance and underwent secondary surgery, may continue to show steady improvement well into the teens. By age 16, none of the children showed completely normal speech, regardless of the type of management. The authors suggested that, although errors were detected at age 16, these errors were minimal and only apparent to trained speech pathologists.

Conclusion

The outlook for the cleft-palate child today is very positive. Current diagnostic procedures are sophisticated enough to allow more specific definition of most parameters of the problem, thus making it possible for more effective treatment procedures to be undertaken. Surgical procedures have been refined to the point that, when these are combined with preventative speech therapy measures, many children can be expected to develop normal speech. Prognosis for children who do have residual speech problems is also good in light of advancements in secondary surgical procedures, available prosthodontic devices, and speech therapy. In order to accomplish the goal of normal speech development, the efforts of a coordinated team of professionals are essential.

SUMMARY

Organic articulation disorders result from physical anomalies that affect the structure and/or function of the articulatory mechanism. These include disorders with a known (dysarthria) or probable (apraxia of speech) neurological basis as well as structural anomalies such as cleft palate. Each of these disorders may require not only special procedures for remediation of the articulatory component but also a team approach to manage all aspects of the problem and counseling for the client and family. The clinician who works with these clients must be knowledgeable about the physical aspects of the problem, possible etiologies, special techniques for differential diagnosis and remediation, and potential associated problems. It may be necessary to set realistic goals that are in keeping with the abilities of the individual client.

REFERENCES

Aram, D. M., & Glasson, C. (1979). *Developmental apraxia of speech*. Mini-seminar presented at the annual convention of the American Speech-Language-Hearing Association Atlanta.

Bennett, M. (1972). The older cleft palate patient. *Laryngoscope, 82,* 1217–1225.

Beukelman, D. R., Yorkston, K. M., & Dowden, P. A. (1985). *Communication augmentation: A casebook of clinical management.* San Diego: College Hill Press.

Bluestone, C. C. (1978). Prevalence of pathogenesis of ear disease and hearing loss. In M. Graham (Ed.), *Cleft palate, middle ear disease and hearing loss.* Springfield, IL: Charles C. Thomas.

Bobath, B. (1967). The very early treatment of cerebral palsy. *Developmental Medicine and Child Neurology, 9,* 373–390.

Bobath, K., & Bobath, B. (1972). Cerebral palsy. Part I: Diagnosis and assessment of cerebral palsy. Part II: The neurodevelopmental approach to treatment. In P. H. Pearson & C. E. Williams (Eds.), *Physical therapy services in the developmental disabilities.* Springfield, IL: Charles C. Thomas.

Boone, D. R. (1972). *Cerebral palsy.* Indianapolis, IN: Bobbs-Merrill.

Bzoch, K. R. (1971). Introduction to section C: Measurement of parameters of cleft palate speech. In W. C. Grabb, S. W. Rosenstein, & K. Bzoch (Eds.), *Cleft lip and palate: Surgical, dental and speech aspects.* Boston: Little Brown.

Bzoch, K. R. (1979). Rationale methods and techniques of cleft palate speech therapy. In K. R. Bzoch (Ed.), *Communcation disorders related to cleft lip and palate.* Boston: Little, Brown.

Canter, G. J., Trost, J. E., & Burns, M. S. (1985). Contrasting speech patterns in apraxia of speech and phonemic paraphrasia. *Brain and Language, 24,* 204–222.

Chappell, G. E. (1973). Childhood verbal apraxia and its treatment. *Journal of Speech and Hearing Disorders, 38,* 362–369.

Chaudhuri, P., & Bowen-Jones, E. (1978). An otorhinological study of children with cleft palate. *Journal of Laryngology and Otology, 92,* 29–40.

Clifford, E. (1979). Psychological aspects of cleft lip and palate. In K. R. Bzoch (Ed.), *Communicative disorders related to cleft lip and palate* (2nd ed.). Boston: Little, Brown.

Cole, R. M. (1979). Direct muscle training for the improvement of velopharyngeal activity. In K. R. Bzoch (Ed.), *Communicative disorders related to cleft lip and palate* (2nd ed.). Boston: Little, Brown.

Connor, F. P., Williamson, G. G., & Siepp, J. M. (1978). *Program guide for infants and toddlers with neuromotor and other developmental disabilities.* New York: Teachers College Press, Columbia University.

Crary, M. (1984). Phonological characteristics of developmental verbal dyspraxia. *Seminars in Speech and Language, 5,* 71–83.

Crickmay, M. C. (1966). *Speech therapy and the Bobath approach to cerebral palsy.* Springfield, IL: Charles C. Thomas.

Cruickshank, W. (1976). The problem and its scope. In W. Cruickshank (Ed.), *Cerebral palsy: A developmental disability.* Syracuse, NY: Syracuse University Press.

Darley, F., Aronson, A., & Brown, J. (1975). *Motor speech disorders.* Philadelphia: Saunders.

Denhoff, E., & Holden, R. (1954). Family influence on successful school adjustment of cerebral palsied children. *Journal of International Council of Exceptional Children, 21,* 5–7.

Dworkin, J. P. (1984). Specific characteristics and treatments of the dysarthrias. In H. Winitz (Ed.), *Treating articulation disorders: For clinicians by clinicians.* Baltimore: University Park Press.

Edwards, M. (1980). Speech and language disability. In M. Edwards & A. C. H. Watson (Eds.), *Advances in the management of cleft palate.* New York: Churchill Livingston.

Estes, R. E., & Morris, H. L. (1973). Relationships among intelligence, speech proficiency, and hearing sensitivity in children with cleft palate. *Cleft Palate Journal, 7,* 763.

Estrem, T. & Broen, P. A. Early speech production of children with cleft palate. Submitted to *Journal of Speech Hearing Research.*

Finnie, N. R. (1975). *Handling the young cerebral palsied child at home.* New York: E. P. Dutton.

Geschwind, N. (1975). Apraxias: Neuromechanisms of disorders of learned movement. *American Science, 63,* 188–205.

Guyette, T. W. and Diedrich, W. M. (1981). A critical review of developmental apraxia of speech. In

N. J. Lass (Ed.), *Speech and language advances in basic research and practice* (Vol. 5). New York: Academic Press.

Hanson, W. R., & Metter, E. J. (1980). DAF as instrumental treatment for dysarthria in progressive supranuclear palsy: A case report. *Journal of Speech and Hearing Disorders, 45,* 268–276.

Harkins, C. S., Berlin, A., Harding, R., Longacre, J., & Snodgrass, R. (1962). A classification of cleft lip and palate. *Plastic Reconstructive Surgery, 29,* 31.

Haynes, S. M. (1978). Developmental apraxia of speech. In D. Johns (Ed.), *Clinical management of neurogenic communicative disorders.* Boston: Little, Brown.

Jones, M., Barrett, M., Olonoff, C., & Anderson, E. (1969). Two experiments in training handicapped children in nursery school. In P. Wolff & R. MacKeith (Eds.), *Planning for better living.* London: Heinemann.

Karnell, M. P., & Van Denmark, D. R. (1986). Longitudinal speech performance in patients with cleft palate: Comparisons based on secondary management. *Cleft Palate Journal, 23,* 278–288.

Kimura, D. (1976). The neural basis of language and gesture. In H. Whitaker & H. A. Whitaker (Eds.), *Studies in neurolinguistics* (Vol. 2). New York: Academic Press.

Koepp-Baker, H. (1971). Orofacial clefts: Their forms and effects. In L. E. Travis (Ed.), *Handbook of speech pathology and audiology.* Englewood Cliffs, NJ: Prentice-Hall.

Kong, E. (1966). Very early treatment of cerebral palsy. *Developmental Medicine and Child Neurology, 8,* 198–202.

LaPointe, L. L. (1982). Neurogenic disorders of speech. In G. H. Shames & E. H. Wiig (Eds.), *Human communication disorders.* Columbus, OH: Merrill.

LaPointe, L., & Wertz, R. (1974). Oral movement abilities and articulatory characteristics of brain injured adults. *Perceptual and Motor Skills, 39,* 39–46.

Lencione, R. M. (1980). Associated conditions. In M. Edwards & A. C. H. Watson (Eds.), *Advances in the management of cleft palate.* New York: Churchill Livingston.

Letcher, L. M., Broen, P. A., Moller, K. T. (1986, November). *A longitudinal study: Phonological changes associated with pharyngeal flap surgery.* Paper presented at the annual convention of the American Speech-Language-Hearing Association.

Logemann, J. A. (1984). Management of acquired articulation disorders in adults. In H. Winitz (Ed.), *Treating articulation disorders: For clinicians by clinicians.* Baltimore: University Park Press.

Longacre, J. J. (1970). *Cleft palate deformation.* Springfield, IL: Thomas.

Martin, A. D. (1974). Some objections to the term "apraxia of speech." *Journal of Speech and Hearing Disorders, 39,* 53–64.

McDonald, E. (1964). *A deep test of articulation.* Pittsburgh: Stanwix House.

McWilliams, B. J. (1982). The cleft palate. In G. S. Shames & E. Wiig (Eds.), *Human communication disorders.* Columbus, OH: Merrill.

Morley, M. E. (1970). *Cleft palate and speech* (7th ed.). London: Churchill Livingston.

Morris, H. L., Spriestersbach, D. C., & Darley, F. L. (1961). An articulation test for assessing competency of velopharyngeal closure. *Journal of Speech and Hearing Research, 4,* 48–55.

Morris, S. E. (1975a). Pre-speech assessment. In S. E. Morris (Ed.), *Pre-speech and language programming for the young child with cerbral palsy.* Wauwatosa, WI: Curative Rehabilitation Center.

Morris, S. E. (Ed.). (1975b). Program guidelines for children with feeding problems. In *Pre-speech and language programming for the young child with cerebral palsy.* Wauwatosa, WI: Curative Rehabilitation Center.

Mysak, E. D. (1980). *Neurospeech therapy for the cerebral palsied.* New York: Teachers College Press, Columbia University.

Nelson, K. B., & Ellenberg, J. H. (1986). Antecedents of cerebral palsy. *New England Journal of Medicine, 315,* 81–86.

Netsell, R., & Cleeland, C. S. (1973). Modification of lip hypertonia in dysarthria using EMG feedback. *Journal of Speech and Hearing Disorders, 38,* 131–140.

Newton, M. (1977). *Cerebral palsy: Speech, hearing and language problems.* Lincoln, NE: Cliffs Notes.

Nober, E. H. (1976). Auditory processing. In W. Cruickshank (Ed.), *Cerebral palsy: A developmental disability.* Syracuse, NY: Syracuse University Press.

Paneth, N. (1986). Birth and the origins of cerebral palsy. *New England Journal of Medicine, 315,* 124–126.

Pearlstone, A. D. (1969). Ocular defects in cerebral palsy. *Eye, Ear, Nose, Throat Monthly, 48,* 36–48.

Perlstein, M. A., Gibbs, E. L., & Gibbs, F. A. (1947). The electroencephalogram in infantile cerebral palsy. *Proceedings of Research in Nervous and Mental Disease, 2,* 377–384.

Peterson, H. A., & Marquardt, T. P. (1981). *Appraisal and diagnosis of speech and language disorders.* Englewood Cliffs, NJ: Prentice-Hall.

Philips, J. (1979). Stimulating syntactic and phonological development in infants with cleft palate. In K. R. Bzoch (Ed.), *Communicative disorders related to cleft lip and palate* (2nd ed.). Boston: Little, Brown.

Phillips, B., & Harrison, R. (1969). Language skills in pre-school cleft palate children. *Cleft Palate Journal, 6,* 108–119.

Ringel, R. L., House, A. S., Burk, K. W., & Dolinsky, J. P. (1970). Some relations between orosensory discrimination and articulatory aspects of speech production. *Journal of Speech and Hearing Disorders, 35,* 3–11.

Riski, J. E., & DeLong, E. (1984). Articulation development in children with cleft lip/palate. *The Cleft Palate Journal, 21,* 57–64.

Riski, J. E., & Millard, R. T. (1979). The processes of speech: Evaluation and treatment. In H. Cooper, R. Harding, W. Krogman, M. Mazaheri, & R. Millard (Eds.), *Cleft palate and lip: A team approach to clinical management and rehabilitation of the patient.* Philadelphia: Saunders.

Rosenbek, J. C., Hensen, R., Baughman, C., & Lemme, M. (1974). Treatment of developmental apraxia of speech: A case study. *Language, Speech and Hearing Services in Schools, 5,* 13–21.

Rosenbek, J. C., & LaPointe, L. L. (1979). The dysarthrias: Description, diagnosis and treatment. In D. F. Johns (Ed.), *Clinical management of neurogenic communicative disorders.* Boston: Little, Brown.

Rosenbek, J. C., & LaPointe, L. L. (1981). Aging communication processes and disorders. In D. Beasley & G. A. Davis (Eds.), *Aging communication processes and disorders.* New York: Grune and Stratton.

Rosenbek, J. C., Lemme, M., Ahern, M., Harris, E., & Wertz, R. T. (1973). A treatment for apraxia of speech in adults. *Journal of Speech and Hearing Disorders, 38,* 462–472.

Rosenbek, J. C., & Wertz, R. T. (1972). A review of 50 cases of developmental apraxia of speech. *Language, Speech and Hearing Services in Schools, 3,* 23–30.

Rosenbek, J. C., Wertz, R. T., & Darley, F. L. (1973). Oral sensation and perception in apraxia of speech and aphasia. *Journal of Speech and Hearing Research, 16,* 22–36.

Ross, R. B., & Johnson, M. C. (1972). *Cleft lip and palate.* Baltimore: Williams and Wilkins.

Ruess, A. (1965). A comparative study of cleft palate children and their siblings. *Journal of Clinical Psychology, 21,* 354–360.

Secord, W. (1981). *C-PAC: Clinical probes of articulation consistency.* Columbus, OH: Merrill.

Skelly, M., Schinsky, L., Smith, R., & Fust, R. (1974). American Indian Sign (Amerind) as a facilitator of verbalization for the oral-verbal apraxic. *Journal of Speech and Hearing Disorders, 39,* 445–456.

Sparks, R., Helm, N., & Albert, M. (1974). Aphasia rehabilitation resulting from melodic intonation therapy. *Cortex, 10,* 303–313.

Sparks, R., & Holland, A. (1976). Method: Melodic intonation therapy for aphasia. *Journal of Speech and Hearing Disorders, 41,* 287–297.

Starr, C. (1979). Dental and occlusal hazards to normal speech production. In K. R. Bzoch (Ed.), *Communicative disorders related to cleft lip and palate.* Boston: Little, Brown.

Trost, J. E. (1981). Articulatory additions to the classical description of the speech of persons with cleft palate. *Cleft Palate Journal, 18,* 193–203.

Trost, J., & Canter, G. (1974). Apraxia of speech in patients with Broca's aphasia. *Brain and Language, 1,* 63–80.

Ventry, I. M. (1980). Effects of conductive hearing loss: Fact or fiction. *Journal of Speech and Hearing Disorders, 45,* 143–156.

Vignolo, L. A. (1964). Evaluation of aphasia and language rehabilitation: A retrospective exploratory study. *Cortex, 1,* 344–459.

Walton, W. K. (1973). Audiometrically "normal" conductive hearing losses among the cleft palate. *Cleft Palate Journal, 10,* 99–103.

Watson, C. G. (1964). Personality adjustment in boys with cleft lips and palates. *Cleft Palate Journal, 1,* 130.

Wepman, J. M. (1958). The relationship between self-correction and recovery from aphasia. *Journal of Speech and Hearing Disorders, 25,* 302–308.

Wertz, R. T. (1978). Neuropathologies of speech and language. In D. Johns (Ed.), *Clinical management of neurogenic communication disorders.* Boston: Little, Brown.

Wirls, C. J., & Plotkin, R. R. (1971). A comparison of children with cleft palate and their siblings on projective test personality factors. *Cleft Palate Journal, 8,* 399.

Woolf, C. M., Woolf, R. M., & Broadbent, T. R. (1963). *American Journal of Genetics, 15,* 209.

Yorkston, K. M., & Beukelman, D. R. (1981a). *Assessment of intelligibility of dysarthric speech.* Tigard, OR: C. C. Publications.

Yorkston, K. M., & Beukelman, D. R. (1981b). Ataxic dysarthria: Treatment sequences based on intelligibility and prosodic considerations. *Journal of Speech and Hearing Disorders, 46,* 398–404.

Yoss, K. A., & Darley, F. L. (1974a). Developmental apraxia of speech in children with defective articulation. *Journal of Speech and Hearing Research, 17,* 399–416.

Yoss, K. A., & Darley, F. L. (1974b). Therapy in developmental apraxia of speech. *Language, Speech and Hearing Services in Schools, 5,* 23–31.

Yules, R. B. (1970). Hearing in cleft palate patients. *Archives of Otolaryngology, 91,* 319–323.

PART THREE

Specific Treatment Programs

In this section, four authors present the specific therapy methods or programs that they have developed. All of the programs are based on the general principles outlined in Part II.

In chapter 11, Bradley describes a multiple-phoneme method that combines the multiphonemic emphasis of the linguistic model with the systematic application of behavioral principles.

Chapter 12 describes Hodson's cycles approach, which facilitates the development of intelligible speech patterns for highly unintelligible children.

The sensory-motor approach, described by Shine in chapter 13, is based on the principles of coarticulation and emphasizes production training while acknowledging the importance of phonology.

Blache's method (chapter 14) incorporates distinctive-feature theory with a minimal pair strategy to help children develop the motor-acoustic characteristics of phonemes and realize the linguistic importance of sound contrasts.

CHAPTER 11 A Systematic Multiple-Phoneme Approach

In recent years, the assessment and management of individuals with articulatory disorders have been influenced by theoretical work on distinctive features and phonological processes (see chapters 2, 3, 4, and 7). These developments have changed many aspects of articulatory therapy and support the idea of dealing with more than one phoneme at a time during therapy sessions (Costello & Onstine, 1976; Ingram, 1981; McReynolds & Engmann, 1975; Mowrer, 1978; Shriberg & Kwiatkowski, 1980; Singh, 1975; Weiner, 1978). Nevertheless, the need for a systematic approach to planning and monitoring therapy remains. There is also need for a clinically feasible means of assessing sound production in conversation. This is even a requirement of law in some states in order to establish the need for speech therapy within a public school system. The multiple-phoneme approach is a program that incorporates the following features: (a) simultaneous teaching of multiple phonemes, (b) systematic application of behavioral principles, and (c) analysis of sound production in conversational speech.

The method was first described by McCabe and Bradley (1973) as an intensive therapy program for

Doris P. Bradley, Ph.D., is a professor of speech and hearing sciences and chairperson of the Department of Speech and Hearing Sciences at the University of Southern Mississippi, Hattiesburg, Mississippi.

individuals with six or more consonant error productions in their articulatory patterns. Since then, various authors (Holtzapple & Marshall, 1977; Schissel & Doty, 1979; Seaton & Bradley, 1978; Van Denmark & Hardin, 1986) have reported its application with different populations and in several settings.

The purpose of this chapter is to explain the multiple-phoneme approach in detail so that students may use it effectively.

RATIONALE

The multiple-phoneme approach to articulation therapy was developed at the University of North Carolina in 1969 with support from grants (GRS RR 05333 USPHS and NIDR DE 42642 01). Its purpose at that time was to document and increase the efficiency of articulation therapy provided to children who had multiple sound errors with etiology of cleft palate and other children who had multiple errors and different etiologies. The development of this method included extensive documentation of articulatory skills prior to therapy and reassessment of articulatory skills after specified amounts of therapy. The success of the procedure has led to its continued use and adoption by others.

Since 1973, a number of authors have established the efficacy of dealing with more than one phoneme at a time (Blache, Parsons, & Humphreys, 1981; Hodson & Paden, 1982) when working with children who have multiple errors (see chapter 7).

The multiple-phoneme approach maintains the traditional steps of therapy but uses them in some different ways (McCabe & Bradley, 1975). It stresses sound production skills at each level without any emphasis on auditory discrimination until after accurate production is well established, because there is evidence that production training also trains discrimination. During the establishment phase, all auditory monitoring is the responsibility of the speech pathologist. After adult forms of sound production are achieved at the word level, the speaker begins to monitor the accuracy of sound productions. Many speech pathologists have

---

NAME: SHANNON

DATE: 3-3-77

B.D.:   3-17-72

C.A.:   4-11

MAMA AND DADDY AND BOB AND SUSAN WAS GOING ON A PICNIC. AND BOB WAS HAPPY ON WHEN HE WAS EATING HIS CEREAL. AND THAT WAS WHEN MAMA AND BOB AND SUSAN AND DADDY WENT FOR A PICNIC. SO MAMA GOT IT READY AND SUSAN PUT A APPLE AND BANANAS. AND MAMA MADE A JELLY AND PEANUT BUTTER SANDWICH AND EGGS SANDWICH. AND DADDY MADE A BIG-WHAT WAS THAT THING AGAIN—THERMOS OF LEMONADE. AND BOB PUT A STUFF OUT IN A CAR. AND THEY WERE ON A WAY TO A PICNIC. SO THEY PUT DOWN THEM BLANKET AND PUT THE BASKET ON THEM BLANKET. SO BOB SAID—WHY DON'T WE PLAY THROW? SO DADDY THROW IT TO ONE TO A OTHER. SOMETIME HE PLAY LAUGHING ON THEM AND DON'T THROW IT. SO A LITTLE LATER DADDY SAID— DO YOU WANT TO GO A BOAT RIDE? AND BOB CRIED YES AND SUSAN CRIED YES. SO DAD AND SUSAN AND BOB WENT ON A BOAT FOR A RIDE.

Total Words: 168

Total Accurate: 110

% Accurate: 65%

FIGURE 11.1

An example of a conversational sample that has been scored for conversational whole-word accuracy. The marked words were produced with at least one phoneme in error.

TABLE 11.1

Comparative Norms of Arizona Articulation Proficiency Scale and Whole-Word Accuracy for Normally Speaking Children

Age	Mean		Standard Deviation		Median		Mode	
	AAPS	WWA	AAPS	WWA	AAPS	WWA	AAPS	WWA
3.0	86.3	68.53	5.5	10.28	85.5	70.5	90	73
3.6	90.93	76.4	5.79	10.72	92.17	75.25	94	72
4.0	90.93	80.0	5.73	10.32	91.83	82.5	96	74
4.6	93.57	83.77	3.58	3.46	93.5	83.0	92	83
5.0	95.13	87.97	3.6	6.04	95.5	90.7	97	91
5.6	96.5	88.6	3.18	7.75	97.3	90.0	100	96
6.0	96.4	91.87	3.27	4.9	97.25	92.83	100	96
7.0	98.57	95.4	1.4	1.1	98.87	95.72	100	96

Note: These data are from "Conversational Speech Sampling in the Assessment of Articulation Proficiency" by L. S. Schmitt, B. H. Howard, and J. F. Schmitt, 1983, *Language Speech & Hearing Services in Schools, 14*, pp. 210–214.

questioned this part of the approach until they have tried it. Then, they have often agreed that undertaking auditory discrimination following the achievement of accurate sound production is beneficial and timesaving.

In keeping with behavioral methods, each step of the program is clearly outlined and sequenced so that increasingly complex behaviors are taught after it has been demonstrated that simpler behaviors have been mastered. Criteria for mastery are provided at each step. Several record-keeping forms are used to make tracking the client's performance in each session easy.

One of the measures used in pre- and post-therapy assessment is whole-word accuracy (WWA) in conversational speech. WWA is illustrated in Figure 11.1. It consists of a sample of a child's tape-recorded conversation typed in standard English form consisting of approximately 150 words. The examiner plays the tape recording and marks on the transcript each spoken word that contains at least one production error. A WWA score is derived simply by calculating the percentage of words spoken correctly. Bradley, Allen, and Clifford (1973) verified the consistency of WWA by testing a group of children during three different conversations. The reported consistency was within 8% across topics and time. More recently, Schmidt, Howard, and Schmidt (1983) reported data from assessments of 3- to 7-year-old children developing speech and language normally. The authors compared scores on the Arizona Articulation Proficiency Scale (Fudula, 1963) and WWA norms from conversational samples. These norms are shown in Table 11.1

WWA can be used effectively to supplement information obtained from single-word articulation tests. The same conversational samples can be used to determine the distinctive features and/or the phonological processes present in the speaker's speech pattern.

METHOD

The multiple-phoneme approach is divided into three phases: (I) establishment, (II) transfer, and (III) maintenance. In each phase, there are steps that lead to the goal for that phase. Each step has specific stimuli, response description, reinforcement schedule, and criterion level.

Phase I

Establishment, Phase I, has the goal that the speaker should produce each consonant sound of English in response to a grapheme or phonetic symbol representing it.

Step 1. Accurate sound production is achieved through Step 1 of Phase I and is facilitated by the use of the sound production sheet (SPS), which appears as Figure 11.2. Consonants are arranged according to place of articulation going across the page. The SPS provides a recording system for each stimulus modality used to achieve accurate production of each sound in isolation. Because sounds cannot be produced in true isolation, a neutral vowel is used in a CV syllable at this step. Each response is recorded. For example, if the client is attempting to produce /k/, the section of the SPS would look like this:

K
A-1 2 3 4 5
B-1 2 3 4 5
C-1 2 3 4 5

The speech pathologist shows the client the grapheme for /k/, which may be an upper- or lowercase letter, and asks "Do you know what sound this letter makes?" If the client indicates yes, the speech pathologist asks the client to attempt production of /k/ in isolation and records the accuracy of five successive attempts in the A modality using / for accurate and − for error.

If the client indicates a lack of knowledge of the sound the symbol /k/ represents, the speech pathologist says "I'll help you" and moves to Level C, which provides the most clues to promote an accurate production.

In this stimulus modality, verbal directions for producing /k/ are provided, along with tactile stimulation or any other technique that will achieve accurate production of the /k/. Assistance is repeated prior to each response until the client can produce at least four accurate /k/ sounds in five

successive trials. Because this procedure is followed for all sounds on the SPS, only five trials are provided for each sound in any session. If a speaker fails to show progress in three sessions, it may be wise to branch to intensive isolation work as shown on the branch index, which is discussed later.

Criterion for movement from one stimulus modality to the next on the SPS is five consecutive accurate productions for one session or four of five for two consecutive sessions. When criterion is reached at Level C, which utilizes auditory, visual, and phonetic-placement stimuli, the shift is made to auditory and visual stimuli only at Level B. Only one auditory-visual stimulus (simultaneous presentation of letter and sound) is modeled for the client, who is then asked to produce five responses. When criterion is reached at Level B, the shift is made to Level A, where only the written (visual) stimulus is provided. When working with children under 5 years of age, one may omit the Level A stimuli and move on to other parts of the therapy because 5-year-old children are not expected to have established symbol-sound associations.

Throughout this phase, reinforcement for correct responses is provided by marking correct and incorrect responses on the SPS. Token or social reinforcement may be provided if appropriate to the client's needs.

Speakers for whom the multiple-phoneme approach is considered appropriate usually have six or more sounds that are not produced accurately on single-word articulation tests or in conversational speech. The SPS is used during the first therapy session with the procedures just described. It is carried out with all consonants—both those produced accurately and those produced inaccurately in conversational speech. Usually, the speaker will reach criterion on all sounds not considered errors during the first or second session. Including non-error sounds on SPS helps provide initial success. The sounds not found to be in error on articulation testing or in whole-word accuracy analysis are not worked with in subsequent steps of therapy. Experience has shown that 20 to 25 minutes are required to go through all the sounds on the SPS if phonetic placement is necessary for several

Name:_____ Code:

Date: _____ A = Visual stim.

Age: _____ B = Aud-Visual

Time: _____ C = Aud-Visual Phonetic Placement

Correct = /

Incorrect = −

p
A - 1 2 3 4 5
B - 1 2 3 4 5
C - 1 2 3 4 5

b
A - 1 2 3 4 5
B - 1 2 3 4 5
C - 1 2 3 4 5

m
A - 1 2 3 4 5
B - 1 2 3 4 5
C - 1 2 3 4 5

w
A - 1 2 3 4 5
B - 1 2 3 4 5
C - 1 2 3 4 5

t
A - 1 2 3 4 5
B - 1 2 3 4 5
C - 1 2 3 4 5

d
A - 1 2 3 4 5
B - 1 2 3 4 5
C - 1 2 3 4 5

n
A - 1 2 3 4 5
B - 1 2 3 4 5
C - 1 2 3 4 5

l
A - 1 2 3 4 5
B - 1 2 3 4 5
C - 1 2 3 4 5

k
A - 1 2 3 4 5
B - 1 2 3 4 5
C - 1 2 3 4 5

g
A - 1 2 3 4 5
B - 1 2 3 4 5
C - 1 2 3 4 5

f
A - 1 2 3 4 5
B - 1 2 3 4 5
C - 1 2 3 4 5

v
A - 1 2 3 4 5
B - 1 2 3 4 5
C - 1 2 3 4 5

s
A - 1 2 3 4 5
B - 1 2 3 4 5
C - 1 2 3 4 5

z
A - 1 2 3 4 5
B - 1 2 3 4 5
C - 1 2 3 4 5

th[1]
A - 1 2 3 4 5
B - 1 2 3 4 5
C - 1 2 3 4 5

th[2]
A - 1 2 3 4 5
B - 1 2 3 4 5
C - 1 2 3 4 5

ch
A - 1 2 3 4 5
B - 1 2 3 4 5
C - 1 2 3 4 5

j
A - 1 2 3 4 5
B - 1 2 3 4 5
C - 1 2 3 4 5

y
A - 1 2 3 4 5
B - 1 2 3 4 5
C - 1 2 3 4 5

sh
A - 1 2 3 4 5
B - 1 2 3 4 5
C - 1 2 3 4 5

zh
A - 1 2 3 4 5
B - 1 2 3 4 5
C - 1 2 3 4 5

h
A - 1 2 3 4 5
B - 1 2 3 4 5
C - 1 2 3 4 5

r
A - 1 2 3 4 5
B - 1 2 3 4 5
C - 1 2 3 4 5

ng
A - 1 2 3 4 5
B - 1 2 3 4 5
C - 1 2 3 4 5

Total Reponses
A_____
B_____
C_____

Total Correct
A_____
B_____
C_____

% Correct
A_____
B_____
C_____

FIGURE 11.2
Multiple-phoneme articulation therapy sound production sheet. (*Source:* Reprinted with permission from C. Denham, R. B. McCabe, and D. P. Bradley (1979), *Multiple Phoneme Articulation Approach.* Tempe, Arizona: Ideas, Inc., page 9)

sounds. After the first two to three therapy sessions, no more than 15 minutes is usually spent on the SPS.

Step 2. This step of Phase I is a holding procedure. This is sometimes necessary if many sounds reach criterion on the sound production sheet at one time but cannot be advanced into the next step of therapy for several sessions. *Holding* requires the client to give one accurate response in Modality A during every therapy session until that sound is advanced to the next level of therapy. This is sufficient to maintain the symbol-sound association and keep the sound in accurate production.

Phase II

Phase II, transfer, has the ultimate goal of using all the error sounds accurately in conversational speech. It includes five conventional steps of therapy. The difference between this procedure and traditional therapeutic methods is that five or more sounds are worked on during each therapy session and each sound may be at a different step. Specific considerations important at each step are discussed next. The plan for each session is recorded on the articulation data sheet, which appears as Figure 11.3.

Step 1: Syllable. This step is used only if the client fails a word probe. If the client is successful in producing the target sound in 6 of 10 monosyllabic words, the syllable step is not necessary, and work proceeds at the word level until 90% accuracy is achieved. It is reasonable to include in the probe five words with the target sound at the beginning and five with it at the end. Selection of words based on frequency of occurrence has been suggested by Denham, McCabe, and Bradley (1979). Another good word probe is the Deep Test of Articulation (McDonald, 1964). If this test is used, an accuracy level of 60% should be achieved before eliminating the syllable step.

In syllable practice, the consonant target sound is produced in conjunction with a variety of vowels. Syllable practice should include a high front vowel such as /i/, a low front vowel such as /æ/, a neutral vowel like /ʌ/, a high back vowel such as /u/, and a low back vowel like /ɑ/. It is helpful to use line drawings of tongue positions appropriate to each vowel along with the standard spelling of the vowel. The consonant target sound is practiced in both initial and final positions of syllables. The clinician may provide one auditory-visual model or one visual stimulus and then the client should produce five syllables. The ratio of stimulus models to the number of syllable productions should be recorded in the comments section of the articulation data sheet if it is necessary to use a ratio other than 1:5. In a typical 1- to 2-minute syllable task, 25 or more responses should be obtained.

Criterion for Step 1, syllable practice, is 80% accuracy in two consecutive sessions or 90% accuracy in one session.

Step 2: Words. At the word step, the objective is accurate production of the target sound in specific words. Appropriate selection of words is critical because the words will be used later in sentences, and it is also important to select a variety of words: verbs, nouns, modifiers, and prepositions. Denham et al. (1979) suggested a core vocabulary based on frequency of occurrence of words. The clinician should also be sure that the words contain a variety of vowels. Clinicians usually make the mistake of choosing too many words for practice at this level. If the client masters 25 to 30 words, that is sufficient to provide a base for producing phrases and sentences.

Criterion for moving from the word step is production of the target sound at 90% accuracy level for one session or 80% accuracy for two sessions. Sounds in the practice words, other than the target sound, may still be in error at this level. Sometimes a client will show 100% accuracy for words beginning with the target phoneme and 10% accuracy for words ending with that sound. In such situations, the clinician should move on to the sentence level with initial-position words while continuing practice at the word level with final-

Patient: _____   Establishment: _____
Clinician: _____   Transfer: _____
Date: _____   Maintenance: _____

Date	Session	Activity	Iso.	Syl.	Words	Sent.	Read	Conv.	Time	Total Error	Total Correct	% Correct	Comments

FIGURE 11.3

Multiple-phoneme articulation therapy articulation data sheet. (*Source:* Reprinted with permission from C. Denham, R. B. McCabe, and D. P. Bradley (1979), *Multiple Phoneme Articulation Approach,* Tempe, Arizona: Ideas, Inc., page 10) position words. The speech pathologist may wish to leave the multiple phoneme program and use minimal contrast therapy (Weiner, 1984) or final consonant deletion phonological process therapy (Hodson and Paden, 1983).

Step 3: Phrase/Sentence. The objective at the phrase/sentence step is accurate word production. This means that the response unit is the word instead of the target sound, and all sounds in the word should be produced accurately. Control of vocabulary may be needed to make accurate word production possible. This is also the step in which the client begins to monitor productions of sounds and words. It is helpful to incorporate the words practiced in Step 2 in the phrase/sentence-level productions along with new words needed to complete the sentence. Clients who are nonreaders can use rebus symbols (Woodcock, Clark, & Oakes, 1979) to aid in sentence productions. Bliss symbols (McDonald, 1980) are useful in the same way. Another approach, used by Denham et al. (1979), is to provide pictures that assist children in remembering sentences.

At first, some children will find it difficult to formulate phrases and sentences. They may be assisted by having them repeat phrases or sentences after the clinician. When possible, reading may also be used. Variety in the types of sentences is also important because it facilitates natural stress and rhythm. The use of imperative, declarative, and interrogative sentence types is essential as a foundation for conversations at the later stages of therapy.

In the phrase/sentence step, errors associated with coarticulation may become evident. In these instances, the client will use target sounds accurately in one sentence and not in another due to the influence of preceding and following phonemes that vary from sentence to sentence. A complete analysis of the phonetic environments in which accurate production occurs may not be necessary if the clinician notes errors and retains exactly the same phonetic environments for additional practice

phrases. It is extremely important to provide additional trials for error words at this step of therapy. Practice may be done on the error word and the word that preceded or followed it, or the clinician may choose to use a phonological process analysis of conversational speech to identify assimilation processes (see chapters 4 and 7). The clinician should vary stress, rhythm, timing, and accent patterns in the auditory models provided to assist the client in achieving normalcy of utterance as well as accuracy of word productions in the context in which the error sound occurred.

Criterion for leaving the phrase/sentence step is 80% accuracy for two consecutive sessions or 90% for one session. In some instances, when calculating accuracy, the clinician must use only the words containing the target sound instead of all words in the sentences because the client who formulates sentences may use many words containing sounds not yet at this level of therapy. This variation should be noted on the articulation data sheet.

Step 4: Reading/Story. The reading step requires several special considerations. Because some clients with articulatory errors are poor readers, material selected for use in speech therapy should be at a comfortable reading level rather than at an instructional level. This enables the client to attend to the accurate production of target sounds without the distraction of word-recognition struggles. Some clients are nonreaders and need a substitute activity. Comic books, picture books, and sequence cards provide this. The objective at this level is accurate production of target sounds in connected speech in utterances of four to six word units. Therefore, any technique that encourages the client to speak long strings of words is useful. Repeating a story read or told by the clinician is also acceptable. Culatta, Page, and Ellis (1983) described a procedure for use of story retelling as a screening tool that is equally useful in therapy. Sometimes this is more efficient than taking the time necessary for a child to formulate a story or struggle with reading aloud.

Storytelling may be facilitated by helping the speaker understand the elements of a story. According to Rumelhart (1975), a story has a setting and an episode. The episode consists of an event and a reaction. The event may be a change of state, an action that people carry out, or a series of events. The reaction may be an internal response, such as emotion or desire, or it may be overt, such as an action or an attempt. Through questions and comments that follow this structure, the clinician is able to assist the speaker in creating a meaningful story.

At the reading/story step, accurate production of the target sounds in words is expected. Whole-word accuracy of every word spoken is the criterion base. Sometimes it is necessary to tape-record responses so that phrases containing errors can be identified and used for additional practice. As at the phrase/sentence level, specific assimilation processes may be identified through analysis of the recording using systems for phonological analysis described in chapter 4.

Criterion at the reading/story step is 80% for two consecutive sessions or 90% for one session. This is whole-word accuracy for all words spoken.

Figure 11.4 is an example of an articulation data sheet that contains the plan for session number 11 of a child who has several sounds at different steps of the program. It is typical for a client at this stage of therapy.

Step 5: Conversation. The objective of this step is accurate production of all sounds used in conversational speech. Sometimes in the early sessions a conversation may be held in which the clinician only monitors one or two sounds that have moved to that level. In such cases, only those words containing the target sounds are counted as responses. Sometimes the clinician finds it necessary to monitor 10 or 12 sounds simultaneously in conversation. In order to accomplish this difficult task, sounds are grouped according to manner of production or place of articulation. The clinician then listens for that group for a designated time period of 3 to 5 minutes. After recording responses, attention is turned to another group of sounds. When most sounds are being monitored at the conversational step, every spoken word is counted as a response. The procedure for determining percentage of accuracy becomes the same as the whole-word accuracy measure of conversational speech.

At the conversational level, it is critical that error words be noted in the context in which they occur so that these phrases or sentences may be used as practice material. Such phrases may be entered on the articulation data sheet as "trouble" phrases. At the conversational level, no single-word practice is needed, because it is usually the phonetic environment of the sound that is causing an error production. Use of the tape recorder enables the client and clinician to recheck some of the errors. It is more time-efficient if the clinician writes the phrase and stops after short segments of 2 or 3 minutes to practice the phrases in which errors occurred.

Conversations should be more than questions and answers. The clinician should use comments to extend the discussion or introduce a related topic. The client should be encouraged to ask questions, clarify meanings, describe events, state cause-and-effect relationships, and identify emotions and desires, as well as state facts. Techniques for developing conversational skills of speakers are not well described in the literature, but recent material on pragmatics contains information that is helpful (Culatta & Horn, 1982; Gallagher & Prutting, 1983; Lucas, 1980).

Criterion for completion of the conversational step is 80% accuracy on all words spoken during the entire session for two consecutive sessions or 90% for one entire session. The criterion suggested in this program is higher than the 75% suggested by Diedrich and Bangert (1980). However, since data are not available to validate the use of 75% with this approach, the criterion previously used has been retained. In view of the whole-word accuracy norms presented by Schmidt, Howard, and Schmidt (1983), some adjustments should be made for age level. For example, 3-year-old children should be held only to a criterion of 69% whole-word accuracy, the level found in children thought to be developing speech normally. Any speaker 6 years or older should reach the 90% accuracy level.

Patient ___Shannon___

Clinician ___KPS___

Date ___1/24/77___
Transfer ___x___
Maintenance ___
Step ___

Date	Session	Activity	Iso.	Syl.	Words	Sent.	Read.	Conv.	Time	Tot. Resp.	Tot. Error	Tot. Corr.	% Corr.	Comments
1/24/77	11	SPS							5					
		/k/			x				3	50	10	40	80	
		/f/				x			3	40	0	40	100	move to read
		/t/					x		5	60	10	50	83	
		/s/		x					3	50	0	50	100	move to words
		/pbm/							10	40	2	38	95	
		/g/			x				5	40	10	30	75	
		/r/	ii*						10	50	40	10	20	

*intensive isolation

FIGURE 11.4
Multiple-phoneme articulation approach articulation data sheet.

NAME: SHANNON
B.D.: 3-17-72
C.A.: 5 yrs.

Date	W.W.A. Percentage	Arizona
9-2-75	12%	40.5
10-6-75	19%	39.5
10-10-75	29%	56.0
12-1-76	30%	56.0
1-17-77	30%	N.A.*
1-24-77	39%	N.A.
1-31-77	35%	N.A.
2-7-77	40%	N.A.
2-14-77	40%	N.A.
2-21-77	66%	N.A.
2-28-77	72%	N.A.
3-7-77	83%	N.A.
One week home.		
3-21-77	91%	N.A.
3-24-77	91%	90.0

*Not available.

FIGURE 11.5
Data on progress of a child whose treatment was relatively inconsistent until an intensive multiple-phoneme approach was instituted covering the last 2 months.

Phase III

Phase III is maintenance, and its purpose is to maintain at least 90% whole-word accuracy in various speaking situations without support from therapy sessions or other external monitoring. It is typical for a speaker to lose about 5% accuracy within 3 months after the termination of therapy. Thereafter, the accuracy level is maintained or moves to around the 95% accuracy level. Most adults have about 97% accuracy in articulatory skills during conversational speech (Faircloth, 1977).

Maintenance can be conducted by return clinic visits, clinician visits to classrooms, telephone conversations, or reports from others who associate with the client. Accuracy should be monitored in various speaking situations during the maintenance phase. The length of time for maintenance used with this approach is 3 months. Since data are not available for other time spans, there is no basis for determining if other intervals would be adequate.

VALUE

The most important advantage of the multiple-phoneme approach is the speed with which intelligibility of speech is improved. In 6 to 8 weeks of daily therapy, consisting of one hour per day, most speakers with multiple articulatory errors can be understood. Whole-word accuracy should increase from a starting point of 10% to 60% or greater.

Figure 11.5 presents data on a child with whom this approach was used. He was evaluated in September of 1975 and showed 12% whole-word accuracy in conversational speech. The following month, he was seen for one week of therapy, which consisted of one-hour individual sessions each day. His whole-word accuracy increased to 29%, and a home program of therapy was initiated. A year later, in December of 1976, little change had occurred and it was decided to provide a 2-month period of intensive therapy. At the end of 2 months, his whole-word accuracy was 91%. When he started to school, the teacher reported no evidence of a speech problem.

At the present time, no research has come to the attention of the author that would allow comparison of results achieved with this approach and with other articulation therapy. Van Denmark and Hardin (1986) reported that children using multiple-phoneme therapy remained highly motivated to improve speech and retained progress whereas articulation skills regressed after traditional therapy.

The multiple-phoneme approach was developed during the years when behavioral or operant programs were fashionable. The current emphasis on the pragmatics of communication does not make it any less desirable to use efficient, effective procedures to change articulatory skills. Neither does current information on phonological process development negate the need for attention to specific sounds in a structured therapy situation for some speakers. Other approaches to articulation should be compared to the multiple-phoneme approach, but needed research has not yet appeared in the literature.

The multiple-phoneme approach is applicable in a number of situations. It is most often used for individual therapy sessions because speakers with severe problems are usually scheduled individually. However, Kasica (1978) described its use in group therapy. It can also be used with clients of various ages. The age range of clients in the report by McCabe and Bradley (1975) was 5 to 14 years. Holtzapple and Marshall (1977) used it with adult aphasic clients. The only age limitations relate to selecting an appropriate criterion for conversa-tional speech accuracy and to the need for modification of the reading level with nonreaders.

LIMITATIONS

Because the multiple-phoneme approach is not a definitive program, some users have indicated that too many decisions are left to the clinician. This might be considered an advantage because it allows the clinician to incorporate other techniques at appropriate steps of the therapy. For example, if a client fails to meet criterion at the word level during several sessions, it is possible to branch to the paired-stimuli technique until criterion is reached (Weston & Irwin, 1971). If sessions are too short to cover all error phonemes, the "wedge" approach suggested by Sommers and Kane (1974) might be used to select two or three phonemes to use with this approach. In a similar manner, a distinctive-feature analysis (see chapter 14) might suggest which sounds should be selected.

For readers who desire more structure, a progression model developed by McCabe and Bradley (1973) is offered in Appendix 11.1. This model suggests the type of stimulus, indicates the target response, states criterion, provides a reinforcement schedule, and indicates points in therapy when branching may be necessary. A branch index appears as Appendix 11.2, which suggests changes in one or more of the variables controlled in establishing the steps of this procedure. Appendix 11.3 contains the key to the symbols used in the progression model and the branch index.

When using the branch for open stimuli, the clinician should use all known techniques to develop the accurate response.

The multiple-phoneme articulation data record that appears as Appendix 11.4 provides a quick way to summarize the information from the data sheets. This facilitates report writing and allows the clinician to report precise information regarding the time required to change error phonemes to correct use in conversational speech.

SUMMARY

The multiple-phoneme approach to articulation therapy is organized to provide therapy on all error sounds during each session of therapy. Each sound may be at a different step of therapy. In a 30-minute session, time allocations should be made for each sound and each therapy step. This ensures some activity on each error sound. The sound productions at Step 1 of Phase I are recorded on the sound production sheet. As soon as a phoneme is moved to Phase II, Step 1, the accuracy of responses is recorded on the articulation data sheet. When sounds are accurate in conversation, the time required for their correction is recorded on the multiple-phoneme articulation data record.

The traditional steps of therapy are used with behavioral criterion and reinforcement schedules. Criterion for moving from each step to the next is provided. Accuracy of all sounds in conversational speech at the 95% level is measured by whole-word accuracy and is the criterion for dismissal from therapy.

Effectiveness of the program is determined through follow-up evaluations 3 months after dismissal from therapy.

The principal advantages of the approach are its comprehensiveness (working on all errors rather than one at a time) and the speed of acquisition of intelligible speech.

REFERENCES

Blache, S. E., Parsons, C. L., & Humphreys, J. M. (1981). A minimal-word-pair model for teaching the linguistic significance of distinctive features. *Journal of Speech and Hearing Disorders, 46,* 291–295.

Bradley, D. P., Allen, G. D., & Clifford, V. V. (1973). Reliability of assessment of articulation skills in conversational speech. *Division of Council on Communication Disorders Bulletin, 11,* 28–31.

Costello, J., & Onstine, J. M. (1976). The modification of multiple articulation errors based on distinctive feature theory. *Journal of Speech and Hearing Disorders, 41,* 199–215.

Culatta, B., & Horn, D. (1982). A program for achieving generalization of grammatical rules to spontaneous discourse. *Journal of Speech and Hearing Disorders, 27,* 174–180.

Culatta, B., Page, J. L., & Ellis, J. (1983). Story retelling as a communicative performance screening tool. *Language Speech & Hearing Services in Schools, 14,* 66–74.

Denham, C. D., McCabe, R. B., & Bradley, D. P. (1979). *Multiple phoneme articulation approach.* Tempe, AZ: Ideas.

Diedrich, W. D., & Bangert, J. (1980). *Articulation learning.* Houston: College Hill Press.

Faircloth, M. A. (1977, November). *Conversational speech analysis.* Short course presented at the meeting of the American Speech and Hearing Association, Chicago.

Fudula, J. B. (1963). *Arizona articulation proficiency scale, revised.* Los Angeles: Western Psychological Services.

Gallagher, T. M., & Prutting, C. A. (Eds.) (1983). *Pragmatic assessment and intervention issues in language.* San Diego: College Hill Press.

Hodson, B., & Paden, E. (1983). *Targeting intelligible speech: A phonological approach to remediation.* San Diego: College Hill Press.

Holtzapple, P., & Marshall, N. (1977). Application of multiple phonemic articulation therapy with apraxic patients. In R. Brookshire (Ed.), *Clinical aphasiology conference proceedings.* Minneapolis: BRK Publishers.

Ingram, D. (1981). *Procedures for the phonological analysis of children's language.* Baltimore: University Park Press.

Kasica, A. (1978). *Multiple phoneme approach to articulation therapy in group setting.* Unpublished manuscript, University of Kentucky, Department of Special Education, Lexington.

Lucas, E. V. (1980). *Semantic and pragmatic language disorders*. Rockville, MD: Aspen Systems.

McCabe, R. B., & Bradley, D. P. (1973). *The systematic multiphonemic approach to articulation therapy*. Short course presented at American Speech and Hearing Association South Eastern Regional Conference, Atlanta.

McCabe, R. B., & Bradley, D. P. (1975). Systematic multiple phonemic approach to articulation therapy. *Acta Symbolica, 6*, 2–18.

McDonald, E. (1964). *A deep test of articulation*. Pittsburgh: Stanwix House, Inc.

McDonald, E. (1980). *Teaching and using Bliss symbols*. Toronto: Bliss Symbolics Institute.

McReynolds, L. V., & Engmann, D. L. (1975). *Distinctive feature analysis of misarticulations*. Baltimore: University Park Press.

Mowrer, D. W. (1978). Phonological processes and articulation therapy. In L. J. Bradford & R. T. Wertz (Eds.), *Communication disorders: An audio journal for continuing education*. New York: Grune and Stratton.

Rumelhart, D. E. (1975). Notes on a schema for stories. In D. G. Bobrow & A. Collins (Eds.), *Representation and understanding*. New York: Academic Press.

Schissel, R. J., & Doty, M. H. (1979). Application of the systematic multiple phonemic approach to articulation therapy: A case study. *Language, Speech and Hearing Services in Schools, 3*, 178–184.

Schmidt, L. S., Howard, B. H., & Schmidt, J. F. (1983). Conversational speech sampling in the assessment of articulation proficiency. *Language, Speech and Hearing Services in Schools, 14*, 210–214.

Seaton, K. P., & Bradley, D. P. (1978, November). *Application of multiple phonemic approach to articulation therapy*. Mini-seminar presented at the meeting of the American Speech and Hearing Association, San Francisco.

Shriberg, L. D., & Kwiatkowski, J. (1980). *Natural process analysis*. New York: Wiley.

Singh, S. (1975). *Distinctive features: Theory and validation*. Baltimore: University Park Press.

Sommers, R. K., & Kane, A. R. (1974). Nature and remediation of functional articulation disorders. In S. Dickson (Ed.), *Communication disorders: Remedial principles and practices*. Glenview, IL: Scott, Foresman.

Van Denmark, D. R., & Hardin, M. A. (1986). Effectiveness of intensive articulation therapy for children with cleft palate. *Cleft Palate Journal, 23*, 215–224.

Weiner, F. (1978). *Phonological process analysis*. Baltimore: University Park Press.

Weiner, F. (1984). *Minimal Contrast Therapy*. State College, PA: Parrot Software.

Weston, A., & Irwin, J. (1971). The use of paired-stimuli in the modification of articulation. *Perceptual Motor Skills, 32*, 947–957.

Woodcock, R. W., Clark, R., & Oakes, D. (1979). *Peabody rebus reading program*. Circle Pines, MN: American Guidance Service.

APPENDIX 11.1 Suggested Progression Model, Multiple Phoneme Articulation

Phase	Step	Stimulus	Target Response	Criterion	Reinforcement Schedule	Branch
I. Establishment	1-SPS	V,V-A, V-A-PP	ph	4/5-2	1:1	ii
	2-H	V	ph	100%	1:1	I, 1-SPS V-A
II. Transfer	1-WP	A	ph	60%	None	+ = II,3 − = II,2
	2-S	V-O	ph	90%-2	1:2	ii
	3-W	V-O	ph	95-100%-1 90%-2	1:3	II,2
	4a-phr/st	V-A	ph	''	1:3	II,3
	4b-phr/st	V-A	ww	''	1:3	II,3
	4c-phr/st	V-O	ph	''	1:3	II,3
	4d-phr/st	V-O	ww	''	1:5	II,3,ww
	5a-R	V	ph	''	1:4	11,4a
	5b-R	V	ww	''	1:10	II,4b
	5c-TW	V	ww	''	1:1	II,5a
	6a-C	A	ph	''	1:10	II,5a
	6b-C	A	ww	''	1:15	II,5b
	6c-TW	A	ww	''	1:1	II,6a
III. Maintenance	I-IC-C	A	ww	90% EX	Var. Int.	II,6b
	2-OC-C	Env.	ww	-	-	-

APPENDIX 11.2   Branch Index, Multiple Phoneme Articulation

Branch	Step	Stimulus	Target Response	Criterion	Reinforcement Schedule
1	I,ii	0	ph	95%-2	1:1
2	I,1	V-A	ph	4/5-2	1:1
3	−II,2	V-O	ph	90%-2	1:2
	+II,3	V-O	ph	90%-2	1:3
4	I,ii	O	ph	95%-1	1:1
5	II,2	V-O	ph	''	1:1
6	II,3	V-O	ph	''	1:1
7	II,3	V-O	ph	''	1:1
8	II,3	V-O	ph	''	1:1
9	II,3ww	V-O	ww	''	1:1
10	II,4a	V-A	ph	''	1:1
11	II,4b	V-A	ww	''	1:1
12	II,5a	V-A	ph	''	1:1
13	II,5a	V	ph	''	1:1
14	II,5b	V	ww	''	1:1
15	II,6a	A	ph	''	1:1
16	II,6b	A	ww	''	1:1

APPENDIX 11.3   Key to Symbols, Multiple Phoneme Articulation

Symbols:

ii	Intensive isolation
V	Visual stimulation
A	Auditory
V-A	Visual-Auditory stimulation
V-A-PP	Visual-Auditory-Phonetic Placement stimulation
O	Open (any type of stimulation needed)
S	Syllable
W	Word
phr	Phrase
st	Sentence
R	Reading
C	Conversation
IC	In clinic
OC	Out of Clinic
ph	Phoneme
ww	Whole word
WP	Word probe
H	Hold
EX	Exit

Criterion:

1. SPS—three days, one response at B and four/five at A, move to Step 2. (Continue on SPS for visual recognition.) Three days with less than three/five at C, move to ii.
2. General:
    1. Below 70% two consecutive days, branch to previous step.
    2. 70–90% two consecutive days, re-program at same step.
    3. 90–95% two consecutive days, move to next step.
    4. 95% and above, one day, move to next step.

APPENDIX 11.4 Multiple Phoneme Articulation Data Record

Name_____   Year_____

Phoneme	Isolation		Syllable		Word		Phrase/Sent.		Reading		Conversation	
	Date Init.	Date Comp.	Date Init.	Date Comp.	Date Init.	Date Comp.	Date Init.	Date Comp.	Date Init.	Date Comp.	Date Init.	Date Comp.

TEST DATA: (Articulation Test Scores and whole word accuracy)

_____

_____

Source: Reprinted with permission from C. Denham, R. B. McCabe and D. P. Bradley (1979), *Multiple Articulation Approach*. Tempe, Arizona: Ideas, Inc., page 11.

CHAPTER 12

Phonological Remediation: A Cycles Approach

The remediation approach described in this chapter was designed explicitly for highly *unintelligible* children. The primary factor that differentiates this approach from phoneme-oriented articulation programs is that *cycles* are used to *facilitate* the development of intelligible speech *patterns*. Cycles are time periods during which all phonological patterns that need remediation are facilitated in succession. Phonemes within the targeted patterns are used to facilitate *emergence* of the respective patterns. Phonological patterns are recycled (i.e., re-presented) during ensuing cycles until each of the targeted patterns begins to emerge in spontaneous utterances. *Complexity* is increased gradually during succeeding cycles by incorporating production-practice words with more difficult phonetic environments and also by grouping phonemes within target patterns.

The length of each cycle varies. Some cycles are 5 or 6 weeks in length; others may be as long as 15 or 16 weeks, depending on the individual child's number of deficient patterns and also on the number of stimulable phonemes within each pattern. The first cycle lays a phonological *foundation* and allows children to experience early success on

Barbara Williams Hodson, Ph.D., is a professor in the Department of Communicative Disorders and Sciences, Wichita State University, Wichita, Kansas.

target patterns in carefully selected production-practice words. Carryover to other words and to other situations is not expected until a later cycle. Three to six cycles of phonological remediation, involving approximately 30 to 40 hours of a speech-language pathologist's time (40 to 60 minutes per week), are usually required for a phonologically disordered client to become intelligible.

RATIONALE

This approach, which is often referred to as the cycles approach, is based on developmental phonology theory (cf. Jakobson, 1941; Macken & Ferguson, 1983; Stampe, 1972) and phonological acquisition research (e.g., Dyson & Paden, 1983; Grunwell, 1987; Ingram, 1976; Preisser, Hodson, & Paden, 1988; Stoel-Gammon & Dunn, 1985). The cycles remediation approach has evolved as a result of formulating and testing clinical hypotheses while working with over 200 highly unintelligible clients between the ages of 2.6 and 14 years.

An underlying premise is that phonological acquisition is *gradual* (Ingram, 1976; Tyler, Edwards, & Saxman, 1987). The cycles approach more closely approximates the way in which normal phonological development occurs than does teaching phonemes one by one (cf. Ingram, 1986). Phonemes are used as a "means to an end" to facilitate the development of intelligible speech patterns. Carefully selected production-practice words incorporating the session's target phoneme(s) are utilized to help clients develop new *auditory and kinesthetic images* for the purpose of eventual *self-monitoring* (cf. Fairbanks, 1954).

Phonological remediation is also based on cognitive psychology principles. The child's *active participation* in the learning process is an integral component of this approach.

REMEDIATION TARGETS

Identifying Target Patterns

The Assessment of Phonological Processes—Revised (Hodson, 1986a) was designed to meet the needs of highly unintelligible children and also their clinicians. The primary goal of this assessment procedure has been to help clinicians obtain phonological data as expeditiously as possible that can provide a framework for designing more efficient and more effective *individualized* remediation programs for children with severe/profound speech disorders. A second goal has been to provide *reliable* and *accountable* post-treatment measures (Hodson, 1985; Hodson, 1986a).

Objects and questions are used to elicit 50 spontaneous naming responses and also continuous-speech samples. Phonological process percentage-of-occurrence scores can be used to calculate phonological deviancy scores and severity ratings. The scores also provide information for specifying goal statements and for planning remediation.

Basic Considerations for Selection and Presentation of Targets

A highly unintelligible client's phonological remediation program should begin with a pattern for which *readiness* is demonstrated. This does not mean that it is appropriate, however, to target patterns/phonemes that the child already produces (even if inconsistent). Rather, the clinician must select the *most stimulable* pattern from the client's phonological *deficiencies* so that immediate and tangible success can be experienced by the child. The next most stimulable pattern is targeted second and so on until all priority patterns (that are deficient) are stimulated during each cycle. The specific patterns/phonemes and the *order* of presentation within a cycle depend, of course, on each individual child's phonological abilities. Target patterns that have not yet begun to emerge in conversational speech by the beginning of each ensuing cycle are recycled.

Each phoneme within a pattern should be targeted for approximately 60 minutes per cycle (i.e., one 60-minute, two 30-minute, or three 20-minute sessions) before progressing to the next phoneme in that pattern and then on to other phonological patterns. Furthermore, it is desirable to provide stimulation for two or more target *phonemes* (in successive weeks) within a pattern before changing to the next target *pattern* (i.e., each deficient phonological pattern is stimulated for two hours or more within each cycle). Only *one* phonological pattern should be targeted during any one session so that the client has an opportunity to focus, and patterns should not be intermingled.

Primary Potential Target Patterns/Phonemes

Early Developing Phonological Patterns. Most normally developing 2-year-olds produce word-initial singleton stops, nasals, and glides and some word-final nasals and voiceless obstruents (Preisser et al., 1988; Stoel-Gammon & Dunn, 1985). Furthermore, 2-year-olds commonly produce utterances that contain two or three syllables, as well as word-initial and word-final consonants. Phonologically disordered children vary greatly in their abilities to produce these early developing word structures and phoneme classes.

Syllableness. Most preschool children sequence at least two syllables. Two- and three-syllable equal-stress word combinations (e.g., *cowboy, ice cream* cone) are appropriate early targets for clients who have not yet learned to produce syllables in sequences. The emphasis during this time is on the appropriate number of syllables (i.e., vocalic elements) rather than on specific consonants. It has been observed that as children learn to sequence two and three syllables in their phonologies, they also simultaneously begin to exhibit two-word utterances in their expressive language samples.

Word-Initial Singleton Consonants (CV). Prevocalic anterior nasals /m,n/, stops /p,b,t,d/, and the labial glide /w/ do not often need to be targeted. If a child completely deletes any of these early developing phoneme classes, however, the missing phonemes/classes are appropriate targets during early weeks of the first cycle. The palatal glide has generally been more problematic for children with severe/profound speech disorders than the labial glide. In fact, some clients have experienced considerable difficulty producing /j/. In such instances, production practice for a deficient palatal glide may need to be delayed for one or more cycles.

Word-Final Singleton Consonants (VC). Postvocalic voiceless stops /p/ and /t/ and/or /k/ (depending on stimulability) and/or word-final anterior nasals /m,n/ (if lacking) are appropriate targets to help children develop their abilities to close syllables. Children with phonological disorders delete word-final obstruents more often than word-final nasals.[1]

Other Word Structures (CVC;VCV). Occasionally a child produces final consonants in some words and initial consonants in others, but fails to produce CVC (initial and final consonants in the same word). Monosyllabic words containing the same initial and final consonant (e.g., *pipe*) seem to help clients learn that consonants can occur at the beginning and also at the end of the same word. Some children produce word-initial and word-final consonants, but delete medial consonants VCV. In such instances, two-syllable words with medial

stop consonants (e.g., *apple*) are useful to help children learn to produce intervocalic singleton consonants.

Posterior/Anterior Contrasts. If a child lacks either velars or alveolars because of *fronting* (e.g., *tea* for *key*) or *backing* (e.g., *key* for *tea*), or because of *omissions,* velar stops (word-final /k/ followed by word-initial /g/ and/or /k/) or alveolar stops (word-final /t/ and word-initial /d/ and/or /t/) should be evaluated next for readiness. The selection, of course, depends on which are deficient and also which are stimulable.

Velars need to be targeted considerably more often than alveolars. Some children demonstrate extraordinary difficulty producing posterior consonants, particularly word-initial /k/ and /g/. It may be necessary in such instances to delay production-practice activities on velar phonemes for a cycle or two until the child is stimulable for velars. The glottal fricative /h/ is another posterior phoneme that some phonologically disordered children need to target.

/s/-Clusters. All of our highly unintelligible clients evidenced consonant cluster/sequence reductions. Furthermore, stridency was particularly lacking in utterances of preschool clients. For children who substitute stops for strident phonemes (e.g., *tea* for *see*), /s/ should be targeted in consonant clusters first rather than as singletons, because clients with phonological disorders tend to produce /s/-plus-stop combinations when clinicians attempt to elicit singleton /s/ (e.g., [s-ti] for *see*). Such clients experience less difficulty producing /s/-clusters initially than an /s/ singleton (i.e., without adding an intruding stop before the vowel).

Moreover, it has been observed that an emphasis on prevocalic singleton /s/ has sometimes created two additional problems for highly unintelligible clients. Children who have been taught to say singleton /s/ and to suppress their inclination to produce an intervening stop have typically experienced difficulty later when they attempt to produce

---

[1]Word-final voiced obstruents (e.g., final /b,d,g,z/) should *not* be targets for highly unintelligible children because phonologically normal children typically do not fully voice utterance-final obstruents.

/s/-clusters. A common phenomenon that has been observed in utterances of children who have had singleton /s/ programming has been the production of /s/-cluster words with only the first element of the cluster (e.g., *sick* for *stick*). A second problem that has occurred has been distortions of /s/. A number of phonologically disordered school-age clients who had received singleton /s/ programming prior to entering the university phonology program produced palatalized or lateralized /s/.

The actual selection order for /s/-cluster targets depends on each client's phonological system. For example, a child who demonstrates velar fronting should not target /sk/ or /ks/ during initial cycles until facility in producing velars is demonstrated. Likewise a child who demonstrates backing should not target /st/ or /ts/ until alveolars have begun to emerge, nor should a child who lacks nasals target /sm/ or /sn/ initially.

Although both word-final and word-initial /s/-clusters should be targeted during each of the first few cycles, they should not be intermingled until final cycles. Thus stimulable word-initial /s/-clusters (/sp/, /st/, /sm/, /sn/, and/or /sk/) should be targeted in succession, then set aside until the next cycle, before (or after) targeting stimulable word-final /s/-clusters (/ts/, /ps/, and/or /ks/).

A carrier phrase (It's a _____) is usually incorporated for /s/-cluster practice words by the third cycle (after a child demonstrates facility in producing the /s/-clusters). During one session the child uses the carrier phrase for words that do not contain /s/ (e.g., It's a *door*). The next session the child is taught how to produce /s/ two times in one utterance (e.g., It's a *star*).

Liquids. The /l/ and /r/ phonemes (if lacking) should also be stimulated during *each* cycle. Although liquid gliding is still relatively common in utterances of normally developing 4-year-olds (Grunwell, 1987; Hodson & Paden, 1981), approximately half of the subjects in recent phonology studies produced liquids appropriately by age 3 (e.g., Dyson, 1988). It is of some interest to note

also that a surprising number of highly unintelligible 3- and 4-year-old clients with extremely limited speech-sound repertoires demonstrated excellent word-final /ɚ/ productions during their initial assessment sessions.

Another clinical observation has been that children who waited to target liquids until all other phonological patterns were established typically required several additional years of intervention programming in order to develop their abilities to produce liquids (particularly /r/). Our clinical records indicate that when stimulation for liquids was provided at the end of each cycle, clients demonstrated closer approximations of liquids during ensuing cycles. Furthermore, some spontaneous productions of liquids began emerging during the period that other targeted patterns (e.g., velars, /s/-clusters) were being generalized into conversational samples.

The goal for early cycles is to develop awareness of liquids and to *suppress* substitution processes (e.g., *gliding, stopping*) rather than for the child to produce perfect /l/ and /r/. When targeting word-initial /r/, the clinician needs to emphasize the vowel and to deemphasize blending during the first couple of cycles in order to suppress productions of /w/. Thus for the target word, *rock,* the clinician models [ɝ], (pauses) and then says [ɑk], stressing and prolonging the vowel. The client must not be allowed to produce a /w/ in the carefully selected production-practice words. At first, most children say [ʊ] rather than [ɝ], which is accepted during the initial cycles as long as the client does not add a /w/.

Velar-liquid clusters (/kl/, /gl/, /kr/, /gr/) can usually be targeted by the third or fourth cycle (provided the client has developed facility for /k/ and /g/). Alveolar-liquid clusters (/tr/, /dr/, /sl/) can also be presented during recycling of liquids. Labial-liquid clusters (/pl/, /bl/, /fl/ and /pr/, /br/, /fr/) should be the *last* liquid clusters to be targeted because of possible labial assimilation effects. School-age clients often need to target postvocalic /ɚ/ and medial /l/ and /r/; however, most preschool clients who have developed a good phonological foundation demonstrate liquid generalization to other word positions on their own.

Additional Potential Targets

Secondary Target Patterns. Secondary target patterns are not targeted until after clients demonstrate that they have acquired all of the early developing phoneme classes (nasals, stops, and glides), basic word structures, and posterior/anterior contrasts. Clients should also demonstrate suppression of the gliding process for production-practice words that contain liquids, as well as emergence of stridency and some consonant clusters in their spontaneous utterances. Preschool clients rarely need to target any of the secondary patterns discussed in this section because they seem to be able to generalize exceptionally well and to develop other components of their phonological systems during the time that they are improving their listening skills and learning to produce the basic priority patterns.

If reassessment following the second or third cycle indicates that *prevocalic voicing* (e.g., *do* for *to*), *vowel neutralization* (e.g., *hut* for *hat, hit,* etc.), *assimilations* (e.g., *numb* for *thumb*), and/or *idiosyncratic* phonological rules (cf. Fey & Gandour, 1982; Leonard, Schwartz, Swanson, & Frome Loeb, 1987) are still prevalent in a child's phonological system, *minimal-pair* contrast words that incorporate the child's actual erroneous production should be used whenever possible to facilitate understanding of the semantic differences between such words.

Singleton stridents may also be targeted (if necessary) after completion of two or three cycles. Preschool clients, however, typically demonstrate generalization to singleton strident phonemes (particularly /f/ and /s/) after several cycles of targeting /s/-clusters. Some school-age clients have needed to target palatal sibilants because of depalatalization (e.g., *sue* for *shoe*) and/or affrication (e.g., *chew* for *shoe*) or deaffrication (e.g., *share* for *chair*), but palatal sibilants should not be targeted until the final cycles, and then only if they have not yet begun to emerge in the client's utterances.

All remaining deficient consonant *sequences* can be targeted during the final phonological cycle. Clusters containing glides (e.g., /kw/, /tw/, /sw/, /bj/, /fj/, /hj/, /kj/, /mj/) are troublesome for some clients, as are certain medial and final consonant clusters. Some school-age clients demonstrate excessive difficulty producing medial /s/-clusters (e.g., *biscuit, boxing*) and final /s/-clusters with the /s/ preceding the stop (e.g., *desk, toast*). Medial and final /s/ + stop clusters and three-consonant clusters (e.g., *string, mixed*) are common targets during the final cycle for school-age clients with phonological disorders.

One of the salient findings of our clinical research has been the realization that targeting consonant clusters is of the utmost importance. Children who are less intelligible in conversational speech than when naming words are usually experiencing difficulty producing consonants in sequences that cross syllable/word boundaries. Word endings are deleted more often in connected speech than when naming isolated words; however, in most instances such deletions are an artifact of consonant sequence reductions rather than simply final consonant deletions. If one word ends in a consonant and the next word begins with a consonant, children who experience difficulty producing two contiguous consonants typically will delete one, particularly if an /s/ is involved. Another clinical observation has been that highly unintelligible school-age clients demonstrate extraordinary difficulty producing /s/-clusters. These older children typically produce the /s/ but delete other consonants in the sequence (e.g., /siz/ for *sneeze*). Teaching such clients to produce and also to incorporate consonant sequences in their speech results in marked intelligibility gains.

Advanced Target Patterns. Some upper-elementary school-age clients experience extreme difficulty producing multisyllabic words (e.g., *aluminum, thermometer*) and complex consonant sequences (e.g., /skj/, /kstr/) especially when they are confronted with textbooks that contain complicated words. Clinicians can develop lists of troublesome words that the client needs to be able to say. Analysis and synthesis techniques for producing such words can be taught to the client, and opportunities for practicing parts and then wholes can be provided.

Inappropriate Targets for Unintelligible Clients

Voiced final obstruents, final /ŋ/, postvocalic/syllabic /l/, "weak-syllable deletion," and the "th" phonemes should *not* be selected as primary targets for unintelligible clients. Phonologically normal children typically prolong vowels slightly, but do not produce fully voiced utterance-final obstruents (Hodson & Paden, 1981). Normally developing 4-year-olds, for example, typically say [peɪtʃ] (with slight vowel prolongation) for /peɪdʒ/. Furthermore, phonologically normal children commonly demonstrate slight pitch alterations for /l/ in words such as *doll, candle,* and *milk,* but do not exhibit tongue tip elevation to the alveolar ridge (for /l/) in such words. Substitutions of /n/ for /ŋ/, particularly in bisyllabic words, and /f/ or /s/ for /θ/ are also common in utterances of young phonologically normal children and do not particularly affect intelligibility. In addition, weak syllable deletion (e.g., [tɛ:vɪʒən] for *television*; [prɑblɪ] for *probably*) is extremely common in conversational utterances of normal speakers. It therefore seems inappropriate for clinicians to ask unintelligible clients to produce patterns that are "superior" to those of their phonologically normal peers.

METHOD

Structure of Remediation Session

The following format for remediation sessions has been used in our university phonology program. The format has also been adapted for use in schools, clinics, and hospitals.

1. The child reviews the preceding session's production-practice word cards. If target patterns are being changed (e.g., velars last session; /s/-clusters this session), the cards from the preceding week are set aside until a later cycle. They can be reused, and new words with more difficult phonetic environments can be added during ensuing cycles to increase complexity. If the phoneme target for this session is for the same target pattern as during the preceding session (e.g., /s/-clusters for both sessions), both sets of cards (e.g., /sp/ words from last session and /st/ words for this session) can be incorporated into some production-practice activities for the current session.

2. The clinician provides auditory bombardment with slight *amplification* for a minute or two. The child listens while the clinician reads the session's listening list of approximately 12 words that contain the target pattern. (The child is *not* to repeat these words, but rather must listen attentively.) The clinician also demonstrates the error and contrasts it with the target while using the amplifier. At the end of the auditory bombardment activity, the clinician may also ask the child to say one or two words into the amplifier's microphone from a second list that contains *potential* production-practice words.

3. The child draws or colors (or pastes on) pictures of three to five carefully selected production-practice words (controlled for phonetic environment) on large (5 × 8 inch) index cards. The child says each word prior to making the picture so that the clinician can evaluate the word for appropriateness/difficulty/possible assimilation effects. (The clinician writes the word on the card so that adults can identify the picture.)

4. The child participates in *experiential-play* production-practice activities. The child names the picture incorporating the target pattern for the day in order to "take a turn." The clinican provides models and/or tactual cues as needed so that the child achieves *100%* success on the target *pattern* for these carefully selected production-practice words. The clinician also provides opportunities for some conversation during each session in order to ascertain when phonological patterns are beginning to emerge in spontaneous utterances.

5. The clinician *probes* for *stimulability* for next session's target phoneme within the selected

target pattern. For example, if /s/ clusters are to be targeted next, the clinician asks the client to say words such as *boats, tops, books,* and/or *spot, stop, smoke, snow,* and *sky.* The most *stimulable* /s/-cluster within the word-initial *or* word-final /s/ cluster pattern is selected to be the target for the following session, the next most stimulable /s/-cluster the next session, and so on.

6. The clinician repeats amplified auditory training. The same listening list of words that was used earlier in the session is read to the child again.

7. The parent (or school aide) participates in a 2-minutes-per-day *home* (or school) *program.* The adult reads the week's listening list and the child names picture cards of production-practice words.

Selecting Production-Practice Words

It is recommended that *words* (rather than nonsense syllables) be used for production practice. Whenever possible, *monosyllabic* words with *facilitative phonetic environments* (Kent, 1982) should be selected during the first few cycles so that clients can experience some immediate success (e.g., Buteau & Hodson, 1989). Words that contain phonemes produced at the same *place* of articulation as the substitute phoneme should be avoided during early cycles. For example, target words such as *cat, can, kiss, kite, goat,* and *gun* would be *inappropriate* for children who evidence velar fronting (i.e., substitute alveolars for velars), and *lamb, lamp, leaf, lip, rope, robe, roof, robot,* and *rabbit* (i.e., words containing labial consonants and/or vowels) should *never* be production-practice words during early cycles for children who substitute the labial glide /w/ for liquids. Care should be taken to reduce opportunities for *assimilation* effects.

Words for which actual *objects* (e.g., *boats* for word-final /ts/) can be incorporated are desirable, particularly for preschool children. In addition, *action* words (e.g., *eats*) should be used to add another dimension. It is also desirable that production-practice words be appropriate for each child's *vocabulary* level.

Remediation Activities

Experiential-play activities (e.g., fishing, bowling) provide motivation for young children. It is especially beneficial to incorporate *pragmatically* appropriate activities. For example, an unloaded camera can be incorporated for the production-practice word *smile.* Opportunities should also be provided for some of the production-practice activities to occur outside the clinician's room.

The *number* of activities varies from session to session. In general, our student clinicians average one activity for every 8 or 10 minutes. The same activities can be repeated week after week. Clinicians are advised to switch to the next activity *before* children lose interest even if a client prefers to continue certain favorite activities.

Phonology clinicians use their skills to select optimal targets and to provide sufficient *cues* so that their clients can experience 100% success on the session's target pattern for the carefully selected production-practice words. Clinicians typically provide *models* (e.g., *Is this a pot or a spot?*) and *tactual cues* (e.g., drawing a finger up the child's arm for /s/ and tapping for a /p/ in an /s/-cluster word) at the beginning of sessions. In some instances, clients wear a portable amplifier for part of the remediation session in order to achieve 100% success for the targeted pattern. Cues and assists are decreased as the client gains facility in producing the session's target. The process of counting and charting errors, which has been found to be counterproductive, is not advocated for this phonological remediation approach. Our observation has been that counting and charting not only interfere with natural interactions between clinician and client, but also allow the child to continue making error productions that provide additional practice and reinforcement for the inaccurate kinesthetic image.

The use of *minimal-pair* words is excellent for children who have sufficient skills to experience success (Tyler et al., 1987). Explanations of minimal-pair differences can be provided even if the child is not yet at a readiness level for productions of the contrasting words. During the final cycles, the use of minimal pairs can be extremely effective in helping children recognize the *semantic* differences between the error and the target productions.

Confrontation activities may be appropriate in some instances for *advanced* school-age clients, especially if perseveration is occurring on specific words. Dean and Howell (1986) discussed providing situations where a child learns through "conflict and reflection." They stated that the child must have an opportunity for discussion with the adult about the "nature of the problem" and that "graded feedback which extends understanding without discouraging" must be provided. They also stressed that the "task must motivate the child."

A 6-year-old client in our clinic who persisted in saying *Wes* for *yes* even after she had learned to produce /j/ in other words was told that she had to respond with a *yes* before receiving a treat. The client was then asked if she wanted an animal cracker. When she answered *"Wes,"* she was given a picture of a boy called *Wes* along with an explanation instead of the cookie. The client's motivation to say *yes* increased noticeably after that experience. Confrontation activities should be used only for those clients who can readily produce the target and who demonstrate *metalinguistic* awareness of the phonological aspects involved.

For school-age clients who can read, a short period of *oral reading* focusing on the session's target pattern should be incorporated during each session. The material for this activity must be at a reading *level* that is *below* that of the child's current reading level so that attention can be directed toward the phonological pattern being targeted rather than on reading skills.

Some children need to begin remediation one step *below* production practice. For clients who lack stimulability or who are unwilling to participate in production-practice activities (e.g., 2-year-olds), it may be best to provide *focused auditory*

input during the first cycle of remediation. Deficient patterns are stimulated by presenting one new phoneme (within a target pattern) during each session. The child participates in activities and listens, but productions are not required during this cycle. The clinician talks about selected objects (e.g., *cup, top* for final consonant stimulation) and incorporates activities (e.g., *jump, up*) related to the week's target pattern. All of the deficient patterns (including liquids) are presented (in succession) auditorally for a cycle. Production-practice activities are incorporated during the second and later cycles (i.e., after the child demonstrates sufficient readiness).

Facilitating Development of Awareness of Phonological Patterns

The purpose of production practice in this approach is *not* to establish a motor pattern. Rather, productions of targets in a limited number of carefully selected words provide opportunities for developing new *kinesthetic* images and for *integrative rehearsal*. At the same time, it is imperative to help the child develop *auditory* awareness of the pattern. Unintelligible children do not seem to hear their own speech. For example, when adults repeat a word exactly as it was said by the phonologically disordered child, the typical response by the child is to correct the adult. This correction is usually followed by the child's identical error production of the word (cf. Berko & Brown, 1960).

Unintelligible children seem to rely solely on their own inaccurate kinesthetic images that "feel right" at the time, and they tend to ignore or negate *auditory feedback* for their inaccurate productions. Combining a limited amount of production practice with amplified auditory training during each session seems to help children improve their self-monitoring skills. The amplifier is also used during production-practice activities whenever a client experiences difficulty with a particular production.

This remediation approach should *not* be used without incorporating amplification, particularly during the first few cycles. Children respond differently when the listening list is presented with amplification than when the clinician simply says the words loudly without amplification. One problem that often accompanies the recitation of words without amplification is that clinicians tend to exaggerate their models, particularly for /s/. It is imperative that a soft, precise /s/ be modeled for two reasons. Young children tend to "over produce" what has been modeled with the common result being distorted sibilants. The second reason is that the more precise /s/ production seems to enable the child to experience a more definitive kinesthetic image.

STRENGTHS/LIMITATIONS

The primary strength of this phonological remediation approach is its efficiency. All treatment approaches appear to help children improve speech (Ingram, 1983), as does maturation; however, the amount of time required for children with phonological disorders to achieve intelligibility varies considerably from one approach to another. Programs that focus on phonemes until a criterion (e.g., 90%) is reached are generally appropriate for a child who misarticulates only two or three speech sounds. For children with extensive speech errors, however, phoneme-oriented approaches have proved to be inordinately time consuming, often requiring 5 or more years of programming. The *longest* period of remediation time required for phonologically disordered clients in our clinic to become intelligible via the phonological cycles approach has been 18 months (i.e., approximately 60 hours of remediation time). Most preschool children required less than a year of phonological remediation.

A second strength of this approach is its adaptability. It has been used effectively with groups (e.g., Montgomery & Bonderman, in press) and with children who have additional etiological com-

plications such as repaired cleft palates (e.g., Hodson, Chin, Redmond, & Simpson, 1983) and developmental dyspraxia diagnoses (e.g., Hodson & Paden, 1983). Furthermore, the approach has been adapted for use with children in mentally retarded classrooms. Time allotments, however, have been doubled for mentally retarded children. Each phoneme per pattern is targeted 2 hours rather than 60 minutes, and 3 years or more may be required before substantial intelligibility gains are observed. Mentally retarded children seem to be especially in need of a comprehensive, system-oriented phonological remediation approach because they lack the normal cognitive abilities requisite for integration of isolated phoneme parts.

Considerably more research needs to be conducted to determine how this remediation approach can be adapted for use with children who speak languages other than English. Phonological analysis procedures can readily be used for other languages (e.g., Hodson, 1986b), but hypotheses need to be formulated and tested to determine remediation implementations for specific languages.

Research also needs to be conducted to develop adaptations for children with profound hearing impairments. This approach has been used successfully for children with recurrent otitis media, the most commonly reported etiological factor noted in case histories of clients with severe speech disorders (Churchill, Hodson, Jones, & Novak, 1988) and for children with moderate-to-severe hearing impairments (Garrett, 1986). Phonological assessment and remediation procedures that incorporate prosodic aspects must be developed and refined for children with profound hearing losses.

This approach was *not* designed for children with mild speech disorders. Phoneme-oriented intervention programs appear to be quite adequate for children who demonstrate only a few essentially intelligible misarticulations (e.g., lisps).

SUMMARY

The phonological remediation approach described in this chapter uses cycles to facilitate the development of intelligible speech patterns in children with severe/profound speech disorders. Phonological patterns are targeted in succession by using carefully selected production-practice words to help unintelligible children develop appropriate auditory and kinesthetic images for eventual self-monitoring. Deficient phonological patterns are recycled as many times as needed until the targeted patterns begin to emerge in the child's spontaneous utterances. The ordering of phonological patterns within cycles is based on developmental and clinical phonology research and on each individual child's phonological abilities.

REFERENCES

Berko, J., & Brown, R. (1960). Psycholinguistic research methods. In P. Mussen (Ed.), *Handbook of research methods in child development* (pp. 517–557). New York: Wiley.

Buteau, C., & Hodson, B. (1989). *Phonological remediation targets: Words and primary pictures for highly unintelligible children.* Danville, IL: Interstate.

Churchill, J., Hodson, B., Jones, B., & Novak, R. (1988). Phonological systems of speech-disordered clients with positive/negative histories of otitis media. *Language, Speech and Hearing Services in Schools, 19,* 100–107.

Dean, E., & Howell, J. (1986). Developing linguistic awareness: A theoretically based approach to phonological disorders. *British Journal of Communication Disorders, 21,* 223–238.

Dyson, A. (1988). Phonetic inventories of 2- and 3-year-old children. *Journal of Speech and Hearing Disorders, 53,* 89–93.

Dyson, A., & Paden, E. (1983). Some phonological acquisition strategies used by two-year-olds. *Journal of Childhood Communication Disorders, 7,* 6–18.

Fairbanks, G. (1954). Systematic research in experimental phonetics: A theory of the speech mechanism as a servosystem. *Journal of Speech and Hearing Disorders, 19,* 133–139.

Fey, M., & Gandour, J. (1982). Rule discovery in phonological acquisition. *Journal of Child Language, 9,* 71–82.

Garrett, R. (1986). *A phonologically based speech-improvement classroom program for hearing-impaired students.* Unpublished manuscript, San Diego State University.

Grunwell, P. (1987). *Clinical Phonology* (2nd ed.). Baltimore, MD: Williams and Wilkins.

Hodson, B. (1985). *Computer analysis of phonological processes.* Stonington, IL: PhonoComp.

Hodson, B. (1986a). *The assessment of phonological processes—revised.* Danville, IL: Interstate.

Hodson, B. (1986b). *The assessment of phonological processes—Spanish.* San Diego: Los Amigos.

Hodson, B., Chin, L. Redmond, B., & Simpson, R. (1983). Phonological evaluation and remediation of speech deviations of a child with a repaired cleft palate: A case study. *Journal of Speech and Hearing Disorders, 48,* 93–98.

Hodson, B., & Paden, E. (1981). Phonological processes which characterize unintelligible and intelligible speech in early childhood. *Journal of Speech and Hearing Disorders, 46,* 369–373.

Hodson, B., & Paden, E. (1983). *Targeting intelligible speech: A phonological approach to remediation.* San Diego: College Hill Press.

Ingram, D. (1976). *Phonological disability in children.* New York: Elsevier.

Ingram, D. (1983). Case studies of phonological disability. *Topics in Language Disorders, 3.*

Ingram, D. (1986). Explanation and phonological remediation. *Child Language Teaching and Therapy, 2,* 1–19.

Jakobson, R. (1941). Child language, aphasia, and phonological universals. (A. Keiler, Trans., 1968). The Hague: Mouton.

Kent, R. (1982). Contextual facilitation of correct sound production. *Language, Speech, and Hearing Services in Schools, 13,* 66–76.

Leonard, L., Schwartz, R., Swanson, L., & Frome Loeb, D. (1987). Some conditions that promote unusual phonological behaviour in children. *Clinical Linguistics and Phonetics, 1,* 23–34.

Macken, M., & Ferguson, C. (1983). Cognitive aspects of phonological development: Model, evidence, and issues. In K. Nelson (Ed.), *Children's language, Vol. 4* (pp. 252–282). Hillsdale, NJ: Erlbaum.

Montgomery, J., & Bonderman, R. (in press). Serving preschool children with severe phonological disorders. *Language, Speech, and Hearing Services in Schools.*

Preisser, D., Hodson, B., & Paden, E. (1988). Developmental phonology: 18–29 months. *Journal of Speech and Hearing Disorders, 53,* 125–130.

Stampe, D. (1972). *A dissertation on natural phonology.* Doctoral dissertation, University of Chicago.

Stoel-Gammon, C., & Dunn, C. (1985). *Normal and disordered phonology in children.* Austin, TX: Pro-Ed.

Tyler, A., Edwards, M., & Saxman, J. (1987). Clinical application of two phonologically based treatment procedures. *Journal of Speech and Hearing Disorders, 52,* 393–409.

CHAPTER 13

Articulatory Production Training: A Sensory-Motor Approach

The contents of this chapter are based on the teachings of E. T. McDonald, who explained the dynamics of articulation/coarticulation and applied the *principles* of coarticulation to assessment and treatment procedures.

Although McDonald (1964a) developed the first comprehensive assessment and treatment approach based on principles of coarticulation, he attributes his basic knowledge to Scripture (1935), Shohara (1939), Stetson (1951) and Kelso and Munhall (1988). *Overlapping speech movements, the original term for coarticulation* described by Scripture and by Shohara, can be traced to others from the early 1900s (McDonald, 1964a). For example, Avery, Dorsey, and Sickels (1928) wrote that ". . . the nature of speech is such that the essential character of any one sound cannot be fully understood without some knowledge of the way it is influenced by those which precede and follow it" (p. 80).

McDonald put the sensory-motor approach into perspective when he wrote in 1964, "although this book will present but one approach, it is not suggested that this is the only effective approach to the

Richard E. Shine, Ed.D., is a professor of speech pathology in the Department of Speech, Language and Auditory Pathology, East Carolina University, Greenville, North Carolina.

diagnosis and treatment of articulatory problems" (p. ix). In fact, no single approach should be used. Rather, principles of treatment common to proven effective approaches should be examined, and selected approaches should be based on empirical *principles of treatment*.

The literature includes numerous approaches demonstrated as effective in the remediation of articulatory/phonological deviancies, and careful examination of any one approach reveals significant overlap of principles of treatment. For example, the final goal of any approach is correct articulation (production) during conversational speech (communicative interaction). Even if one stresses the use of a phonological process approach, success is measured by correctness of articulatory production determined by "phonetic analysis." Production is thus recognized as an essential part of treatment. The clinician who understands and incorporates rules of the dynamics of coarticulation in addition to phonological process, distinctive-feature, and multiphonemic rules is potentially more effective in attaining success. Thus, it is suggested that the following detailed description of the principles involved in the sensory-motor approach (McDonald, 1964a, 1980, in press) be applied as part of a comprehensive approach incorporating, at the very least, principles of distinctive features, multiphonemics, and phonological processes. The sensory-motor approach emphasizes production training but acknowledges the importance of phonology (language) as well as other approaches and principles of treatment.

The foresight of McDonald (1964a) in differentiating articulation and phonology may be seen in the following:

> The word "speech" might be defined from several different points of view, e.g., a definition might be cast in *semantic, or physiologic, or acoustic terms* (italics added). Often, however, users of the word "speech" leave it undefined. Many textbooks dealing with "speech", "speech" pathology, and "speech" correction offer no definition of the word "speech." It is not uncommon to hear the word "speech" used to mean "language" or for "speech" to be confused with some of the processes by which speech is produced, as when defective articulation is labeled "defective speech." Since our purpose is to develop a point of view which can provide a rationale for assessing and correcting defective articulation, it is essential that we *distinguish between speech and language* (italics added) and that we differentiate between "speech" and the processes by which it is produced. . . . Language is portrayed as an accumulation of concepts which exists in some symbolic form. Speech is regarded as one of several modalities through which language is utilized. Articulation is viewed as one of several interrelated processes by which speech is produced.
>
> Further, for our purposes, we find that a physiologically oriented definition of speech provides the most effective basis for developing rationales for the diagnosis and treatment of articulatory defects. (p. 71)

In order to understand the principles of the sensory-motor approach, it may be helpful to review some terminology that was explained in chapter 2. As early as 1951, Stetson differentiated between phonetic (phone) and phonemic (phoneme). He indicated "the terms 'phonetic,' 'sound,' 'articulation' refer to articulate processes of speech *without regard to meaning*" (italics added) and that phonemic ". . . has to do primarily with meanings. . . ." The following con-

cepts are important for differentiating articulation and phonology.

Phonology is a linguistic term that refers to *the sound system of language*. Phonology is *language specific* and as such *finite*. The terms *phoneme, phonemic, morphophonemic,* and *position* can be used in reference only to phonology. Phonology deals with the *linguistic rules of phonemes* used to effect *changes in meaning*. Word-initial (I) and word-final (F), and at times word-medial (M), are linguistic terms used to designate *position of phonemes*. Generally, initial and final are used with reference to single syllable lexical units (CV, VC, CVC) and medial with reference to multisyllabic lexical units (CVCVCVC) as in the word *bicycle*. As Johnson, Darley, and Spriestersbach noted years ago (1963), "the Articulation Test Form provides for entries derived from the testing of the single consonant sounds in three positions—initial, medial, and final. We recognize that the traditional concept of three positions of consonants in words is artificial—an artifact growing out of orthography in disregard of the dynamics of speech production" (p. 89).

Articulation is a physiologic term that refers to the *motor gesture system* through which the phonology of language is produced. The terms *phonetic, phone, allophone,* and *function* can be used in reference only to articulation. Function acknowledges the dynamic nature of coarticulation and implies the existence of allophonic variation. Articulation deals with *production rules* used to *produce the phonology of language*. Articulation is *infinite* in nature as reflected in *allophonic variation*. Articulation is *dynamic* and consonants function either *prevocalicly* or *postvocalicly* in the *syllable movement pattern*. Articulation cannot refer to position (the orthography of sounds).

A basic understanding of the dynamics of articulation/coarticulation is presented by analysis of the sentence, *I have a cat dish.* Lexically, the sentence contains 3 word-initial consonant phonemes (have, cat, dish) and 3 word-final consonant phonemes (have, cat, dish). Syllable production analysis (motor phonetics) reveals 4 prevocalic consonant phones (ha, va, cat, dish) and 2 postvocalic consonant phones (cat, dish). Lexical terminology,

TABLE 13.1
Examples of Lexical Items Produced with Highly Similar Stress Patterns

Lexical Items	Context	IMF Lexical Analysis	Pre-/Postvocalic Syllable Analysis
yesterday	CVC/CV/CV	y(I); s,t,d(M)	y,t,d(pre); s(post)
gas today	CVC/CV/CV	g,t(I); d(M); s(F)	g,t,d(pre); s(post)
come to pay	CVC/CV/CV	c,t,p(I); m(F)	c,p,t(pre); m(post)

such as word-initial and word-final, does not accurately describe the articulatory/syllable production of "have" when it is produced with secondary stress or without a pause after it. The "v" is lexically a word-final consonant phoneme but becomes a prevocalic consonant phone during production in the syllable "va" (as will be shown). With regard to IMF and production (incompatible terms), the only initial sound is "I" and the only final sound is "sh"; all other sounds are medial. The sentence contains 5 lexical syllables (I / have / a / cat / dish) and 5 articulatory syllables (I / ha / va / cat / dish). Note that the articulatory syllable juncture is different from the lexical division.

Another example of the incompatibility of IMF terminology in describing production is provided in Table 13.1, which lists lexical items produced with highly similar syllable stress patterns. Lexically, in "yesterday" the word-initial consonant phoneme is "y"; however, in "gas today" there are two word-initial consonant phonemes and in "come to pay" there are 3 word-initial consonant phonemes *even though the contextual configuration is identical in all 3 examples*. With regard to production, the analysis of pre-/postvocalic function reveals that all 3 lexical items are produced in a similar, predictable manner. Semantically, there is total difference in the 3 items but motorically they are highly similar. It seems obvious that the IMF analysis is limited and totally invalid with reference to production.

A linguistically based approach provides knowledge and principles for the assessment and treatment of phonological process deviancies understood or evaluated from a linguistic point of view. However, a phonologic process analysis is based on misarticulations (a phonetic analysis) and

is merely a linguistically based interpretation of misarticulations. Both the linguistic and the production principles involved must be considered. Ignoring semanticity or production with children who lisp or children with a minimal number of error phones/phonemes seems inappropriate because both phonological and articulation principles are a part of the deviancy. Articulation and phonology are interrelated aspects of communication, that is, the production of language. The phonology of a language is produced via articulation and the analysis of simplifying phonological processes is an analysis of misarticulations.

RATIONALE

The principles of the sensory-motor approach are universally applicable in the production of articulate speech. The syllable is identified as the primary "unit" of production. Articulatory/coarticulatory production is dynamic, not static, and the influence of movement patterns is crucial in assessment and treatment. Sensory-motor production training is initiated with the correct production of error phones in coarticulatory contexts. Training procedures target allophones of error phones. Even though the syllable is the primary unit of production, the bisyllable is the smallest unit of production recommended in the initiation of training.

Production training for each error phone involves systematically shaping the correct coarticulation of a representative sample of contexts in progressively more complex language. Manipulation and control of the influence of coarticulation at the syllable juncture is emphasized as critical in intra-extratherapy generalization. Generally, because principles of coarticulation and natural prosodic patterns are stressed, generalization of correct production occurs spontaneously across phones that are physiologically and acoustically similar (Blaustein, 1973; Mariani, 1975). Treatment emphasizes expansion of the number of correct contexts within more and more variable coarticulatory patterns. Assessment and treatment principles recognize the concept of "function of consonants" within the syllable movement pattern as opposed to the linguistic terminology, which recognizes "position" of consonants in words.

The adaption of McDonald's (1964a) sensory-motor approach as outlined by Shine and Proust (1982) includes six phases: evaluation, awareness, establishment, intratherapy generalization, transfer/extratherapy generalization, and maintenance.

EVALUATION PHASE

Too often the clinician initiates remedial procedures (including identification of error phones and selection of target phones) after administering only one single-word picture articulation test or phonological process test. Decisions about remediation based on the accuracy of production of consonant phones based on assessment in only two or possibly three positions in a single word picture articulation test is a questionable practice. Some clinicians indicate that in their particular situation time does not permit completion of a comprehensive assessment protocol. Such statements as "I don't have time to do a complete evaluation in this environment" may be based on incorrect assumptions, e.g., (1) the evaluation has to be completed in one session and only 20 to 30 minutes of testing time is available per patient and (2) testing, particularly comprehensive testing, is a waste of time. Assessment is considered as ongoing; several sessions can be used over a period of weeks. After the necessary formalized procedures are completed,

diagnostic treatment can be introduced to determine appropriate antecedent stimuli at new levels of language and coarticulatory complexity. Testing beyond what is necessary to appropriately describe the problem is a waste of time (Schultz, 1972), but a comprehensive assessment protocol will potentially save significant time in the overall duration of treatment.

Data Needed for a Comprehensive Articulatory/Phonological Assessment

The objective within the evaluation phase is to administer assessment procedures necessary for a differential and comprehensive diagnosis. Assessment should be terminated when the articulation/phonology deviancy has been sufficiently defined to enable development of appropriate therapy direction and strategies.

In the administration of all articulation/phonology tests, one should phonetically transcribe in narrow transcription the entire stimulus word if any phone within the word is misarticulated, whether or not it is the target phone. For example, in administering the Arizona Articulation Proficiency Scale (Fudala, 1974), the /p/ is the target phone in the word *cup*. If, for example, a 5-year-old child produces *tup/cup,* the entire word is transcribed $[t^h \Lambda p^-]$ (X^h = aspirated production; X^- = held plosive/not exploded) revealing a substitution that is acoustically similar (voiceless plosive) but physiologically dissimilar (place of production). A fronting phonologic process is noted. The presence of a CVC context suggests development of a complex syllable pattern versus a simplified open syllable which would have been indicated by $[t^h \Lambda]$. Although a t/k fronting substitution is present in this context, narrow transcription may reveal /k/ was produced correctly in a different test word, functioning prevocalicly in the word *monkey.* Such data suggest inconsistencies of articulatory production potentially influenced by the child's level of articulatory development as well as the context in which the sound occurred. The narrow phonetic transcription provides valuable information for the analysis and interpretation of production data. Such data include syllable movement patterns, correct and incorrect contexts, variability of articulatory accuracy, presence of phonological processes, the presence or absence of distinctive-feature patterns, phonetic and phonemic inventories, and/or error phones and "mastered," correct phones.

Assessment Instruments

All of the assessment and interpretation procedures to be discussed are typically followed with children who exhibit significant articulatory/phonologic deviancies. They are considered minimal requirements for determining the nature and scope of treatment. Not all tests will be necessary for all individuals and other assessment procedures can replace those listed, providing the necessary articulation data are obtained. For individuals with a minimal number of error phones (five or fewer) a comprehensive assessment may be completed with fewer tests. Generally speaking, if the patient is cooperative and capable, *administration and interpretation* should not exceed 45 minutes to one hour.

1. Administer an articulation test (AAPS, Fudala, 1974) to assess production of all English phones in the context of single words. The sentence test may be administered to older individuals.

2. Sample varied contexts by administration of the Screening Deep Test of Articulation (McDonald, 1968) to (a) determine the influence of context on the accuracy of production of the nine commonly misarticulated phones and (b) identify correct contexts of error phones.

3. Obtain a connected speech sample to (a) assess intelligibility, (b) assess the influence of prosody and coarticulation on accuracy of production, (c) identify additional correct contexts, and (d) further assess phonological process and distinctive-feature patterns.

4. Administer phonological process analysis to determine patterns of misarticulations.

5. Administer other assessment procedures deemed necessary to comprehensively assess communicative deviancies.

Interpretation of Phonetic/Phonemic Data

The phonetic/phonemic data can be interpreted to determine treatment direction and strategies as follows.

1. *Compile a list of all error phones* from the data obtained during evaluation. Test data are interpreted to indicate the degree of consistency or percentage of accuracy with which each phone was produced, generally based on samples of 10 or more contexts. This permits identification of three levels of phone production: (1) *correct or "mastered"* (80% to 100% accuracy), (2) *inconsistent but emerging* (50% to 80% accuracy), and (3) *error phones* requiring remediation (0% to 40% accuracy). Consistency data of nine consonant phones each in 10 contexts is provided in Figure 13.1, the record of a Screening Deep Test of Articulation (SDTA).

Based on results of the SDTA in Figure 13.1 and other test instruments, error phones identified for JJ, our example patient, were: [s, z, ʃ, ʒ, tʃ, dʒ, r, ɹ, ɹ, k, g].

2. *Complete a phonetic inventory*, that is, an inventory that "includes all the sounds that the patient produces, regardless of whether these sounds are correct or incorrect relative to the target sound" (Elbert and Gierut, 1986). Thus, if the patient produced [fʌm] for /θʌm/ but never produced /f/ correctly in an appropriate lexical context ("fish or fan or leaf"), the [f] would be a part of the phonetic inventory but not the phonemic inventory.

The place/manner sheet, as illustrated in Figure 13.2, is used to complete a "coded" phonetic inventory that can be used in developing clinical stimulus contexts. In "coding" the phonetic inventory a check mark (√) is used to designate correct production and a zero (0) for incorrect production. The check mark or zero (correct or incorrect) is placed to the left of the target phone to code prevocalic production and to the right to code postvocalic production. The entire phone is circled

FIGURE 13.1

Individual record sheet for a screening deep test of articulation with JJ's error phones identified.

Place of articulation

Manner of articulation			Bi-labial	Labio-dental	Lingua-dental	Lingua-Alveolar	Lingua-Palatal	Lingua-velar	Glottal
Plosive	vL		(p)			(t)		o X✓	
	v		(b)			(d)		o X✓	
Fricative	vL		✓(ŋ)	(f)	(θ)	✓ X✓	X o X✓		✓(h)
	v			(v)	(ð)	o X o	X X		
Affricate	vL						✓ X		
	v						X		
Glide	VL								
	v		✓(w)				✓(j)		
Resonants	Lateral	v				(l)			
	Median	v					X		
	Nasal	v	(m)			(n)		(ŋ)✓	

○ "Mastered" or inconsistent but emerging phones
X Error phone
✓ Correct contexts; pre/postvocalic
o No correct production identified

FIGURE 13.2
Correct and error phones for example patient JJ. (*Source: A Workbook in Phonetics* by M. Downes, 1985, Winston-Salem, NC: Communication Development Products. Adapted from Buchanan, 1963.)

if produced correctly both pre- and postvocalicly. Circled phones would include both "mastered" and "emerging but inconsistent" phones. An X is placed over the phone if the phone is designated as an error phone (see Step 1) and a potential target phone (see Figure 13.2). A different marking procedure could involve circling each correct prevocalic consonant in green and each correct postvocalic consonant in red (or other contrasting colors) on the place/manner sheet.

Figure 13.2 presents the "coded" correct and error phones for our example patient, JJ. The place/manner sheet listing the correct and error phones is closely followed in developing stimulus contexts for heightening awareness training and in facilitating correct production of the error phones during intratherapy generalization.

3. *Identify correct contexts* for each error phone. Generally there will be error phones for which correct contexts are not found. However as therapy progress is made, reassessment often reveals correct contexts. A *correct context* is one in which *each phone within the context including the error phone is correctly articulated.*

List all correct bisyllable and monosyllable correct contexts of lexical items (CVC-CVC; CVC-CV; CVC-VC; VC-CVC; CV-CVC; CVC; CV; CCV; etc.) for each of the designated *error phones*. Correct contexts are listed to facilitate development of stimulus contexts. The following examples depict the variety of potential contexts available for initiating a comprehensive sensory-motor approach. List correct contexts for each error phone (E = error phone) that functions either prevocalicly or postvocalicly.

1. in a bisyllable abutting consonant context (consider [s] as the target phone): CVC-EVC (*cat-sun*); CVE-CVC (*house-cup*)
2. in a bisyllable at the syllable juncture in a context adjacent to a vowel: CV-EVC (*cow-sun*); CV-EV (*my-saw*); CVE-VC (*house-on*)
3. in a bisyllable but not in an abutting context at the syllable juncture: EVC-CVC (*sun-cup*); CVC-CVE (*big-house*); CV-CVE (*my-house*)
4. in a monosyllabic context: EVC (*sun*), EV (*saw*), CVE (*house*), VE (*ace*)
5. as a segment of a cluster within a bisyllabic or monosyllabic context (consider [r] as the target phone): CEVC (*trip*), CEV (*tree*), CVCCEVC (*big-trip*), CVC-CEV (*one-tree*)

Procedures for the formulation of abutting pair contexts are discussed in Appendix 13.1.

4. *Complete additional testing of varied contexts* as is necessary to identify correct production for phones with 0% accuracy or to identify additional bisyllable correct contexts for use in initiating training. Assessment instruments could include (a) Deep Test of Articulation: Picture Form (McDonald, 1964b); (b) Deep Test of Articulation: Sentence Form (McDonald, 1964c); and (c) Clinical Probes of Articulation Consistency (Secord, 1981).

5. *Select target phones* from the list of error phones (see Step 1) and correct contexts (see Step 3). Potential target phones are identified by listing all correct contexts for each error phone.

Phones produced correctly more frequently than incorrectly may continue to emerge without clinical intervention but they can be incorporated as part of the intervention stimuli on a trial basis. Inclusion would be beneficial if the phones enhanced development of distinctive-feature patterns or diminished phonological process patterns. Additionally, because the sensory-motor procedures are initiated by having the patient imitate modeled speech production, a phone misarticulated during spontaneous production but produced correctly with stimulation may provide excellent success for the patient and thus be an appropriate phone on which to initiate training.

As was seen in Figure 13.1, JJ produced correct contexts for each of the following error phones: [s, r, ɚ, tʃ, ʃ, k, g]. Additional assessment revealed that *duck-sun* was produced correctly on the DTA:PF (McDonald, 1964b). The correct contexts for each error phone are given in Table 13.2.

TABLE 13.2
Correct Contexts For Each Error Phone Produced by Example Patient JJ

/s/	/tʃ/	/ʃ/	/k/	/g/
bʌs–fɪʃ	bɔl–tʃeɪn	bʌs–fɪʃ	lak–fɪʃ	glʌv–θʌm
haʊs–flæg		lak–fɪʃ	tiθ–lak	
sɔ–tuθ	*Consonant and*		dʌk–sʌn	
	Vowel "r"			
dʌk–sʌn	ɪɚ–bɛl			
	tɹi–θʌm			

Adhering to a strict sensory-motor approach, without appropriate consideration of principles of distinctive-feature or phonological processes, one would consider the following principles in the selection of a target phone. (1) The target phone must be produced consistently correct in the context selected. (2) The target phone must occur at the syllable juncture in a bisyllable context to emphasize coarticulation and naturalness of production to facilitate generalization. (3) The phone selected should potentially generalize to other physiologically and acoustically similar error phones. *The ideal context for initiating training is a bisyllable CVC-CVC in which the target phone functions as an abutting consonant either pre- or postvocalicly at the syllable juncture.* Abutting consonant contexts typically evoke significant coarticulatory patterns of the target phone and thus facilitate generalization to spontaneous, coarticulatory speech patterns. It is extremely rare for treatment to be initiated with anything less than a bisyllable context.

Selection of an Appropriate Context and Target Phone

The /s/ phone was produced correctly in four different contexts, two of which (*duck-sun, bus-fish*) were CVC-CVC contexts with /s/ as an abutting consonant. In addition, *bus-fish* contained the /ʃ/ error phone and *duck-sun* contained the /k/ error phone. Selection and production practice with either of these contexts would potentially facilitate improvement of the error phone not targeted. The /ʃ/ in *bus-fish* would emphasize frication, which is already a target for /s/. Either context could be selected for initiation of training, but *duck-sun* seems the more ideal context because the /k/ phone occurs at the syllable juncture and it is dissimilar in manner and place of production. Generalization could occur with frication and plosion.

The context *ball-chain* could also be a good choice but it has less to offer in generalization. The affricate may be an excellent choice for the second or third target phone selected. Neither of the /ʃ/

contexts is ideally appropriate because the /ʃ/ is not one of an abutting pair.

The *lock-fish* context could be excellent with its inclusion of the /k/ error phone and the inclusion of frication with both /f/ and /ʃ/. The vowel "r" phone could also be targeted but generally the VV-CVC context can be included later when the patient is more familiar with the technology involved.

The first choice for initiation of treatment was the /s/ target phone in the correct context *duck-sun*. The second choice was /k/ in the correct context *lock-fish*. Because correct production of the plosive would be firmly established in the *duck-sun* context, generalization would be rapid. The /tʃ/ target phone in *ball-chain* was the third phone to be included in our now budding multiphonetic approach. Targeting /tʃ/ would stress affrication and midpalatal place of production. The "r" phones would be incorporated next.

Additional Assessment and Interpretation

1. *Complete a distinctive-feature interpretation* of the error phones. Analyze the patient's error phones based on Blache's distinctive-feature analysis (see chapter 14), which emphasizes place and manner aspects of *production*. List phones in error and, as discussed by Blache, outline the "developmental sequencing for feature selection" and the "natural training order" of phones. This procedure takes into account an "optimal remedial order" of error phones based on perception and production of distinctive features (see Blache's section on "Review of Clinical Procedure"). Following this procedure, distinctive-feature principles can be integrated with principles of the sensory-motor approach and a strategy for remediation developed. Additionally, *verbal feedback* of the correctness and incorrectness of each response made by a patient can emphasize parameters of distinctive-feature production and enhance the patient's awareness of correct sound production.

2. *Complete a phonemic inventory* that includes "only those sounds that are used contrastively, or those sounds that signal meaning" (Elbert and Gierut, 1986, p. 53). Analyze the patient's *phonological process patterns* and identify the error phones that account for the significant proportion of the phonological process patterns used. This allows for selection of target phones that will eliminate significant process patterns while integrating sensory-motor and distinctive-feature principles as part of the selection process.

Management of Antecedent and Consequent Stimuli

It is strongly recommended that a strict stimulus-response-stimulus (S—R—S) paradigm be incorporated with the initiation of remedial procedures (see chapter 6).

In following strict procedures, the speech-language pathologist provides one stimulus and expects one response. If no response (NR) is given, NR is noted on the score sheet and a new stimulus given. Multiple stimulations for a single response should be avoided. Often such procedures train the patient to respond only after multiple stimulations. If the frequency of NRs is significant, the appropriateness of the antecedent stimuli as well as probable reasons for a lack of response are evaluated and necessary changes made.

In the S—R—S paradigm, the antecedent stimulus is considered more important than the consequent stimulus. One cannot administer a consequent stimulus without a correct or incorrect response that is evoked by the antecedent stimulus, which is thus considered to be the more important stimulus. In treatment, the first task of the clinician is to identify a "discriminative" antecedent stimulus (S^D), one that *consistently evokes the desired response*.

Consequent stimuli are of two types: (1) token reinforcement and (2) verbal feedback. Token reinforcement is not limited to "chips" but rather includes tally marks such as X, /, or 0 or any other visible notation system. Verbal feedback, which *specifically describes the correctness or incorrectness* of each response, is the *most important consequent event*. Often inappropriately referred to as verbal "reinforcement," verbal feedback provides the patient with information that theoretically facilitates metalinguistic knowledge and results in articulatory preprogramming changes. The primary purpose of tokens or the token reinforcement system is to motivate the patient to continue to strive for success.

Passing and Failure Criteria

The following criteria are suggested for use throughout the training procedures. Passing criterion is 20 consecutive correct responses at one step. Failure criteria is twofold: 10 consecutive incorrect responses at one step (failure to reach passing criteria) or less than 80% accuracy at one step for two successive sessions.

AWARENESS PHASE

Orientation to Speech Helpers

Terminal Objective. The patient will be able to spontaneously name or otherwise identify 8 of 10 speech helpers following imitative articulation of a variety of phones, speech movements, or other vocal behaviors. The speech helpers include the lips, teeth, tongue, gum ridge, alveolar ridge, hard palate, soft palate, voicebox/larynx, nose, ears, and expired breath stream. This procedure generally takes no more than 30 to 40 minutes.

The identification of speech helpers is *optional*. It is necessary to determine the value of this procedure based on the needs of the patient. Clinical experience suggests that, typically, children with multiple misarticulations (7 to 10 error phones) benefit from the orientation procedures. This orientation phase can be completed within one and rarely more than two 20- to 30-minute sessions,

Identification of Speech Helpers. The procedures for identifying speech helpers are as follows.

1. Permit the patient to "discover" his own speech helpers during production of speech movements or other vocal behaviors. Awareness of speech helpers can be enhanced by expecting self-discovery following minimal cueing. Cues may include lips touching while saying *mama*, the breath stream moving a small strip of paper during production of /p/, tactile stimulation on the back of the hand during production of /p/, or pinching the nostrils closed during production of /m/. Awareness is indicated by having the patient point directly to his own speech helper or by self-identification in a mirror or on a line drawing or other illustration of the speaking mechanism. Routine use of the mirror may not be beneficial or it may cause confusion. If the patient continues to have difficulty in spontaneous discovery of some of the speech helpers, use additional self-generated stimulus procedures, such as placing a narrow strip of paper between the patient's lips during production of bilabials. The paper heightens awareness of the use of the lips in the production of speech.

2. A stimulating procedure developed by Taylor & Shine (1978) involved use of a *shadow-gram profile*. Using a bright light, reflect a shadow of the patient's profile on a poster board or paper and trace an outline. Draw in sagittal representation of speech helpers (tongue, teeth, soft palate, etc.) for the patient to identify. The drawing has personal significance and theoretically is stimulating and rewarding for the patient. The drawing can be sent home with instructions for the patient to identify and explain the use of speech helpers to family members.

3. After speech helpers have been identified, review those initially not known to determine the patient's awareness. Individuals who continue to experience difficulties in spontaneous identification, especially of the lips, tongue, teeth, breath stream, nose, and "voice box," may be excellent

candidates for heightening awareness training. Initiate training at the "establishment phase" for patients with good awareness skills and minimal articulatory deviancies.

Heightening Awareness of Auditory, Tactile, and Proprioceptive/Kinesthetic Sensations Associated with Correct Articulatory Movements

Terminal Objective. The patient will be able to correctly imitate the production of those consonants within his phonetic inventory in CVCV bisyllable and disyllable contexts, CVCVCV trisyllable contexts, and VCCV abutting consonant contexts in variable stress patterns. Additionally, the patient may be instructed to identify verbally or by pointing or self-touch the articulatory contacts that were made during production of selected consonants. Passing criterion is 20 consecutive correct responses for each context or level of production.

The heightening awareness procedure is *optional* and generally recommended for individuals with multiple misarticulations; these may be patients with 7 or more error phones, a severe articulatory deviancy, or poor intelligibility. The procedure may also be of benefit to individuals exhibiting minimal motor speech involvement and may be used in conjunction with the speech motor training program for apraxia of speech developed by Logue (1976a, 1976b, 1978). The clinician is referred to McDonald (1964a, pp. 138–142) and McDonald (in press) for an additional explanation of heightening awareness training. The *primary objective,* as stated by McDonald (1964a), is to heighten the patient's awareness of *patterns* of auditory, tactile, and proprioceptive/kinesthetic sensations associated with correct coarticulatory movements. All phones in the phonetic inventory are used, specifically those phones produced correctly spontaneously or with stimulation in at least a CV or VC context. The procedures progress from production requiring minimal coarticulatory skills in which a single correctly articulated consonant and a variety of vowels are produced in a bisyllable context (/bibi/) to bisyllable contexts combining all correct consonants with vowels to form bisyllables (/fɑfi/), to disyllables (/hubeɪ/), trisyllables (/mɑlijæ/), and consonant abutting pairs (/ɪfdu/). The patient is additionally required to produce varied stress patterns by imitating the speech-language pathologist's primary stress pattern on the first or second syllable with bisyllables and on the first, second, or third syllables with trisyllables. Following correct imitation the patient may also be required to tell (a) which articulators touched and/or where they touched and (b) the direction of movement of the articulators, front to back, back to front, back–front–back. Finally, maximum coarticulatory complexity is required by having the patient imitate production of abutting contexts.

An Example. The heightening awareness procedures allow assessment of the patient's auditory and tactile discrimination abilities as well as prosodic and coarticulatory skills within a "diagnostic teaching" format. The patient's ability to respond appropriately within the clinical setting to antecedent and consequent stimuli will also be determined. The general success criteria of 20 consecutively correct responses at each step may be reduced to 10 responses for patients with excellent skills.

Information from the evaluation phase (see Figure 13.2) revealed that patient JJ can produce the consonants [p, b, t, d, ʌ, f, v, θ, ð, h, w, j, l, m, n, ŋ] and all vowels with the exception of "r" vowels. The phonetic inventory includes 16 phones that are "mastered" or produced correctly more frequently than incorrectly. Error phones produced correctly by this patient included [s, r, ɹ, ɚ, tʃ, ʃ, k, g]. Correctly produced error phones are rarely used as stimulus consonants in the heightening awareness procedures. Phones for which no correct productions were noted included [z, ɹ̥, ɝ], other vowel "r" phones, [dʒ], and [ʒ].

Step 1. Combine one correctly articulated consonant with a representative sampling of vowels to form *bisyllables*. In our example, the bilabial /b/ phone is selected. Model the production of each bisyllable with near equal stress on each syllable. Move from maximally (approximately 10 responses) to minimally (approximately 10 responses) contrasted coarticulatory movement patterns *between* bisyllable presentations.

The first stimulus presentation, /bibi/, is repeated by the patient. The correctness of the consonant and vowel production is evaluated by the speech-language pathologist, and verbal feedback, specifically but briefly explaining the correctness or incorrectness of production, is provided to the patient. *The second stimulus* presentation, /bɑbɑ/, is managed in an identical fashion. In our example a high front vowel /i/ and a low back vowel /ɑ/ were coarticulated with /b/ in successive imitative productions by the patient (see Figure 13.3). The vowel stimuli were selected to provide "maximally" different coarticulatory movement patterns *between* succeeding stimuli (S1 and S2, S2 and S3, etc.). The task is to maximally contrast movement patterns *between* syllable productions and to gradually incorporate minimal contrasts.

Steps 2 through 8. Combine all correct consonants with all vowels to form bisyllables or disyllables in which the phones provide a wide variety of places and manners of production. The objective is to emphasize the patient's production of highly variable coarticulatory patterns.

Step 2. Vary both consonants and vowels from maximally to minimally contrasted coarticulatory movement patterns *between bisyllable* presentations (see Figure 13.3). The maximally contrasted presentations provide greater differences in coarticulatory movement patterns between succeeding stimuli than minimally contrasted presentations. Experience has demonstrated that individuals having difficulties in vowel discrimination or general sound discrimination have progressively more difficulty with correct imitation as contrasts become more minimal (see Figure 13.3). The patient's successful progression from maximum to minimum contrasts can be enchanced if the change is gradual.

FIGURE 13.3
Suggested syllable presentations for JJ during Steps 1 through 4 of the heightening awareness phase. The vowel diagram and place/manner chart, on which the patient's phonetic inventory is coded, are viewed during development of the syllable stimuli. Once the process is understood, little or no preparation time is needed to use this procedure.

Maximal Contrast	Minimal Contrast
Step 1. Between Bisyllable Presentations	
1. bibi	11. bibi
2. bɑbɑ	12. bɪbɪ
3. beɪbeɪ	13. beɪbeɪ
4. bubu	14. bɛbɛ
5. bæbæ	15. bæbæ
. . . .	. . .
. . .	. . .
. . .	. . .
10. boʊboʊ	20. bubu
Step 2. Between Bisyllable Presentations	
Step 3. Randomly stressed first or second syllable	
1. bibi	11. bibi
2. haha	12. weɪweɪ
3. teɪteɪ	13. pɪpɪ
4. juju	14. fɛfɛ
5. wæwæ	15. vævæ
. . .	. . .
. . .	. . .
. . .	. . .
10. fɪfɪ	20. hoʊhoʊ
Step 4. Within Disyllable Presentations	
1. piha	11. bipɪ
2. joʊteɪ	12. weɪmɛ
3. wihu	13. fævʌ
4. loʊvæ	14. pɑtoʊ
5. nɛwu	15. joʊlʊ
. . .	. . .
. . .	. . .
. . .	. . .
10. tæmu	20. pitɪ

Step 3. Continue the progression from maximal to minimal contrast of *bisyllables*. However, in this step randomly stress the first or second syllable. The patient must imitate the identical stress for a correct response (see Figure 13.3). This procedure recognizes that English is a stress language and stress skills are necessary for effective communication.

Step 4. Vary consonants and vowels to provide maximally to minimally contrasted coarticulatory movement patterns *within disyllables*, randomly stressing first or second syllables. In this procedure one can present a front consonant and vowel in the first syllable followed by a back consonant and vowel in the second syllable, systematically changing from maximal to minimal contrasts (see

Figure 13.3). In a correct response the patient is required to produce correctly the four phones as well as the modeled syllable stress pattern. Again, the procedure can provide excellent diagnostic teaching data pertinent to the patient's coarticulatory, imitative, and discriminatory abilities.

Steps 5 and 6. After the client correctly imitates each production of a *bisyllable* in Step 5 (*disyllables* in Step 6), ask him to identify which speech helpers touched. For example, the clinician says /bibi/; the patient repeats the context and if evaluated as correct, then states, "My lips touched or came together." If imitated incorrectly, a new stimulus item is presented. In the disyllable /tɑpeɪ/, the patient would state, "My tongue touched behind my teeth on top and then my lips touched" (or something similar). A patient's success in developing awareness of which speech helpers touched based on auditory, tactile, and proprioceptive/kinesthetic sensations can be beneficial to the remedial process.

Steps 7 and 8. Use *disyllables* in Steps 7 and 8. Ask the patient to identify the direction of movement of the articulators, front to back, back to front, or other appropriate statements depending on the context produced. In this procedure the patient repeats the modeled stimulus context /fɪdoʊ/ and then states, "My lips touched in front and then my tongue touched behind my teeth—front toward the back."

Steps 9, 10, and 11. Introduce *trisyllables* in Step 9. Present contexts with a variety of stress patterns. In the modeled context /pulɑbi/, the patient is required to correctly imitate all consonants and vowels while producing the primary stress on the second syllable. In step 10 ask the client to identify the speech helpers that are touched with trisyllables, naming them in the correct sequence. In Step 11 ask the client to indicate the general direction of movement involved in producing the trisyllable.

Steps 12 and 13. Introduce *abutting consonant pairs*, such as: /ibdɑ/, /vinpɑ/, /oʊfli/, etc. Present

maximum coarticulatory movement pattern contrasts in Step 12 and minimal contrasts in Step 13. Ask the patient to repeat what he hears.

The minimum number of responses in the 13 steps would be 260. However, if the patient experiences significant difficulty with some steps, time has to be weighed against the value that could be obtained from the procedures. Pre- and posttesting following heightening awareness training procedures have revealed progress in the correct production of a patient's error phones even though training involved only correct phones. Results suggest that heightening awareness to the sensations associated with correct production can bring about progress with error sounds not practiced.

Patients whose problems dictated inclusion of heightening awareness training can now progress to the establishment phase.

ESTABLISHMENT PHASE

Reinforcing Correct Articulation of the Error Phone

Terminal Objective. The patient will be able to correctly articulate the target phones of each error phone either prevocalically or postvocalically in an abutting bisyllable correct context (CVC-CVC). Success criterion is 20 consecutively correct responses in short phrases and sentences following auditory modeling, prompting, or visual stimulation.

Outline of the Establishment Phase

During the evaluation phase the target phone /s/ and the correct context *duck-sun* were selected for the initiation of treatment. Only the correct context *duck-sun* is used in the seven steps of the establishment phase. Potentially the correct context will be repeated 140 times in a variety of contexts and prosodic speaking patterns. These include patterns characteristically found in conversational speech. For example, the correct context is produced with near-equal stress, at a slow rate, with a prolongation of the target phone when appropriate, stressing the syllable containing the target and then not containing the target and, in short sentences, with a variety of natural prosodic patterns.

Stimulus Procedures

In the initiation of treatment, a picture of a duck and the sun should be presented. Artistic and creative clinicians may draw or create an imaginary picture of the sun that includes features of a duck. It can then be labeled a *duck-sun*. A duck-sun is bright and shiny, and it flies in the sky and makes us warm (creative semanticity). The sensory-motor approach has been criticized because stimulus items are nonlexical. However, clinical experience reveals that during the establishment phase stimulus items such as *duck-sun* do not have to be used in a nonlexical manner. They can be used as nouns during bisyllable productions and particularly during sentence construction. Note that the following sentences are grammatically correct and they can be used in a linguistically meaningful manner by preschool through young school-age children: *I have a duck-sun. The duck-sun is warm. Duck-sun is a funny word.*

Step 1. Produce *duck-sun* with near equal stress and firm coarticulation without a pause between the syllables. Have the patient imitate. Remember that *duck-sun* is a correct context and as such the patient will not improve knowledge or skills unless specific verbal *feedback* is provided. A phonological process contrastive procedure could be included as Step 1a, as follows: Contrast a creative drawing of *duck-sun* with one of *duck-thun* if the patient exhibited an interdental lisp. Use contrastive procedures as outlined in chapter 7 and during production take advantage of place and manner parameters and other production parameters to teach the patient.

Step 2. Produce the correct context at a slow rate to provide extended duration of tactile, auditory, and proprioceptive/kinesthetic feedback. During the child's production, call attention to the articulators that are touching or identify acoustic features involving manner of production. Teach the patient as much as possible about correct production.

Step 3. Produce the correct context, prolonging the target phone, as in *duck-sssssssun*. The clinician models the appropriate production, holding an index finger up or covering the "un" with a card for readers during the entire duration of the /s/ and dropping the finger down or suddenly uncovering the rest of the word "un" to complete the bisyllable. While the patient is prolonging the production of the target phone, the clinician provides continuous verbal feedback pertinent to auditory, tactile, or other parameters that will result in cognitive awareness. This procedure is used only with continuant phones or phones that can be prolonged, such as the fricative aspect of an affricate.

Steps 4 and 5. Model the correct context, first stressing the syllable containing the target phone to obtain 20 consecutively correct responses, and then repeat the procedure stressing the syllable not containing the target phone. The rationale for this step is to use stress to influence a variety of allophonic productions of the target phone in order to facilitate generalization to conversational speech. Stress is a major factor in effective communication and as such is introduced early in the training sequence.

Steps 6 and 7. Model the production of the correct context in phrases and short sentences for the patient to imitate. Include sentences like the following: "I have a *(duck) (sun)*. I want my *(duck)* (sun). *(Duck) (sun)* can go. The *(duck) (sun)* will shine." In the construction of sentences, use only phones that are part of the patient's phonetic inventory to the degree that it is feasible.

During Step 7, contrastive stress patterns can be introduced and the patient can engage in composing sentences using the correct context. Model a sentence such as "I have a duck-sun." As explained by McDonald (1964a), have the patient repeat the sentence. If production is *incorrect* provide appropriate verbal feedback and model a new sentence. If production is *correct* then ask, "Do you have a duck-moon?" The patient should reply, "No, I have a duck-SUN," providing appropriate contrastive stress on the word *sun*. The word "I" can be changed to "we," resulting in stress of "I." Additionally, *have* can be changed to *want* and *duck* can be changed to *dog*. This can be a creative procedure requiring behavior that results in spontaneous generalization to conversation.

The completion of the establishment phase results in stabilization of production of the target phone within one context but, importantly, in a variety of rate, stress, and intonation patterns that are characteristically present in spontaneous conversational speech. It is important to recognize that the sensory-motor rationale specifies beginning with error phones for which correct productions have been identified, thus beginning at the patient's level of functioning, and progressing to higher levels of complexity. Note that requiring 20 consecutively correct responses at each of the seven steps described would result in a minimal total of 140 responses (rarely more than 200 responses), which ideally can be completed within a 20- to 30-minute session (7 responses to 5 responses per minute). The overall time will depend on the skills and accuracy of both the patient and the speech-language pathologist and certainly the cooperative nature of the patient.

Introduction of Multiphonemic/Phonetic Principles

Upon completion of the establishment phase for one target phone, the principles of the multiphonemic/phonetic approach (McCabe & Bradley, 1973, 1975; chapter 11 of this text) are incorporated. A new target is selected. A part of the next session is devoted to intratherapy generalization for the /s/ target phone and a part is devoted to stabilization of a new target phone and correct context within the establishment phase. At this point,

principles of distinctive features and/or phonological processes are used to select a new target phone. In principle, efforts will be made to select a new target that is acoustically and/or physiologically dissimilar to the initial target phone (/s/ in our example). Generalization is expected for similar phones. Additionally, *phonological process patterns* are examined to determine if simplification patterns are present that might appear more important to remediation than the distinctive-feature principles. For example, a patient might exhibit a significant postvocalic deletion pattern (open syllable pattern) that could take precedence over selection principles involving distinctive features. The ideal situation would be one in which the correct context production approach, distinctive features, and phonological process patterns would all point to the selection of a single consonant phone out of two or three possible phones. As the establishment phase is completed for each target phone, that phone is moved to the generalization phase and a new target phone is selected for establishment. Eventually a session might incorporate training with four, five, or even more target phones. A comprehensive approach will evolve if multiple target phones are selected on the basis of distinctive-feature and phonological process principles and incorporated as part of the sensory-motor production approach.

GENERALIZATION PHASE

Terminal Objective. The patient will be able to correctly articulate the target phone in a wide variety of bisyllable contexts progressing to spontaneous production in connected speech in response to visual, auditory, and conversational interactive stimulation. Success criterion is 20 consecutive correct responses in structured communicative interaction and at least 80% accuracy in conversational speech.

The primary objective of the intratherapy generalization phase is to facilitate, within therapy, generalization of the correct articulation of the target phone to a wide variety of, but systematically varied, contexts. The sensory-motor approach stresses the importance of production training of *allophones* of each designated target phone. In the example, the correct context *duck-sun* is identified as a *facilitating context,* facilitating correct production of the /s/ phone. The target phone /s/ *functions* prevocalicly in the syllable movement pattern, at the syllable juncture of the bisyllable abutted by the postvocalic *functioning* /k/ phone. The facilitating context is modified to structure systematic minimal changes in the movement patterns from one stimulus context to the next. The objective is to enhance the maintenance of correct production by requiring minimal variation of the coarticulatory movement patterns from one context to the next. As contexts are manipulated, the patient obtains practice and develops awareness of correct allophonic production. The variety of coarticulatory patterns demanded tends to *facilitate automatic generalization to natural conversational coarticulatory patterns*. In many instances transfer to real-life situations is automatic, particularly when principles of distinctive-feature (place/manner) and phonological process approaches (semanticity) are acknowledged and taught.

Training involves a series of steps in which the contexts are expanded and varied with the target phone functioning either prevocalicly or postvocalicly. In our example the /s/ functions prevocalicly in the CVC context *sun*. Once generalization is complete prevocalicly, similar steps are followed to generalize the /s/ within a postvocalic context. Once intratherapy generalization with a prevocalic phone is complete, facilitation and typically generalization of the postvocalic phone occurs rapidly and at times automatically. Clinical experience has revealed that redundant practice of the prevocalic function does not lead to interference in learning the postvocalic function. It is postulated that this is because natural coarticulatory production is emphasized and practiced in the sensory-motor approach. Possibly coarticulatory complexity at the syllable juncture (sometimes referred to as word-medial, Wolfe, Blocker, & Prater, 1988) results in the development of skills that facilitate rather than hinder generalization. If a correct context for the postvocalic phone was not

identified during the initial assessment, the DTA:PF (McDonald, 1964b) is readministered to identify the postvocalic target phone. If the percentage of accuracy of the postvocalic phone is 50% or greater, production training may not be necessary. Therapy time can then be devoted to other target phones.

Outline of the Generalization Phase

To facilitate correct articulation of the target phone in systematically varied contexts, training is initiated with the correct context used during the establishment phase (*duck-sun* in our example). There are five levels of training. In each of the first four levels there are two training steps. Contexts are *systematically* varied in the first step and *randomly* varied in the second step. At level one and level two (Steps 1 through 4), the abutting consonants of the correct context are maintained. In level one, the vowel and consonant in the syllable not containing the target are varied systematically in Step 1, then randomly in Step 2. In level two, the vowel and consonant in the syllable containing the target are varied systematically (Step 3) and then randomly (Step 4). In level three the consonant abutting the target phone is modified systematically in Step 5 then randomly in Step 6. Finally, in level four, all of the modified contexts are produced in sentences, following a model in Step 7 and spontaneously generated in Step 8. Level 5 has three steps. The first step is optional as it incorporates contexts from homework assignments that may or may not be available. The two additional steps incorporate practice with variable rate and stress patterns in sentences to facilitate generalization to connected spontaneous speech.

The vowel diagram (Figure 13.4) and the place/manner chart (Figure 13.2) are used to develop contexts. In the systematic variation of contexts, vowels and consonants are selected on the basis of similarity to those being replaced. In the context ['dʌk·sʌn], the ['dʌ] in *duck* could be replaced by

FIGURE 13.4

Variation of vowels (using vowel diagram) and consonants (using place/manner chart in Figure 13.2) for Steps 1, 2, 3, of Generalization Phase.

a. Systematic variation of consonant and vowel in syllable not containing target.

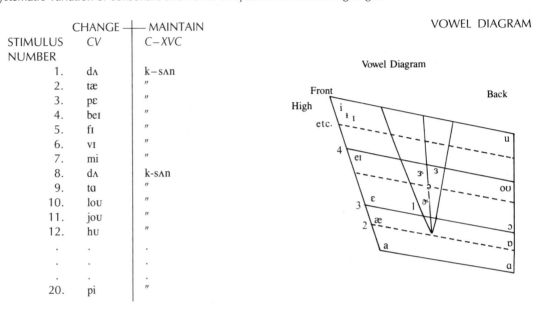

STIMULUS NUMBER	CHANGE CV	MAINTAIN C–XVC
1.	dʌ	k–sʌn
2.	tæ	"
3.	pɛ	"
4.	beɪ	"
5.	fɪ	"
6.	vɪ	"
7.	mi	"
8.	dʌ	k–sʌn
9.	tɑ	"
10.	loʊ	"
11.	joʊ	"
12.	hʊ	"
.	.	.
.	.	.
.	.	.
20.	pi	"

Note the attempt to provide minimal change in tongue hump height and the coarticulatory pattern with vowels. Consonants are also shifted minimally as is feasible.

b. Random variation of consonant and vowel in syllable not containing target.

STIMULUS NUMBER	CHANGE CV	MAINTAIN C–XVC
1.	dʌ	k–sʌn
2.	mi	"
3.	tæ	"
4.	loʊ	"
5.	beɪ	"
6.	dæ	"
7.	tæ	"
8.	fɪ	k–sʌn
9.	bɛ	"
10.	doʊ	"
11.	ju	"
.	.	.
.	.	.
.	.	.
20.	fɪ	"

Note maximal changes between stimulus presentations.

FIGURE 13.4 (continued)

c. Systematic variation of consonant and vowel in syllable containing target.

MAINTAIN	CHANGE	
CV C-X-	VC	
1. dʌk-s	ʌn	
2. "	ad	
3. "	oʊp	
4. "	um	
5. "	up	
6. "	oʊf	
7. "	ɑŋ	
8. dʌk-s	ʌn	
9. "	ʌm	
10. "	æm	
11. "	æl	
12. "	ɛt	
13. "	eɪv	
14. "	ɪf	
15. "	ɪp	
. .	.	
. .	.	
. .	.	
20. "	æb	

VOWEL DIAGRAM

Vowel Diagram

[A vowel diagram showing Front/Back, High, with positions i, ɪ, eɪ, ɛ, æ, a, ɝ, ə, ɚ, u, oʊ, ɔ, ɒ, ɑ; numbers 2, 3, 4 and "etc." labeled]

[tʰæ] or [tʰɑ] recognizing that the vowels [æ-ʌ-ɑ] all have low tongue hump height (front, mid, back) and that the consonant cognates [t] and [d] differ only in voicing. The *principle* is to vary the context but to do so knowledgeably with respect for coarticulatory demands. Minimal distinctive-feature place and manner variation generally demands minimal changes in coarticulatory movement patterns from stimulus to stimulus. Random place and manner variation may demand maximal coarticulatory changes in movement patterns from stimulus to stimulus and thus random contexts are introduced only after stabilization of a wide variety of minimally varied patterns. The planned systematic variation enhances continuous accuracy of production and, in many instances, enables the speech-language pathologist to identify and modify contexts that evoke incorrect production of the target phone and then gradually and systematically incorporate contexts that are more complex relative to the uniqueness of each pa-

tient's system. *Word lists* and other procedures that order contexts randomly can potentially evoke misarticulations. The speech-language pathologist often attributes the misarticulation to a patient's lack of motivation or carelessness rather than to the complexity or uniqueness of the coarticulatory contexts being produced. Thus, the selection of stimulus contexts is vitally important in procedures requiring correct production but emphasizing distinctive features or phonological processes as the main remedial strategy. Incorporating principles of context selection in other approaches could potentially increase their effectiveness.

Stimulus Procedures

There are potentially 22 steps in the intratherapy generalization phase: 11 steps for the prevocalic function and 11 steps for the postvocalic function of each target phone. Correctness of production at each step is facilitated by structuring minimal shifts in vowel and consonant change and using only correctly articulated consonants. The objective is to require minimal coarticulatory change from stimulus to stimulus. Additionally the discrimination/perceptual abilities of the patient are sampled by meaningless items like /tæk·soun/. However, clinical experience demonstrates that nonlexical word pairs become meaningful in sentences, and a minimal-pairs contrastive procedure can also interject meaning. The inclusion of nonlexical items facilitates being able to systematically vary coarticulatory production demand and avoids random context presentations that may result in misarticulations. Additionally, nonlexical items avoid the negative stimulus value sometimes associated with known words that evoke habitual simplification patterns or compensatory misarticulation patterns.

Step 1. The correct context is *duck-sun* [ˈdʌk·sʌn] and the target phone is /s/. Systematically vary the consonant and vowel in the syllable not containing the target. Use the vowel diagram (Figure 13.4) and place/manner chart (Figure 13.2) to develop word pairs involving minimal shifts of movement (Figure 13.4a). The /dʌ/ prevocalic consonant and the vowel in *duck* are systematically changed and the abutting /k/ consonant and second syllable containing the target /sʌn/ are maintained. Changing the C and V in the syllable not containing the target and maintaining the abutting consonant /k/ theoretically results in minimal but possibly important allophonic change of the target and abutting phone at the syllable juncture. Correctness of the target is maintained in a variety of different coarticulatory patterns.

Step 2. Randomly vary the consonant and the vowel within the syllable not containing the target as shown in Figure 13.4b. In this procedure stimuli from Step 1 are randomly selected. Upon completing this step or when appropriate, introduce a homework assignment (see Figure 13.5).

Step 3. Systematically vary the consonant and the vowel in the syllable containing the target as shown in Figure 13.4c. The /ʌn/ in *sun* is systematically changed to develop word pairs involving minimal shifts of movement. The allophonic variation is theoretically more significant than in Steps 1 and 2 because of the adjacency of the vowel to the target phone.

Step 4. Randomly vary the consonant and vowel in the syllable containing the target. Introduce a homework assignment (Figure 13.5). Generally the patient will complete Steps 1 through 4 during one session and thus two homework assignments may be given.

Step 5. Randomly vary the consonant and vowel in both syllables (randomly select contexts from Step 1 and Step 3).

Step 6. Systematically vary the consonant abutting the target to develop word pairs with minimal shifts of movement (see Figures 13.2 and 13.6).

Step 7. Randomly vary the consonant abutting the target to develop word pairs. Stress patterns may also be varied (use contexts from Step 6).

Step 8. Randomly modify contexts from Steps 1 through 7 to develop variable word pairs. The patient may enjoy spontaneously developing his own word pairs.

Step 9. This is an optional step involving homework completed by the patient. Using the patient's homework lists, present items for imitation or allow the patient to spontaneously produce items. The clinician may need to screen items to avoid contexts containing error phones.

Step 10. Develop sentences using any and all contexts practiced as well as many not practiced in Steps 1 through 9. Introduce meaningful lexical contexts similar to those presented in Figure 13.3. The patient may enjoy developing his own meaningful contexts. Practice contrastive stress as a major requirement of this step. See Step 7 of the Establishment Phase for examples of contrastive stress procedures that function to introduce vari-

FIGURE 13.5
Homework Program (HP).

The four procedures outlined below are designed to involve the client in developing clinical materials. Worksheets are to be completed at home with the help of significant others when desirable or necessary.

Obtain parent help if necessary.

1   Instruct the client to develop a list of 10 to 20 words with the consonant abutting the target. Place worksheet 1 in notebook.

X = /s/ as a prevocalic phone   X = /s/ as a postvocalic phone
CC = cat sun   CC = bus tie

_____ t   t _____
_____ t   t _____
_____ t   t _____
_____ t   sun   bus   t _____
_____ t   t _____
_____ t   t _____
_____ t   t _____

              s _____   _____ s
              s _____   _____ s
    cat   s _____   _____ s   tie
              s _____   _____ s
              s _____   _____ s

2   Instruct the client to develop additional lists of words in which abutting consonants are maintained. Place worksheet 2 in notebook.

X = /s/, CC = cat-sun   X = /s/, CC = bus-tie

_____ t s _____   _____ s t _____
_____ t s _____   _____ s t _____
_____ t s _____   _____ s t _____
_____ t s _____   _____ s t _____
_____ t s _____   _____ s t _____
_____ t s _____   _____ s t _____
_____ t s _____   _____ s t _____

3   Instruct the client to develop a list of words in which the target is maintained but abutting phone is randomly varied. Same contexts as in 2 above.

_____   s _____   _____ s   _____
_____   s _____   _____ s   _____
_____   s _____   _____ s   _____
_____   s _____   _____ s   _____
_____   s _____   _____ s   _____
_____   s _____   _____ s   _____

4   Instruct patient to develop 10 to 20 sentences using word pairs developed in 1 through 3.

	MAINTAIN	CHANGE	MAINTAIN
Stimulus Number	CV	C	XVC
1.	dʌ	k	sʌn
2.	"	g	"
3.	"	d	"
4.	"	n	"
5.	"	t	"
6.	"	p	"
7.	"	b	"
8.	dʌ	m	sʌn
9.	"	f	"
10.	"	v	"
11.	"	θ	"
12.	"	l	"
13.	"	n	"
14.	"	m	"
.		.	.
.		.	.
.		.	.
20.	"	p	"

FIGURE 13.6
Systematic variation of consonants abutting the target.

able coarticulatory production practice and to facilitate generalization to natural spontaneous connected speech.

Step 11. Assist or instruct the patient to compose sentences using modified contexts previously practiced (Steps 1 through 10) and use each word pair in a sentence. Stress development of meaningful lexical word pairs.

Upon completing Step 11 with the prevocalic consonant (*duck-sun* in our example), complete the assessment procedures necessary to identify a correct context for the postvocalic /s/ phone (*house-cup* could logically be correct). Readminister the contexts that assess the postvocalic /s/ in the Deep Test of Articulation: Picture Form or Sentence Form (McDonald, 1964b, 1964c) to identify correct contexts and particularly to assess the percentage of accuracy to determine if training procedures are necessary.

By the time the generalization phase for a particular target phone is complete, two, three, four or even more phones may have been introduced and may be at various levels within the approach. The time of the clinical session will thus be divided into three or four sections allowing work on each of the different target phones. The multiple target phones and the incorporation of principles from various approaches will result in overall improvement in the patient's intelligibility and create generalization to error phones not practiced as well as facilitate generalization to conversation speech (the true target of treatment).

Intratherapy generalization can be expanded to include reading materials, stories, action or sequence pictures, and conversation. Each of these stimulus conditions can be used as probes to determine the necessity of continuing to target any one phone. If the patient achieves at least 80% accuracy in spontaneous connected speech that is truly communicative in nature, additional treatment is probably unnecessary.

TRANSFER PHASE

Terminal Objective. The patient will be able to correctly articulate the pre- and postvocalic target phones during spontaneous conversation with at least 80% to 90% accuracy in a wide variety of environments and speaking conditions or situations. Using paper and pencil or hand counters, the clinician and the patient when appropriate will independently collect and chart data on the accuracy of production of target phones.

The primary objective of this extratherapy generalization phase is to determine the patient's accuracy of target phone production by means of observation or tape recordings in a wide variety of everyday speaking situations. In the schools the speech-language pathologist can talk with the child in the hallway, the back of the classroom, library, cafeteria, the playground, or any other feasible environments.

MAINTENANCE PHASE

With individuals who have been discharged from regularly scheduled treatment sessions, periodic stability checks can be an excellent reminder. A probable schedule could include conversational sampling of 2 to 5 minutes of ''talking time'' (actual time client is engaged in conversing) initially once per week for one month, then twice per month for two months, and finally once per month for two or three months. Of course, after the first three or four stability checks, the client may exhibit sufficient progress to be terminated permanently.

SUMMARY

The sensory-motor approach emphasizes sound production training based on the principles of coarticulation. It is suggested that this approach be used in conjunction with other linguistically based methods such as phonological process and distinctive-feature approaches in order to facilitate acquisition of the sound system as well as correct production of phones. At the same time, it is important for the clinician to clearly distinguish between linguistic and articulatory concepts in determining treatment procedures.

The syllable is considered to be the primary unit of production, but the bisyllable is the smallest unit recommended for training. Production training for the target phone involves systematically shaping the correct coarticulation of selected contexts in progressively more complex language. Natural prosodic patterns are stressed.

This sensory-motor approach includes six phases: evaluation, awareness, establishment, intratherapy generalization, transfer/extratherapy generalization, and maintenance. A comprehensive *evaluation* is required, drawing from traditional and linguistically based procedures. Selection of target phones and appropriate contexts is based on in-depth analysis of correct and incorrect productions. The *awareness* phase is optional, to be used primarily with children who exhibit multiple misarticulations. If needed, it can include orientation to ''speech helpers'' and heightening awareness of sensations associated with correct articulatory movements in progressively complex contexts. In the *establishment* phase, the target phone is produced in an already identified correct phonetic context throughout seven steps that serve to firmly establish the correct production in this context. At the end of this phase, a new target is selected that will be established while the first phone is being generalized to new contexts. The *generalization* phase is characterized by systematic and then random variation of contexts in which the target is produced. The varying phonetic contexts must be carefully designed to assure continued correct production as new contexts are introduced. When generalization within therapy is achieved, data regarding *transfer* to natural communication outside of therapy is collected by both clinician and client. Periodic stability checks are suggested to assure *maintenance*.

REFERENCES

Avery, E., Dorsey, J., & Sickels, V. A. (1928). *First principles of speech training.* New York: Appleton-Century.

Blaustein, S. (1973). *Generalization across phones as a result of programmed sensory-motor articulation therapy.* Unpublished master's thesis, Pennsylvania State University, University Park, PA.

Elbert, M., & Gierut, J. (1986). *Handbook of phonology: Approaches to assessment and treatment.* San Diego: College Hill Press.

Fudala, J. (1974). *Arizona articulation proficiency scale, revised manual.* Los Angeles: Western Psychological Services.

Johnson, W., Darley, F. L., & Spriestersbach, D. C. (1963). *Diagnostic methods in speech pathology.* New York: Harper & Row.

Kelso, J. A. S., & Munhall, K. G. (1988). *Motor phonetics: Stetson reassessed.* Boston: College Hill Press.

Logue, R. D. (1976a). *Motor-speech disorder in children.* Short course, ASHA Convention, Houston.

Logue, R. D. (1976b). *Monitoring articulatory postures (MAP): A speech motor training program.* Greenville, NC: East Carolina University.

Logue, R. D. (1978). Disorders of motor-speech planning in children: Evaluation and treatment. In L. J. Bradford (Ed.), *Communication disorders: An audio journal for continuing education* (Vol. 3). New York: Grune & Stratton.

Mariani, F. (1975). *Generalization across phones following sensory-motor treatment.* Unpublished master's thesis. Pennsylvania State University, University Park, PA.

McCabe, R. B., & Bradley, D. P. (1973). The systematic multiphonemic approach to articulation therapy. Short course presented at American Speech and Hearing Association South Eastern Regional Conference, Atlanta.

McCabe, R. B., & Bradley, D. P. (1975). Systematic multiple phonemic approach to articulation therapy. *Acta Symbolica, 6,* 2–18.

McDonald, E. T. (1964a). *Articulation testing and treatment: A sensory motor approach.* Pittsburgh: Stanwix House.

McDonald, E. T. (1964b). *Deep test of articulation: Picture form.* Pittsburgh: Stanwix House.

McDonald, E. T. (1964c). *Deep test of articulation: Sentence form.* Pittsburgh: Stanwix House.

McDonald, E. T. (1968). *A screening deep test of articulation.* Pittsburgh: Stanwix House.

McDonald, E. T. (1980). Disorders of articulation. In R. J. Van Hattum (Ed.), *Communication Disorders: An Introduction* (pp. 159–209). New York: Macmillan.

McDonald, E. T. (in press). *Articulation Testing and Treatment: A Sensorimotor, Diagnostic Teaching Approach.* Phoenix, AZ: Communication Skill Builders.

Schultz, M. (1972). *An analysis of clinical behavior in speech and hearing* (pp. 10–44). Englewood Cliffs, NJ: Prentice-Hall.

Scripture, E. W. (1935). Overlapping of speech sounds. *Nature, 136,* 759.

Secord, W. (1981). *C-PAC: Clinical probes of articulation consistency.* San Antonio, TX: Psychological Corp.

Shine, R., and Proust, J. (1982). *Clinical treatment manual: Articulatory production training: A programmed sensory-motor approach.* Greenville, NC: East Carolina University.

Shohara, H. (1939). *Significance of overlapping movements in speech.* Proceedings of the Second Central Zone Conference of the American Society for the Hard of Hearing, St. Louis.

Stetson, R. H. (1951). *Motor phonetics: A study of speech movements in action.* Amsterdam: North Holland.

Taylor, R., & Shine, R. (1978). *Primary and secondary stress factors influencing the diphthongization and/or monophthongization of the /r/ vowel.* Laboratory research, East Carolina University, Greenville, NC.

Wolfe, V., Blocker, S., & Prater, N. (1988). Articulatory generalization in two word-medial, ambisyllabic contexts. *Language, Speech and Hearing Services in Schools, 19,* 251–258.

APPENDIX 13.1 Formulation of Abutting Pair Contexts

The procedures outlined here are designed to elicit a correct context in which the target phone is one of an abutting consonant pair.

If the target functions prevocalicly in the first syllable or postvocalicly in the second syllable of the correct context, follow procedure 1. If the target is adjacent to a vowel at the syllable juncture, follow procedure 2. If the target is an element of a cluster, follow procedure 3. With each procedure, as a CVC-CVC context is developed, initiate training at Step 1 of the establishment phase.

Procedure 1. Example contexts are *saw-teeth* and *fish-house*. Pair the syllable containing the target with another CV, VC, or CVC so that the target occurs at the syllable juncture. With *saw-teeth* begin with a CV, such as *toe-saw*. If the X is produced correctly, have the patient produce the context imitatively or spontaneously and provide verbal feedback pertinent to production parameters. Practice with varied stress patterns. If incorrect try another CV. Introduce CVCs in which the abutting C logically would facilitate correct production of the target, such as *cut-saw, fun-saw,* or *won-saw*. Progress to *won-sock* and initiate training at Step 1 of the establishment phase.

With *fish-house* begin with a VC such as *house-out*. Note if produced with significant coarticulation and an appropriate stress pattern, /hau·saut/ may be produced.

Systematically vary the V and C in the syllable not containing the target and gradually work toward production of a CVC-CVC.

Procedure 2. Example contexts are *my-saw* and *house-on*. Progress as suggested in procedure 1 above. Experiment with contexts and abutting consonants using the vowel diagram and the patient's phonetic inventory as "coded" on the place/manner sheet (Figure 13.2).

Procedure 3. Example contexts are *tree-thumb* and *star-thumb*. Develop a bisyllable context in which the first element of the cluster, /t/ in *tree*, occurs postvocalicly in the first syllable and the second element /r/ occurs prevocalicly in the second CVC syllable. Obtain several imitative productions of each context that follows, providing verbal feedback to heighten awareness of parameters of correct production: *tree, treed, cat-treed, bat-treed,* and eventually *cat-read*. Produce the context with a stress pattern that causes the target to be produced as a cluster within the bisyllable context. Follow similar procedures with other clusters.

Conversely, if a patient cannot produce an "st" cluster but can produce a postvocalic /s/ and a prevocalic /t/, imitative production with variable stress patterns can quickly result in the development of clusters. For example, have the patient produce *loose-top* and work toward *you-stop*.

CHAPTER 14 A Distinctive-Feature Approach

Since the publication in 1952 of *Preliminaries to Speech Analysis: The Distinctive Features and Their Correlates* by Roman Jakobson, Gunnar Fant, and Morris Halle, momentum has been generated to discover the true nature of the entities called *phonemes*. While Jakobson, Fant, and Halle's book is very technical and difficult to apply clinically, it was preceded by a more pertinent book called *Child Language, Aphasia and Phonological Universals* (Jakobson, 1941/1968). This work contained an explanation of the manner in which children acquire speech sounds—in a step-by-step fashion. In *The Acquisition of Distinctive Features* (Blache, 1978), the distinctive-feature theory of these texts was applied to the establishment of a clinical method to correct speech sound errors. This chapter is devoted to a presentation of the manner in which distinctive-feature principles may be used to correct deviant articulation.

This discussion presumes no prior knowledge of distinctive-feature theory. It is organized in such a way that basic concepts are introduced first. This is followed by a discussion of the application of these basic principles in the clinical setting. A variety of ways in which the basic teaching format

may be modified so that it may be integrated into existing remedial approaches are discussed. Finally, the strengths and limitations of the approach are commented upon.

While the term *theory* may be disconcerting to some, it should be remembered that a theory is nothing more than speculation in the process of becoming scientific law. Today the scientific community is fairly certain of those sound properties that are used in human communication. Computers are being programmed to produce and recognize human speech. While arguments do develop concerning some aspects of the communication process, enough information is readily available to outline the basic elements of speech sound acquisition. From this perspective, it is possible to infer a remedial program.

RATIONALE

Basic Concepts

The term *distinctive feature,* as described in chapter 2, is a by-product of the idea that a speech sound or phoneme is a complex unit. Each speech sound has component parts, i.e., manner features, place features, voicing features, etc. At the same

Stephen E. Blache, Ph.D., is a professor of communication disorders and sciences at Southern Illinois University, Carbondale, Illinois.

time, these component parts have a linguistic function: They are *used to make words different*. A speaker must have enough articulatory control to stabilize her sound gestures so that they result in an acoustic end product that is recognizable to other listeners in the culture (Jakobson, 1932/1962).

The terms *distinctive* and *feature* should be given equal weight. In this discussion, *feature* implies the physical postures used to generate the utterance and the subsequent acoustic properties. *Distinctive* indicates the psycholinguistic use of these properties, i.e., making words different. It implies a speaker and a listener from the same language, exchanging ideas using a motor-acoustic code. In all, the transmission of an idea involves a code that is physiologically generated, acoustically transmitted, psychologically perceived, and culturally standardized.

The Training Unit

Formally, a phoneme is *a set of concurrent motor-acoustic properties that are used to differentiate words in a given language*. While the set of properties constitutes the phoneme's structure, the use of the properties to distinguish utterances constitutes its function. The distinctive-feature approach places a great deal of emphasis on the importance of isolating a single sound property as a training goal rather than training phonemes as a whole. Because the phoneme is so complex, it is considered easier to work with the component parts, one at a time, rather than confuse the child with several different challenges at the same time. This strategy also permits the therapist to concentrate on one goal at a time.

In many traditional articulation approaches, the child has been expected to produce an ideal sound as an all-or-nothing task. Irrespective of the subtle shifts in place or manner of articulation, the therapist reinforces the child on the basis of standard articulatory ideals. The current approach, however, uses a form of progressive approximation, in

which the child is reinforced for articulatory changes that represent significant shifts toward the target phoneme. By concentrating on the features, rather than the sound, the therapist is able to concentrate on one phonemic property at a time. Because of the nature of the sound system, a significant shift in a distinctive-feature property signals a sound that is different from the original utterance. The therapist is expected to assess whether or not the new sound represents phonemic progress.

The Phonemic System

The sound properties or features that separate the consonantal phonemes of American English are illustrated in Figure 14.1. Each of the lines represents a distinctive feature and a possible training goal. To organize the consonantal phonemes, the child must control six distinctive features: velopharyngeal movement (*nasality*), laryngeal vibration (*voicing*), labial/lingual production (*front*), front/back lingual production (*back*), the duration of the utterance (*continuation*), and turbulent dental friction (*stridency*). Although these concepts may seem simple, the manner in which the properties may be combined to produce 19 different phonemic units results in a complex learning task. The physiological requirements of the system are substantial. Also, the acoustic signals that result from the feature combinations represent difficult learning goals. The average child takes between 4 and 6 years to gain mastery over such a system.

Using the Phonemic Model

The phonemic model in Figure 14.1 may be used in several ways. For example, it can be used to analyze the nature of sound substitution errors. If a child substitutes an [m] for an [n] sound, the child is confusing the lips with the tongue. The model can also be used to assess the severity of the substitution. A child who substitutes an [m] for [b] has a milder problem than a child who substitutes [m] for [ʃ]. The former child has forgotten to close the velum, the latter has additional problems with la-

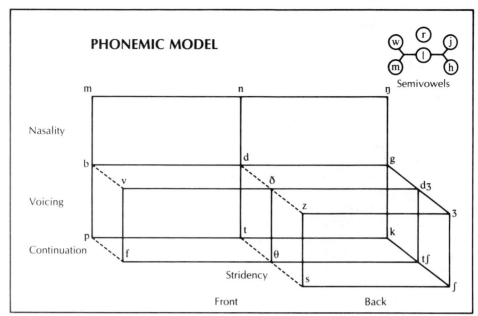

FIGURE 14.1

Configuration used to display the distinctive features that separate the consonants of American English. Each line on the city-block model represents one of the six distinctive features. (*Source: "Minimal Word-Pairs and Distinctive Feature Training"* by S. E. Blache, in *Phonological Intervention: Concepts and Procedures* (p. 67), M. Crary (Ed.), 1982, San Diego: College-Hill Press, Inc. Copyright 1982 by College-Hill Press. Reprinted by permission.

ryngeal inhibition, dental approximation, prolonging the signal, and two place-of-articulation errors. If one counts the lines from intersection to intersection that separate the two different substitutions, it will be noted that the former substitution involves one line; the latter, six lines. This model is called a *city-block* model. It represents the type and number of distinctive features that separate any 2 of the 19 phonemes.

In clinical practice, the model is used to assess the appropriateness of new speech sound approximations. For instance, if one is trying to teach the child the importance of the front/back lingual contrast due to a [t] for [k] substitution, the following might happen. Once the child abandons production of the [t] in attempting to produce [k], the child sometimes opts for [tʃ]. It can be noted on the model that to get from [t] to [k], the child must generate *back place*. The [tʃ] represents back place plus *continuation*. The child, then, has produced

the correct feature, back tongue position, plus an extra one. As was noted earlier, the child would be reinforced at this stage, and then would be taught the significance of not prolonging the back lingual utterance. We have found that children who are not reinforced for creative, though imperfect, utterances tend to stop experimenting with sound properties. The stimulation of discovery behavior is the main focus of this therapeutic approach.

Stimulating Creative Phonemic Behavior

The main vehicle for stimulating new sound properties is the *minimal word-pair*. We define a *minimal word-pair* as any two phonetically equivalent words that only differ by a *single sound property*. Therapy consists of teaching the motor-acoustic characteristics and the linguistic importance of each of these sound-pair contrasts.

To develop word-pairs, the therapist must have two words with an equal number of segments. The words may be of any length, but they both must have the same number of phonemes. In addition to this requirement, in all but one position, the words must contain the same sounds in the same order. The contrast may be in any position in the words, but all other segments must be identical. Some examples are given in Table 14.1.

As noted, it is possible to have two matching words that are not minimal distinctive-feature contrasts. While *pea* and *me* have an equal number of segments and the contrast is prevocalic, the sound-pair involves two features, nasality and voicing. If a sound contrast such as this is used during discrimination testing, it will not be possible to determine which feature is being used. The child may use one or both features to perceive the difference between the pronunciation of the two words; hence, the therapist will not be sure if the child is detecting the target feature. Because of this ambiguity, it is suggested that all minimal word-pairs used in this method be restricted to single distinctive-feature contrasts.

The Semantic Referent

Once the two words have the proper phonetic balance, it is important to make sure that the child understands the ideas behind the words. If the child does not have the concept to be labeled, it is extremely difficult for the child to associate the motor-acoustic utterance with meaning. Although

it is possible to teach the child the lexical concept in question and then do phonemic training, it is often much easier to choose other words from the child's lexicon to obtain the desired feature contrast. In cases such as organically based semantic retardation, the therapist may need to develop one or both of the concepts prior to or simultaneously with the phonemic/word contrast.

METHOD

The minimal word-pairs teaching approach is organized into four basic steps (see Figure 14.2—B. *Presentation Phase*). The therapist first determines whether the child knows the concept to be used, i.e., the words to be transmitted (Step 1). In Step 2, the therapist checks to see if the child can perceive the difference in pronunciation that separates the two words. In Step 3, the therapist stimulates the child to experiment with new utterances and shapes the behavior. Finally, the therapist integrates the acquired feature into longer and longer verbal utterances and different social situations (Step 4). Because of the importance of each of these steps, they will be discussed in detail.

Step 1: Discussion of Words

Once a minimal word-pair contrast has been chosen to teach a particular distinctive feature, it is important to determine whether the child understands the words. If she does not, the feature properties may not be retained because the words will not be used in everyday speech. In other words,

TABLE 14.1
Examples of Minimal Word-Pairs

[pi /bi]	pea/bee	2 segments, prevocalic contrast
[pɪt/bɪt]	pit/bit	3 segments, prevocalic contrast
[slæp/slæb]	slap/slab	4 segments, postvocalic contrast
[nɪpəl/nɪbəl]	nipple/nibble	5 segments, intervocalic contrast

MINIMAL WORD-PAIRS ORIENTATION

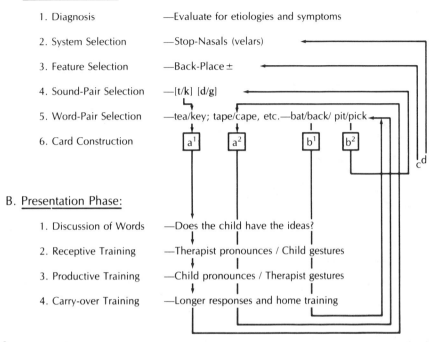

A. Preparation Phase:

    1. Diagnosis   —Evaluate for etiologies and symptoms

    2. System Selection   —Stop-Nasals (velars)

    3. Feature Selection   —Back-Place ±

    4. Sound-Pair Selection —[t/k] [d/g]

    5. Word-Pair Selection   —tea/key; tape/cape, etc.—bat/back/ pit/pick

    6. Card Construction

B. Presentation Phase:

    1. Discussion of Words   —Does the child have the ideas?

    2. Receptive Training   —Therapist pronounces / Child gestures

    3. Productive Training   —Child pronounces / Therapist gestures

    4. Carry-over Training   —Longer responses and home training

FIGURE 14.2

Protocol procedure for organizing a minimal word-pairs therapy program. (a = change in word-pairs; b = change in position of contrast and/or sound-pair context; c = change in distinctive feature; d = change in sound system.) (*Source: "Minimal Word-Pairs and Distinctive Feature Training"* by S. E. Blache, in *Phonological Intervention: Concepts and Procedures* (p. 72), M. Crary (Ed.). 1982, San Diego: College-Hill Press, Inc. Copyright 1982 by College-Hill Press. Reprinted by permission.)

the child must possess a need to make a feature distinctive.

To check on the child's understanding, she is asked simple, either-or questions that can be responded to by pointing. If, for instance, a therapist is trying to teach a child the distinctive difference between the expressives *T* and *key* (front/back lingual contrast), the therapist must determine whether the pictures are relevant to the child (see Figure 14.3a). The child is asked:

"Which one opens the door?"
"Which one is a letter of the alphabet?"
"Which one goes into a lock?"
"Which one do you write?", etc.

If it is known that the child can understand the questions and she points to the wrong picture, the child simply may not know the word ideas, or the pictures may be inappropriately drawn.

If a child does not know the letters of the alphabet, *T* may be a poor choice. By using a cup and saucer with a tea bag, the therapist can use the same phonetic contrast with a different semantic referent, or [t] and [k] can be put into other pairs to serve the same function, i.e., to elicit the front/back lingual contrast. Word contrasts such as *tape/cape, ten/Ken,* and *told/cold* will serve just as well because the ultimate training goal is the distinctive feature.

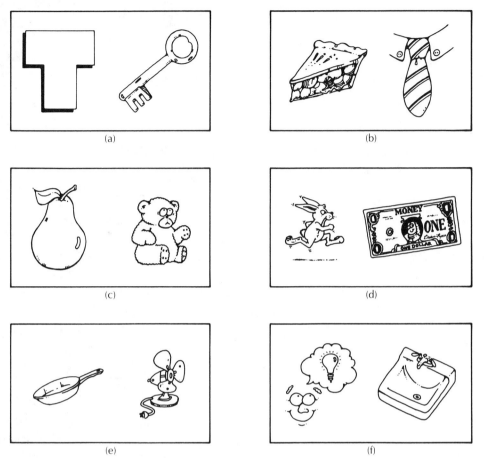

FIGURE 14.3
Exemplars illustrating six different distinctive feature contrasts. (a = front/back lingual; b = labial/lingual; c = voiced/voiceless; d = nasal/nonnasal; e = continued/interrupted; f = strident/mellow.) (*Source:* "Minimal Word-Pairs and Distinctive Feature Training" by S. E. Blache, in *Phonological Intervention: Concepts and Procedures* (p. 65), M. Crary (Ed.), 1982, San Diego: College-Hill Press, Inc. Copyright 1982 by College-Hill Press. Reprinted by permission.)

Step 2: Discrimination Testing and Training

Once the therapist is sure the child knows the ideas to be labeled phonetically, the child is examined for perceptual awareness of the distinctive feature. The therapist speaks the two words, repeating them in random order. Each time the word is spoken, the child is asked to point to the word that has been said. If the child points correctly *seven consecutive times*, the therapist can be fairly sure that the child hears the distinctive feature difference.

The probability of a child simply guessing the correct words is so low that this possibility can be discounted. However, it should be remembered there may be more than one perceptual cue for some phonemic distinctions, such as voiced-voiceless. For final consonants, vowel duration will be different in the voiced and voiceless context, so that cues may be provided even in the absence of the final phoneme. For example, the words *bat* and *bad* are produced as /bæt/ and /bæ:d/ and may remain /bæ/ and /bæ:/ when /t/ or /d/ is omitted.

Caution. Children seem to have an almost standard reaction to this test. If the therapist uses a criterion much beyond seven consecutive correct responses, they tend to become bored with the task and may not attend. As attention wanders, discrimination errors will appear to occur. However, these errors are due to attention span and not discrimination ability. Once children demonstrate that they can perform correctly, seven times in a row, they have proved their skill. They are ready to move ahead to a more challenging task.

All things being equal, a child will only guess *seven consecutive* correct responses at the chance rate of 7 in 1000 times; *six consecutive* correct responses, 3 in 200 times; *five consecutive* correct, 3 in 100 times. Seven consecutive correct responses is actually very conservative. Probability theory would indicate that there is no way to absolutely eliminate a very lucky situation, but it is fairly safe to conclude the child hears a distinctive difference with 5, 6, or 7 consecutive responses. The approach is designed to compensate for an occasional stroke of luck.

Program Modifications. Sometimes a child will not be able to reach criterion levels. When this occurs, the therapist uses other word-pair contrasts with the same distinctive feature. If this happens repeatedly, poor discrimination skills are being revealed. The child should be encouraged to become a better listener through use of the minimal word-pairs as training items in a discrimination program. In this case, correct discrimination responses are reinforced, as with other auditory discrimination programs.

On occasion, a child will exhibit poor auditory memory span. The child does not remember significant linguistic information. In cases like this, the therapist pronounces one of the two words, but delays the visual presentation of the pictures. In the interim period, the child must remember the target word, and then demonstrate this retention when the two pictures are displayed. The delay times may be set to fit the needs of the individual child. Correct auditory memory responses are reinforced, as with other auditory memory programs.

Summary. In the second step of the technique, the child is channeled into feature production training after demonstrating perceptual awareness, or the program is modified to strengthen auditory discrimination and/or auditory memory skills. The minimal word-pair that isolates the distinctive feature can be used in three ways: (a) discrimination testing, (b) discrimination training, and/or (c) auditory memory training. The important thing is to isolate the goal behavior, i.e., the feature to be perceived, discriminated, and/or retained.

Step 3: Production Training

There is a fourth use for the minimal word-pair: the elicitation of creative articulatory behavior—new sound gestures. Once the child demonstrates that she perceives the distinctive feature, the child is expected to demonstrate the use and control of the feature.

In this step, the child is told that she is to "be the teacher." The child is instructed to say the words, and the therapist is to point to the word that has been said. Due to the feature selection process, the child always can pronounce one of the words, but is unable to pronounce the alternate word. The child can be expected to exhibit the following standard pattern.

Demonstrating Deficit. The child begins by pronouncing the word she can say. The therapist points to the word. Then the child attempts to say the word she is unable to produce correctly. The child expects the therapist's finger to move to the other picture. However, the second utterance sounds like the first. The therapist indicates this fact by touching the first picture again. The child, in most cases, will immediately point to the other picture and say that the therapist is wrong. The therapist then indicates that the first word was heard. The therapist offers to help the child say the other word so that the finger will move. The therapist is helping her "play the phonemic game."

Working at the Word Level. Most children are motivated to get the finger to move to the other picture. The therapist then uses traditional cues to elicit the distinctive feature property. However, it is important to elicit a word response because a sound spoken in isolation is unnatural and too abstract. Furthermore, connected speech is extremely rapid. The sentence *Joe took father's shoe bench out,* a 17-segment expression, is generally said in less than 2 seconds. A sound spoken in isolation produces gestures of abnormal length. In the distinctive-feature approach, the child is being taught to say words that communicate meaning. When the therapist has cued the child properly, and the word is spoken correctly, the child often exhibits satisfaction in the accomplishment with a broad smile.

Immediate Reinforcement. Immediately upon hearing the correct pronunciation of the feature, the therapist reinforces the child. This is done by a smile, praise, and the movement of the finger to the picture the child intended. The child is encouraged to practice the utterance while it is fresh in her mind. The child then alternates the pronunciation of the two words. When the therapist is certain the child has the proper articulatory control, the program is expanded to ensure transfer into syntactical and social situations.

Isolating the Articulatory Goal. It should be noted that the therapist must develop a sensitivity for the object of reinforcement, i.e., the distinctive feature. In this approach, a decision based on correct versus incorrect sound approximations is not accurate enough. The therapist must isolate the goal behavior with great precision. The child's creative attempts must be analyzed for their implications. If the utterance contains the desired property, it is reinforced. The therapist must think in terms of the features instead of the target sound.

Building Rapport. This approach crystallizes the learning objectives. It isolates distinctiveness in a very immediate manner. It is very challenging and direct. For this reason, the therapist must establish rapport prior to the initiation of this treatment program. Prior to any form of direct therapeutic training, much preparation should be done to build a sense of trust between child and therapist. The person with whom the child can play a game is, many times, just as important as the game she plays. Take time to win the child's respect. The minimal word-pairs approach tells 'how' the therapist will be pleased, *rapport* is 'why' the therapist should be pleased. Indirect activities that are fun should compliment those direct activities that are real work.

Step 4: Carryover Training

Once the child demonstrates the ability to control the articulatory system and pronounce the desired word, the target word is put at the end of longer and longer expressions. Beginning with two-word expressions, the child is encouraged to say the target word in conjunction with the indefinite article *a*, and then the definite article *the*. This can be done by using an orthographic representation of the words *a* or *the* and placing them next to the minimal word-pair pictures. Both the target word and the distinctive-feature "lure" word are elicited in the practice session. The child practices saying "*a T*" and "*a key*." Using both minimal pair-words keeps the negative practice component in the task.

The indefinite article *a* is generally introduced before the definite article *the* because the former is less complex segmentally than the latter, i.e., V versus CV. If a child has difficulty at this stage, consideration should be given to modifying the program to include standard coarticulatory sequencing in the position of the definite and indefinite articles (McDonald, 1964). Words that end with all the basic sounds of American English are introduced in place of *a* or *the* preceding the target word and the lure. Therapists should concentrate on two considerations: (a) making the two-word expressions as natural as possible and (b) reinforcing only the feature in the target word.

After the child pronounces two-word expressions, longer and longer utterances are tried. The three-word carrier *Touch the . . .* and the four-word carrier *Point to the . . .* permit the child to speak in a meaningful way and still practice the production of the feature. As the expressions become longer and longer, the child must remember to use the appropriate feature in an automatic way. This device has also been used in traditional therapy.

The Social Situation. While children are learning to talk in a meaningful way in the clinic, it is expected that they will also practice at home. Each child has a word book containing all the target words that the child has learned. Parents are encouraged to set aside family time for the recitation of the words—generally at the end of the evening meal. Parents serve as motivators and monitors of the child's speech. At no time are they encouraged to correct the child's speech. Rather, they are instructed to praise the child for good word pronunciation. If words are said incorrectly, parents are asked to say nothing to the child, but are requested to report the situation to the clinician at the next therapy session.

Modifying Home Programs. In general, parents are not equipped to perform a phonetic analysis on a particular utterance. They do not know when a creative utterance represents phonemic progress. After the parents report unusual articulations, the therapist analyzes the utterance(s) and informs the parents whether to reinforce or not. At the same time, parents are encouraged to provide positive reinforcement whenever possible. At the beginning of each therapy session, the clinician asks the parents about the child's progress. If parents lack the motivation or concern to help the child, an educational counseling program is instituted to develop better motivational reinforcement for the child and improve monitoring behavior on the part of the parent. Sometimes children learn skills in the clinic and do not use them at home. The in-

volvement of parents is seen as crucial to avoid this type of carryover problem.

Relationship to Current Approaches

The minimal word-pairs technique isn't really an alternative to current practice. Rather, it is an integration and streamlining of traditional techniques. The procedure highlights the importance of using a holistic approach to therapy. It stresses the psycholinguistic function of the feature, but also emphasizes the development of proper placement and auditory discrimination skills. The therapist serves as a representative of the linguistic culture and provides feedback as to the adequacy of phonetic skills—in a phonemic context.

Stimulation Versus Training. The distinctive-feature approach is a stimulation program rather than a complete training program in that it provides a context in which learning can occur, but does not teach the child how to produce the sound. It is assumed that given the proper circumstances, children will seek to discover articulatory skills. This concept has its roots in Montessorian education. When the underlying problem is due to inadequate learning, the minimal word-pairs discovery process tends to be reinforcing in and of itself because the child can immediately use what she has learned for communication.

However, some children are prevented from developing natural articulatory skills by organic or structural problems. In such cases, the minimal word-pairs technique tends to be converted to a training program. The therapist implements management procedures to correct structural/organic defects. The basic program is modified to strengthen general motoric skills, improve auditory retention skills, and develop better listening habits, and when the child lacks the capacity to learn simply through discovery, reinforcement paradigms are introduced and/or augmented.

The distinctive feature encapsulated in the minimal word-pairs contrast is the cornerstone of the system. A distinctive-feature orientation forces the therapist to select one articulatory behavior at a time (feature) and teach the distinctive function of that feature.

Organizing the Distinctive-Feature Program

Before a distinctive-feature program is instituted, the therapist should check for a variety of factors that may necessitate modifications in the program. As a minimum, the therapist should check for a second language in the home, a regional dialect, a poor speech model, and the possibility that a child is using an idioglossia. In addition to this, each child should be evaluated for inadequate hearing and functionally inadequate articulatory structures. The therapist should have some indication of the child's intellectual capacity and the motivation to develop communication skills. Finally, it is often helpful to test the child's discrimination skills and auditory memory span. Deficits in any of these areas call for program modifications. Experience has shown that approximately two of every five children seen will require special programming.

Getting Started. In the past, it has been popular to select a single distinctive feature for training and attempt to teach this feature in many different sound-pair contexts. The current approach restricts the feature selection process to specific sound classes. Developmental studies have shown that certain sound classes stabilize before others. Stops and nasals, for instance, stabilize in the child's repertoire before sibilants. The features are grouped by sound-pair contrast into six major sound classes: primitive, vocalic, stop/nasal, semivowel, continuant, sibilant. However, problems with only four of these classes tend to be seen in the age range between 4 years 9 months and 8 years. The earlier two classes represent children

who have not begun to develop speech, or those that have significant problems with vowels. Both of these levels of development are expected to be completed by the third year. This discussion will concentrate on the four later developing stages.

To develop a distinctive-feature program, the therapist must determine the level of development of the phonemic system. Once this is accomplished, sound-pairs and features are selected to rebuild or extend the existing phonemic system. Minimal word-pairs are selected and picture cards are drawn to elicit the desired distinctive features.

The Quick Test. Level of development may be determined through the Quick Test (see Table 14.2). In this test, the child is asked to pronounce 67 words elicited through picture stimuli. The words represent the vocabulary items most commonly used in articulation testing. These 67 words represent a prevocalic, intervocalic, and postvocalic sampling of 25 consonantal and semivowel sounds (cf. Blache, 1978, Appendix J). By design, each of the 25 sounds is tested one to three times. The child is graded on the number of times a sound is misarticulated, and the number is compared to the performance of other children of the same age. If the child misarticulates a sound more often than other children of the same age, the sound is considered defective—until evidence is exhibited to the contrary. This operation is repeated for each of the 25 sounds. This permits the formulation of some idea about the adequacy of the entire phonemic system.

Determining the Level of Development. It is this overall pattern that is of greatest importance in the establishment of a level of phonemic development. The 25 sounds and the 67 words used to test those sounds are shown in Table 14.2. The sounds have been categorized and arranged in developmental order, i.e., stop/nasals then semivowels, continuants then sibilants. The therapist will determine what is the earliest sound system that needs stimulation.

Scoring Sounds. To make this decision, the child is asked to pronounce the test words. Only one sound

TABLE 14.2
The Quick Test

				Age Groups																			
				4:9–4:11				5:0–5:11				6:0–6:11				7:0–7:11				8:0–8:11			
Class	Symbol	Spelling	Test Words / Errors	0	1	2	3	0	1	2	3	0	1	2	3	0	1	2	3	0	1	2	3
	[m]	m	monkey, hammer, broom	p	*	*	*	p	*	*	*	p	*	*	*	p	*	*	*	p	*	*	*
	[n]	n	knife, penny/money, moon	p	*	*	*	p	*	*	*	p	*	*	*	p	*	*	*	p	*	*	*
	[ŋ]	ng	finger, ring	p	p	p		p	p	?		p	?	*	*	p	?	*	*	p	?	?	*
Stops and	[p]	p	pig, paper, cup	p	*	*	*	p	*	*	*	p	*	*	*	p	*	*	*	p	*	*	*
Nasals	[t]	t	table, potato, boat	p	p	*		p	?	*	*	p	?	*	*	p	?	*	*	p	?	*	*
	[k]	c,k	cat, cookie, duck	p	*	*	*	p	*	*	*	p	*	*	*	p	*	*	*	p	*	*	*
	[b]	b	bicycle/bike, baby, bathtub	p	?	*	*	p	?	*	*	p	?	*	*	p	?	*	*	p	?	*	*
	[d]	d	dog, ladder, bed	p	?	*	*	p	p	*	*	p	?	*	*	p	?	*	*	p	?	*	*
	[g]	g	gun, wagon, egg	p	?	*	*	p	?	*	*	p	*	*	*	p	*	*	*	p	*	*	*
Semivowels	[hw]	wh	whistle	p	p			p	p			p	p			p	p			p	?		
	[w]	w	window, flowers	p	p	*		p	p	*		p	*	*		p	*	*		p	*	*	*
	[l]	l	lamp, balloon, ball	p	p	p	?	p	p	?	*	p	*	*	*	p	*	*	*	p	*	*	*
	[r]	r	rabbit carrot, car	p	p	p	p	p	p	p	?	p	p	?	?	p	?	?	*	p	*	*	*
	[j]	y	yellow, yoyo	p	?	*		p	*	*		p	*	*		p	*	*		p	*	*	
	[h]	h	horse	p	*			p	*			p	*			p	*			p	*		
Continuants	[f]	f,ph	fan, telephone, leaf	p	*	*	*	p	*	*	*	p	*	*	*	p	*	*	*	p	*	*	*
	[v]	v	vacuum, television/TV, stove	p	p	?	*	p	p	p	*	p	p	p	*	p	p	*	*	p	*	*	*
	[θ]	th	thumb, toothbrush, mouth	p	p	p	p	p	p	p	p	p	p	p	p	p	p	p	?	p	p	p	*
	[ð]	th	this/that, feathers, smooth	p	p	p	?	p	p	p	?	p	p	*	*	p	p	*	*	p	*	*	*
	[tʃ]	ch	chair, matches, watch	p	p	p	?	p	p	?	?	p	?	*	*	p	?	*	*	p	*	*	*
	[dʒ]	j,g	jumping, pajamas/P/s, orange	p	p	p	?	p	p	?	*	p	?	*	*	p	*	*	*	p	*	*	*
Sibilants	[s]	s,c	sun, glasses, house	p	p	p	p	p	p	p	p	p	p	p	p	p	p	p	?	p	p	?	?
	[z]	z	zebra, scissors, eyes	p	p	p	p	p	p	p	p	p	p	p	p	p	p	p	?	p	p	?	?
	[ʃ]	sh	shoe, dishes, fish	p	p	p	?	p	p	?	*	p	?	*	*	p	?	*	*	p	*	*	*
	[ʒ]	g	measure, beige	p	p	p		p	p	p		p	p	?		p	p	*		p	p	*	

Note: Speech sounds are tested only in the contexts given. (P = appropriate for age, i.e., pass; * = performance equal to the lower 5% of population, i.e., failure; ? = performance equal to lower 6% to 10% of population, i.e., questionable.)

in each word is scored. The therapist notes the number of times the child misarticulates the sound. Referring to the appropriate age group, the therapist circles the symbol beneath the number of times the sound is in error. This is done for each of the 25 speech sounds. If a (*) is circled, it indicates a performance equivalent to that of the lower 5% of the age group. If a (?) is circled, it indicates a performance equivalent to that of the lower 6% to 10% of the age group. The (P) symbol indicates a performance that is appropriate for the child's age.

Estimating Phonemic Level. After the performance on each of the 25 sounds has been evaluated, the therapist looks for two or more significant errors in the earliest sound class, the stop/nasals. If two or more significant errors are present, this is where therapy is begun. If no significant defect is found with the stop/nasal system, the therapist proceeds to the next developing sound system, i.e., the semivowel system. This operation is repeated until a level of development has been selected.

Mild Phonemic Problems. In those cases where only one defective sound is found in a system, or there is a limited number of defective sounds, the therapeutic goal becomes one of sound stabilization rather than system reconstruction. In cases such as these, it is often helpful to deep-test the defective sound in many different coarticulatory contexts. The therapist can then determine which features in the defective sound are most often in error and rank them. If there are several defective sounds, the earliest developing sound is evaluated first. A therapy program is designed for the particular sound. At the completion of the first speech sound program, the child's phonemic system is reevaluated and the former evaluation process repeated.

The Sound Systems. After the completion of the Quick Test, the therapist has a good idea of where the child stands developmentally. Those children who have difficulty with two or more sounds in the stop/nasal system, [m n ŋ b d g p t k], are treated

according to Therapeutic Model 1 (see Figure 14.4). Children with two or more errors in the semivowel system, [hw w l r j h], are taught with reference to Therapeutic Model 2 (see Figure 14.5). Children with difficulties with the continuant system, [f v θ ð tʃ dʒ], or the sibilant system, [s z ʃ ʒ], are treated in accordance with Models 3 and 4, respectively (see Figures 14.6 and 14.7). Before each of these models is discussed in detail, some general comments about the nature of the models are in order.

The Developmental Models. Each model represents a progressive step in distinctive feature organization. Models 1, 3, and 4 represent an expansion of the consonantal system. Model 2 represents the stabilization of the semivowel system. It is envisioned that the consonantal structure and the semivowel structure are similar in character, but the sound systems are used sequentially in speech, and tend to be somewhat independent of one another.

Infantemes. On each model, the distinctive-feature development has been illustrated by means of lines that separate the circles. The circles represent vague phonemic classes called *infantemes* (Albright & Albright, 1958). The *infanteme* is a set of motor-acoustic properties that are used to make words different *in the language of the child.* In other words, infantemes are childlike phonemes. When a child has incomplete mastery over the distinctive-feature system of the adult, the child appears to substitute one sound for another. Actually, when a child does not understand a distinctive feature, two or more sounds tend to be interchangeable. One of the sound elements is more probable than another, i.e., is more natural. This gives the appearance of a purposeful action of replacing one sound with another. However, careful examination of such behavior in repeated samples reveals confusion, rather than replacement. The two or more sounds tend to be in what linguists call *free variation.* Those sounds that are likely to be in free variation are grouped within the circle.

As will be noted in Model 1 (Figure 14.4), the voiceless, front-lingual infanteme has three free-

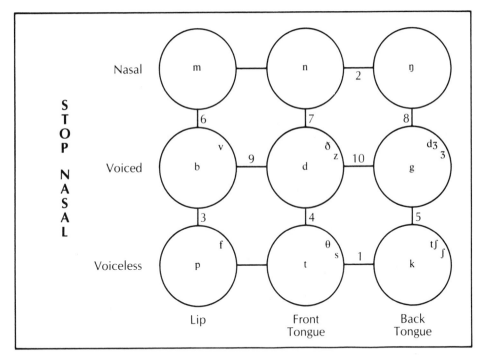

FIGURE 14.4
Model 1: The stop nasal system. The nine different infantemes of this system are organized by means of four different distinctive features: labial/lingual, front/back lingual, voiced/voiceless, and nasal/non-nasal. The arabic numerals represent the most typical training order. (*Source:* "Minimal Word-Pairs and Distinctive Feature Training" by S. E. Blache, in *Phonological Intervention: Concepts and Procedures* (p. 85), M. Crary (Ed.), 1982, San Diego: College-Hill Press, Inc. Copyright 1982 by College-Hill Press. Reprinted by permission.)

varying elements, [t θ s]. Before the child understands the importance of continued production and dental airflow, these three sounds tend to be interchangeable. The sound element that is underlined is the most probable gesture to be stabilized, for it represents the most pertinent or natural utterance for the class. It can be seen that phonemes become progressively separated as we move through the models.

Acceptable Free Variation. It can also be noted that the free-varying elements represent acceptable creative gestures for a given level of development. For instance, if the child is learning the importance of the use of the lips versus the use of the tongue in a voiceless context, [p] may be contrasted with any of the three sounds in the front-lingual class. The child is more likely to use [t], but [θ] and [s]

are also lingual utterances. As each system becomes better developed, greater rigor is applied when accepting variants. When the system is fully developed, as in the completion of Model 4, no free variation is expected; all the distinctive features have been learned. At this point the child's infantemes have become phonemes.

Order of Reconstruction. Small arabic numerals may be noted next to the specific feature lines. These represent an optimal order for distinctive-feature selection. However, it is not necessary to teach each feature. The therapist begins by selecting the appropriate model for the child's level of development. The defective sounds in the center of the circles, as noted on the Quick Test, are circled in contrasting color. Each line that connects a defective infanteme to another infanteme is marked.

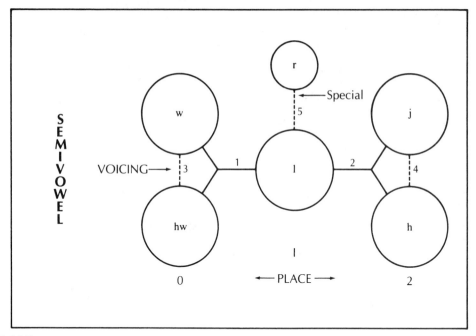

FIGURE 14.5
Model 2: The semivowel system. The six different infantemes of this system are organized by means of four different distinctive features: labial/lingual, front/back lingual, voiced/voiceless, and retroflex/nonretroflex. The arabic numerals represent the most typical training order. (*Source:* "Minimal Word-Pairs and Distinctive Feature Training" by S. E. Blache, in *Phonological Intervention: Concepts and Procedures* (p. 87), M. Crary (Ed.), 1982, San Diego: College-Hill Press, Inc. Copyright 1982 by College-Hill Press. Reprinted by permission.)

After all the appropriate lines have been noted, the arabic numerals are recorded, from smallest to largest. This is the order of the first, provisional distinctive-feature program.

Maximal Contrast. In general, the features are taught on a continuum beginning with the greatest physiological and acoustical contrast and moving to finer distinctions. This technique is called *maximal contrast.* The features and feature combinations have an inherent or natural hierarchy (Jakobson, 1941/1968) in which the pairs are ordered in such a way as to minimize changing the distinctive features. This is done by using similar sound-pair contrasts that are based on the same differential property. When therapy programs have been revised due to a lack of progress, carrier words are changed before sound-pairs, sound-pairs before features, and features before sound systems.

Interactive Therapy. In interactive therapy the child is expected to develop initial command over a word utterance within a maximum period of 5 minutes. If progress has not been demonstrated by this point, another word-pair should be chosen and trained. Stimulation of the feature in a particular sound-pair contrast should continue in enough word-pair contexts until the therapist is confident the speech sounds are consistently differentiated.

Modifying a program within the confines of the models is strongly encouraged. If the therapist has a phonetic rationale for changing the prescribed order, she is generally thinking in distinctive-feature terms and considering the needs of a particular child. Therapeutic progress, of course, is the bench mark at all times. In this approach, top priority is given to rational rather than rote behavior for both the clinician and the child.

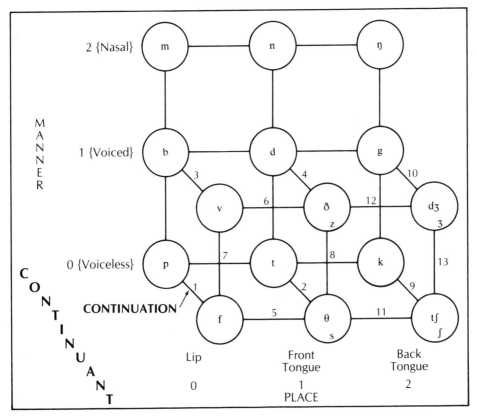

FIGURE 14.6
Model 3: The continuant system. The six new infantemes of the consonantal system are organized by means of four different distinctive features; continued/interrupted, labial/lingual, front/back lingual, and voiced/voiceless. The arabic numerals represent the most typical training order. (*Source: "Minimal Word-Pairs and Distinctive Feature Training"* by S. E. Blache, in *Phonological Intervention: Concepts and Procedures* (p. 88), M. Crary (Ed.), 1982, San Diego: College-Hill Press, Inc. Copyright 1982 by College-Hill Press. Reprinted by permission.)

Synopsis. Each line that has been noted represents a distinctive-feature contrast to be learned in a specific sound-pair context. The entire procedure is quite simple. It can be outlined as follows:

1. Administer the Quick Test.
2. Note the earliest sound system that has two or more errors.
3. Refer to the appropriate model and circle the defective sounds.
4. Note all the distinctive-feature lines that join and connect to the defective sounds.
5. Note the arabic numerals on those lines to develop an order for training.

6. Apply the basic minimal word-pairs technique and monitor progress by means of the model.

These models are designed to help the therapist think in distinctive-feature terms. They yield a complex perspective for the individual speech sounds, provide a developmental sequencing for feature selection, and give a natural training order.

Model 1: The Stop/Nasal System. This system has nine infantemes developed through the comprehension and control of four distinctive features

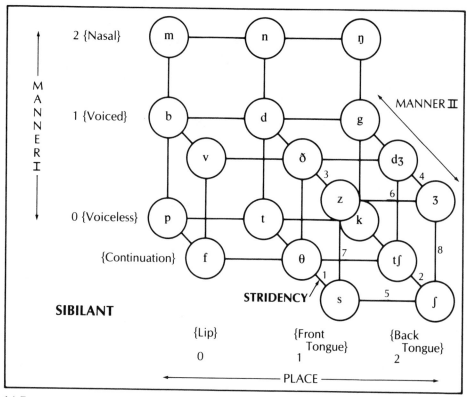

FIGURE 14.7

Model 4: The sibilant system. The four new infantemes of the consonantal system are organized by means of three different distinctive features: strident/mellow, front/back lingual, and voiced/voiceless. The arabic numerals represent the most typical training order. (*Source:* "Minimal Word-Pairs and Distinctive Feature Training" by S. E. Blache, in *Phonological Intervention: Concepts and Procedures* (p. 89), M. Crary (Ed.), 1982, San Diego: College-Hill Press, Inc. Copyright 1982 by College-Hill Press. Reprinted by permission.)

(see Figure 14.4). The nasal/nonnasal contrast and the voiced/voiceless contrast establish a three-point manner-of-articulation dimension, i.e., nasal, voice, voiceless. The labial/lingual contrast and the front/back lingual contrast establish a three-point place of articulation dimension, i.e., labial, front-lingual, back-lingual.

Acoustic Standards. In this level of development, the child is expected to be aware of the acoustic properties that represent the positioning of the velopharyngeal port mechanism and the vibratory state of the larynx. In addition to this, the child must be sensitive to those acoustic properties that

signal place-of-articulation characteristics, i.e., formant transitions.

Physiological Standards. Physiologically, the child must develop control of sound gestures that could be characterized as labial, apico-lingual, and dorso-lingual in character. In other words, the child must use three distinctive positions to signal place characteristics. In addition to that, the child must be able to control voice onset time (VOT) with enough skill to make the presence or absence of voicing readily identifiable. Finally, the child must be able to open and close the velopharyngeal port with purposeful regularity.

Sound-pair order for the stop/nasal class is shown in Table 14.3.

If significant deviations are found with [p t m n], the child's vowel system should be examined. Any vowel error is considered significant past 3 years of age. If significant vowel errors are apparent and/or the child does not distinguish between the lips and the tongue, refer to the early developmental programming described in *The Acquisition of Distinctive Features* (Blache, 1978, pp. 327–331).

Model 2: The Semivowel System. This system has six infantemes developed through the comprehension and control of four distinctive features (see Figure 14.5). The labial/lingual contrast and the front/back lingual contrast establish a three-point place-of-articulation dimension, i.e., labial, front-lingual and back-lingual. The voiced/voiceless contrast and the retroflex/nonretroflex contrast serve as the manner-of-articulation dimension.

Acoustic Standards. Acoustically, the semivowels have much in common with the diphthongs and continuants. At this stage the child is expected to be able to perceive formant changes that signal extreme vocal-tract closure in a front-mid-back position of the oral cavity (see Figure 14.5). In addition to that, the child must be aware of the acoustic properties associated with the special tongue

motions for the [r] sound and the vibratory state of the larynx.

Physiological Standards. The child is expected to partially close, then open the vocal tract with enough regularity to signal labial closure, front-lingual closure and back-lingual closure. At the same time, the child is expected to be able to control laryngeal tone in conjunction with these movements. This must be done with enough regularity to signal a voiced/voiceless distinction. This latter component, however, is of limited importance to the language and seldom produces significant difficulties for this sound class. Finally, the child has to be able to curl the tongue in a rapid fashion with no lingual-alveolar contact.

Clinical Correlates. The features are taught in a front-to-back direction, already observed with the stop/nasal class. Some 85% of the problems with this class tend to be internal in nature; i.e., sounds within the class tend to be confused with each other, rather than with sounds outside of the class. At times, some children will leave this system in an incomplete state of development and then develop the consonantal system in full. These children are sometimes referred to by the clinical label

TABLE 14.3
Stop/Nasal Sound-Pair Order

No. Pair	Feature	Sample Words
1. [t–k]	front/back lingual	tea/key, tape/cape, ten/Ken
2. [n–ŋ]	front/back lingual	win/wing, fan/fang, ton/tongue
3. [p–b]	voiced/voiceless	pea/bee, pig/big, pat/bat
4. [t–d]	voiced/voiceless	toe/doe, time/dime, tot/dot
5. [k–g]	voiced/voiceless	curl/girl, coat/goat, cap/gap
6. [b–m]	nasal/non-nasal	beet/meat, bat/mat, bike/Mike
7. [d–n]	nasal/non-nasal	D/knee, deck/neck, dot/knot
8. [g–ŋ]	nasal/non-nasal	wig/wing, bag/bang, log/long
9. [b–d]	labial/lingual	big/dig, bark/dark, bow/dough
10. [d–g]	front/back lingual	deer/gear, date/gate, doe/go

"lallers." This label is unfortunate because it does not specify the nature of the phonetic deviation. The often-heard statement "All I see are /l/, /r/, and /s/ problems" indicates that all /l/ or /s/ problems are alike. This may betray a lack of in-depth differential testing for causal agents and a sketchy understanding of phonetics—especially in the area of close transcription.

Sound-pair order for the semivowel class is shown in Table 14.4.

Kantner and West (1969) indicate that there are nine different types of "r" sounds in American English. If one wishes to take such a microscopic view of this sound, the therapist has only to define the exact nature of the difference between the variants, and integrate these differences into the semivowel system. As will be noted, the models are very broad in nature. They are designed to illustrate the most prominent phonetic properties used in everyday communication. This should not prevent the therapist from developing finer models to eradicate unpleasant distortions. It should be noted that, at this microscopic level of training, the child is being trained to be more than a linguistic communicator. She is being trained to be a phonetician in the most subtle sense. Modifying pictures of speech sound targets to indicate correct versus incorrect approximations of the same word has been a traditional technique in the field and will not be expanded on here.

Model 3: The Continuant System. This system has six infantemes appended to the previous nine infantemes of the stop/nasal system. These six new utterances are developed through the introduction of a new distinctive feature, continued/interrupted, and the generalization of place and manner features already observed in the stop/nasal system (see Figure 14.6; Figure 14.4).

Acoustic Standards. The continuant system is acoustically similar to the stop/nasal class in that it makes use of voicing and place-of-articulation properties. This entire class has a prolonged voicing marker through a sustained noise signal. Acoustically, the child is expected to detect place-of-articulation characteristics on the basis of the dominant spectral features in conjunction with the presence or absence of a periodic tone.

Physiological Standards. The child must learn to sustain a physical posture and force air through a particular vocal-tract constriction. Unlike the stop/nasals, the continuants require a dominant secondary vibrator (noise source) that results in sustained aspiration. At the same time, this effect must be maintained in the presence or absence of voicing. While the distinctive-feature properties common to the stop/nasal and continuant/noncontinuant system are very similar, it would be incorrect to consider them identical. The physiological and acoustical manifestations of voicing and place of articulation have more in common with each other within the respective systems than they do across the systems. This is one major reason why the

TABLE 14.4
Semivowel Sound-Pair Order

No. Pair	Feature	Sample Words
1. [w/hw–l]	labial/lingual	wet/let, weed/lead, win/Lynn
2. [l–j/h]	front/back lingual	Lou/you, less/yes, limb/him
3. [w–hw]	voiced/voiceless	we/Whee!, nonsense words (optional)
4. [j–h]	voiced/voiceless	you/who, Yah!/hay, yellow/hello
5. [l–r]	retroflex/nonretroflex	led/red, low/row, list/wrist

distinctive features are taught within sound classes, rather than throughout the system, one feature at a time.

Clinical Correlates. Children who have not mastered the continuation feature (and the concomitant need to reevaluate voicing and place properties) tend to replace the continuants with the stop/nasal sounds. In process terminology, this is referred to as *stopping*. Children who exhibit this form of replacement have been called "baby talkers." While the speech is recognizable it retains many infantile characteristics. By the time this system has been fully stabilized, only the sibilants tend to be replaced or confused.

Unlike the stop/nasal development that required the learning of four distinctive features, the continuant system requires the acquisition of one new feature and the generalization of phonemic concepts that have been previously acquired. In essence, the development of the stop/nasals is seen primarily as feature acquisition; the development of continuants, primarily as feature generalization.

Sound-pair order for the continuant class is shown in Table 14.5.

A careful examination of the training order of the distinctive features and sound-pairs will reveal

two internal stages of stabilization. This training order presumes that children will introduce the continuation feature in the anterior place position. The anterior [f], [v], [θ] and [ð] sounds are integrated before the posterior affricates, [tʃ] and [dʒ]. Some children, however, will stabilize the latter sounds before the former.

Model 4: The Sibilant System. The sibilant system has four infantemes appended to the previous stop/nasal/continuant system. These four new utterances are developed through the introduction of a new distinctive feature, strident/mellow, and the generalization of place and manner features already observed in the continuant system (see Figure 14.7; cf. Figure 14.6).

Acoustic Standards. The final step in the organizational process is reflected in Model 4. Acoustically, the sibilants require highly variable noise to make them distinct from their counterparts in the continuant system. Sibilants must vary in terms of frequency and intensity. This variability is detected by the ear as noisy and unpleasant. It has

TABLE 14.5
Continuant Sound-Pair Order

No. Pair	Feature	Sample Words
1. [p–f]	continuant/interrupted	pin/fin, pan/fan, pour/four
2. [t–θ]	continuant/interrupted	tree/three, tie/thigh, torn/thorn
3. [b–v]	continuant/interrupted	bee/V, base/vase, bat/vat
4. [d–ð]	continuant/interrupted	doze/those, ladder/lather, D/thee
5. [f–θ]	labial/lingual	free/three, fin/thin, fought/thought
6. [v–ð]	labial/lingual	Vs/these, van/than, nonsense words
7. [f–v]	voiced/voiceless	fat/vat, fan/van, face/vase
8. [θ–ð]	voiced/voiceless	teeth/teethe, nonsense words
9. [k–tʃ]	continuant/interrupted·	keys/cheese, kick/chick, cane/chain
10. [g–dʒ]	continuant/interrupted	Gail/jail, goose/juice, ghoul/jewel
11. [θ–tʃ]	front/back lingual	thief/chief, thick/chick, thin/chin
12. [ð–dʒ]	front/back lingual	nonsense words
13. [tʃ–dʒ]	voiced/voiceless	cello/jello, cherry/Jerry, chunk/junk

been given the name *stridency*. To hear this difference, compare a prolonged utterance of [θ:] and [s:]. The former is mellow; the latter is strident.

Physiological Standards. Stridency is produced by air being forced through constricted dental gaps. As the air passes through these small openings at a high rate of speed, the air particles bounce against each other in random fashion, resulting in a great deal of acoustic irregularity. When the tongue initiates or obstructs this airflow, the acoustic signal produced is less variable, and the sound is perceived as mellow.

Clinical Correlates. The inability to stabilize the sibilant system has a clinical counterpart, i.e., lisping behavior. In Figure 14.7, it can be seen that the interdental lisp [θ/s] and the lateral lisp [ɬ/s] or [ʃ/s] have distinctive-feature definitions. The former type of lisp is based on a stridency error; the latter, on place of articulation. Again, as with the [r], it is possible to develop more microscopic models to attack the [s] at the fine-transcription level. However, consideration should be given to the ultimate goal of the clinical program, the production of sound properties of sufficient quality to carry differential information in an undistracting manner.

Sound-pair order for the sibilant class is shown in Table 14.6.

The stabilization of the sibilant system represents the completion of the consonantal system. At this stage, all the distinctive features should be salient and under formal motoric control. Sound substitutions are no longer observed because the child's infantemes have the same phonetic definition as the adult phonemes.

Individual Differences. As in everything else, individual differences do exist. The models are not considered canonical but tenative in nature. At present, there are no data to support the concept of one sequential order of sound acquisition. What is apparent is a general unfolding organizational process. This natural unfolding is reflected in the sequential sound system models.

Review of Clinical Procedure. To summarize, before the models are used, the therapist administers the Quick Test. She develops a hypothesis as to which training model is most appropriate. Because of the differential testing that has gone on beforehand, the therapist is prepared to modify the program for the individual. Using one of the models, the clinician determines which areas need to be rebuilt. She decides which distinctive features are the most likely candidates for therapy by noting the lines on the model that stabilize the defective sounds. The lines represent the distinctive features and have been numbered for optimal remedial order. After features have been chosen, minimal word-pairs are constructed. The child is taught to perceive and produce the distinctive features,

TABLE 14.6
Sibilant Sound-Pair Order

No. Pair	Feature	Sample Words
1. [θ–s]	strident/mellow	think/sink, thick/sick, thumb/sum
2. [tʃ–ʃ]	strident/mellow	chip/ship, chop/shop, chew/shoe
3. [ð–z]	strident/mellow	teethe/tease, nonsense words
4. [dʒ–ʒ]	strident/mellow	legion/lesion, nonsense words
5. [s–ʃ]	front/back lingual	sip/ship, seat/sheet, sell/shell
6. [z–ʒ]	front/back lingual	Caesar/seizure, nonsense words
7. [s–z]	voiced/voiceless	sip/zip, Sue/zoo, see/Z
8. [ʃ–ʒ]	voiced/voiceless	nonsense words

which are incorporated into longer and longer verbal expressions. The words are practiced in different social settings. Throughout this entire process, the child is being taught a linguistic task—to make words different.

STRENGTHS AND LIMITATIONS

As has been alluded to before, this approach is primarily directed toward the functional articulation problem, i.e., the slow phonemic learner. The approach, which is flexible, must be modified to meet the particular needs of the individual child. This is particularly true of structurally or organically based problems. The distinctive feature and the minimal word-pair are given central focus; they are considered the keys for transforming a sound into a functional linguistic tool.

Although the approach is flexible, it does have certain natural limitations. The ability to perceive and produce the phonemic system is only one aspect of word production. Children not only have to make sounds, they must learn to sequence them over time. The distinctive-feature approach is not designed to aid in this aspect of training. Distinctive features are taught in prevocalic, intervocalic, and postvocalic positions, but there is not a strong data base available to dictate when or how this phonemic sequencing process should be taught. It is assumed that the capacity to produce different phonemic utterances has priority over the ability to sequence phonemic utterances.

However, this does not mean that the latter ability is trivial. The priority of the capacity to gener-

ate the features over the capacity to sequence the features is a slight one. Some sequencing problems can be accounted for by an inability to generate the features, and these problems are not sequential problems at all. This is why the current approach was developed first. A second type of program is envisioned for sequential feature development within the word. However, more time is needed to research and develop such a program.

Integrating Jakobson's distinctive feature theory into a developmental paradigm for the articulation skills needed to produce the stream of speech is only one matter for future concern. Harnessing the microcomputer to simplify the management, diagnosis and therapy of articulation problems using a distinctive feature approach is currently underway. As this approach continues to evolve, it will be possible to have computers adjust the minimal word-pairs program—taking into consideration factors such as audiometric threshold configuration, sociolinguistic environmental background, levels of socio-emotional and intellectual development, and the structure and operation of the articulatory apparatus. However, no matter how powerful the therapy program may become, it is the therapist that is the most important catalyst in the learning process. Motivating the child to learn must be given priority in any clinical approach. If the program cannot be modified to fit a child, change the approach. Therapeutic success, being able to speak sounds distinctively different, should be the ultimate goal.

SUMMARY

Distinctive-feature theory provides the foundation for this program. Distinctive features are those components of phonemes that discriminate meaning. A failure in acquisition of a specific distinctive feature results in a phonological disorder that affects an entire class of speech sounds—all sounds that contain that feature as one of their component

parts. For example, if a child does not acquire the voiceless feature, then all phonemes that include voicelessness in their composition will not be used, producing a phonological disorder that is perceived as defective speech.

Distinctive features are abstract concepts, yet their acquisition and use are essential to normal speech production. Teaching a child an abstract feature that she may lack presents a major challenge to the professional who hopes to help the child develop normal speech. The system explained here provides a method to teach features that is easy for children to learn and effective in its results. Essentially, the program uses pairs of words that are alike in every way except for one feature. These pairs of words are called minimal word-pairs. Examples are *pea* and *bee* which, when spoken, differ only by the voice-voiceless contrast in the initial consonant. Minimal word pairs are used to teach any feature requiring training. Meanings inherent in the words used bring the abstract nature of features to a level of concreteness that a child can grasp. An obvious strength of this procedure is that multiple sound errors may be corrected by teaching the correct use of a single missing feature that is responsible for the several errors.

As mentioned, minimal word-pairs that illustrate single distinctive-feature contrasts are used to stimulate the use of the necessary feature. Therapy is organized in steps permitting successive approximations toward correct productions, including discussion of words, auditory discrimination of the distinctive feature in the word-pairs, production training, and carryover. The program represents a holistic approach to therapy that integrates and streamlines elements of traditional methods.

REFERENCES

Albright, R., & Albright, J. (1958). Application of descriptive linguistics to child language. *Journal of Speech and Hearing Research, 1*, 257–261.

Blache, S. (1978). *The acquisition of distinctive features*. Baltimore: University Park Press.

Jakobson, R. (1962). Phoneme and phonology. In R. Jakobson (Ed. and Trans.), *Selected Writings. Vol. I: Phonological Studies*. The Hague: Mouton. (Original work published 1932)

Jakobson, R. (1968). *Child language, aphasia and phonological universals* (A. Keiler, Trans.). The Hague: Mouton. (Original work published 1941)

Jakobson, R., Fant, G., & Halle, M. (1952). *Preliminaries to speech analysis: The distinctive features and their correlates*. Cambridge, MA: MIT Press.

Kantner, C., & West, R. (1969). *Phonetics: An introduction to the principles of phonetic science from the point of view of English speech*. New York: Harper.

McDonald, E. (1964). *Articulation testing and treatment: A sensory-motor approach*. Pittsburgh: Stanwix House.

Glossary

The terms in this glossary are defined as they are used by the authors of the chapters in this text.

acoustic feature   distinctive feature that is based on the physical characteristics of the sound. For example, a sound that has a high frequency hissing quality is characterized as sibilant.

acoustic property   perceptual characteristic of a sound that can be heard

adaptation   variation in the way in which articulators move and the extent to which vocal tract configuration changes shape according to preceding and following sounds

affricate   speech sound formed as a stop followed by a fricative release; a manner of articulation

affrication   phonological process in which fricatives are produced with a stop initiation

allomorph   variation in the production of a meaningful segment that does not change its meaning, i.e., plural markers can be produced as /s/, /z/, or /ɪz/

allophone   articulatory gesture, or phone (speech sound), that is a variant of a phoneme category within the language. Allophones do not affect meaning.

alveolar   refers to speech sounds made with the tongue coming in contact with or moving close to the alveolar ridge; denotes place of articulation

antecedent event   stimulus that immediately precedes the client's response

anterior   refers to speech sounds in which the point of constriction is anterior to the point for the production of /ʃ/; denotes place of articulation

aphasia   acquired language disorder caused by brain damage, resulting in partial or complete impairment of language comprehension, formulation, and/or use in communication

apraxia of speech   motor disorder of speech programming that may be characterized by inconsistent substitutions, oral searching behavior, greater articulatory breakdown in connected speech than in single sounds or words

articulation   actions of the organs of speech that modify the breath stream resulting in speech sounds

articulators   physical structures in the oral cavity that are responsible for or engaged in the production of speech sounds (i.e., lips, tongue, teeth, lower jaw, palate)

articulatory feature   distinctive feature that is based on the actions of the organs of speech. For example, front refers to a sound that is made in the front of the mouth.

aspirate   audible burst of air accompanying the opening of the closure after a stop

assimilation   modification in the audible characteristics of a phone (speech sound) due to the characteristics of another phone in the utterance. An earlier phone in a word may affect a latter phone, resulting in progressive assimilation, or a later phone may affect an earlier one, resulting in regressive assimilation. The phones do not need to be contiguous. Furthermore, the influencing phone may be deleted in the actual utterance.

assimilatory processes   phonological processes that result from modification of one phoneme to match the characteristics of a neighboring phoneme

augmentative communication   any approach designed to support, enhance, or augment the communication of individuals who cannot use speech for independent verbal communication in all situations

babbling   prespeech behavior characterized by syllables that may be initiated or terminated by consonant-like sounds

back   refers to speech sounds made with the tongue retracted; denotes place of articulation

backing   phonological process in which posterior consonants are substituted for anterior ones

baseline   record of the rate of a behavior before training or conditioning procedures are initiated

behavioral probe   sample of the client's behavior as measured by a testing procedure

bifid uvula   division or cleft in the small oval-shaped process extending from the lower border of the velum at midline

bilabial   refers to speech sounds made with partial or complete closure of the lips or of the lips and teeth; denotes place of articulation

carryover   in articulation training, the ability to use a target sound during functional speech outside of the therapy setting

categorical perception   listener's classification of a speech sound as belonging to a specific phonological category. A unit of speech is not classified as belonging partially to one category and partially to another, but categorically to a single category.

cerebral palsy   developmental disability in which the main clinical feature is lack of motor control

cleft palate   structural anomaly that can affect the tissues, muscles, and bony processes of lip, alveolar process, hard palate, soft palate, and uvula

cluster reduction   phonological process in which one or more members of a consonant cluster are omitted, i.e., /pr/ for /spr/ or /b/ for /bl/

coalescence   form of assimilation that occurs when the features of two sounds are combined to form a third sound; also called *reciprocal assimilation*

coarticulation   the simultaneous movement of the muscles and articulators to produce two different phones in connected speech. This movement modifies the production of adjacent phones.

cognates   two sounds made with the same place and manner of articulation, differing only in whether they are voiced or unvoiced, e.g., /t,d/, /f,v/

communication   process of encoding, transmitting, and decoding signals in order to exchange information and ideas between participants

compensatory speech production   substitution of a perceptually similar phoneme for a phoneme that cannot be produced normally by the speaker

consequent event   stimulus that immediately follows the client's response

consonant   speech sound made by marked or complete constriction in the vocal tract. Consonants may initiate and terminate syllables.

consonant cluster   two or more adjacent consonants occurring within the same syllable

consonant harmony   phonological process in which the production of one consonant is modified to match the characteristics of another consonant in the utterance

consonant sequence   two or more consonants not separated by a vowel; the two consonants can cross syllable boundaries. See *consonant cluster* for comparison.

consonant singleton   single consonant separated from other consonants by a vowel or silence

continuant   refers to speech sounds that can be maintained in a steady state; denotes distinctive feature

contrastive items   speech sound pairs of which one sound is the target sound and the other is the error sound

conversational juncture   in articulation training, the transition between words in conversational speech

coronal   refers to speech sounds made with the tongue blade raised; denotes distinctive feature

cue   hints or suggestions provided to the client to assist in the production of the correct response

cycle   time periods during which all deficient phonological patterns are targeted in succession

deaffrication   phonological process in which affricates are produced without the stop initiation or without the fricative release

deep test   an articulation test designed to identify phonetic contexts in which a target speech sound is produced incorrectly as well as those in which it is produced correctly (facilitating contexts). The target sound is assessed in a variety of phonetic environments.

dental prosthesis   artificial device that substitutes for missing teeth and maintains correct dentition

dentition   form and arrangement of the teeth in the dental arch

devoicing   phonological process in which voiceless sounds are substituted for voiced sounds

diadochokinetic rate   rate of movement of the articulators (tongue, lips, etc.) as measured by ability to repeat syllables rapidly

diffuse   refers to speech sounds produced forward in the oral cavity including labials, dentals, and alveolars in contrast to palatals and velars; denotes distinctive feature

diphthong vowel created by a change in the configuration of the vocal tract during vowel production that alters the resonating characteristic of the tract. Two vowels are fused together within a single syllable.

dissimilation phonological process in which one of two similar sounds is produced in a manner to make it less similar to the other

distinctive feature articulatory or acoustic element that defines a phoneme. Each phoneme can be thought of as a unique combination of features.

distributed refers to the length of the constriction of the vocal tract that exceeds the narrow constriction produced by the teeth for /f/, /v/, /θ/, and /ð/; denotes distinctive feature

dysarthria faulty production of speech caused by nervous system damage. If may involve impairment of resonation, articulation, phonation, or prosody.

ear training see *sensory perceptual training*

epenthesis insertion of a sound between two others. This insertion would generally make the sequence easier to say, e.g., /wɑrmpθ/ for warmth.

extinction return of a response that has been conditioned using positive reinforcement to its preconditioned rate (base rate) after the reinforcer has been eliminated

facilitating context phonetic environment in which a sound usually produced incorrectly is more easily produced correctly

feedback in articulation training, the sensory (auditory, visual, tactile, or kinesthetic) information that is utilized to monitor the production of speech

fixed ratio schedule of reinforcement reinforcers provided following a fixed number of responses, i.e., one reinforcer following every correct response, or every third correct response, or whatever number is chosen

flowchart taxonomy of objectives arranged from easy to more difficult

fricative consonant produced by forcing the voiced or voiceless breath stream through a constriction formed in the vocal tract. Turbulence in the airstream produces friction noise or aperiodic sound.

fronting phonological process in which sounds are produced farther forward in the oral cavity (usually at the alveolar ridge) than for the standard production

glide prevocalic consonant characterized by a rapid movement of the articulators from a high front or back tongue arch to a vowel that follows. Although glides are resonants, they are considered to be consonants because they initiate syllables.

gliding phonological process in which glides are substituted for another class of sounds (usually liquids)

glottal refers to speech sounds made by closure of the vocal folds with no characteristic resonant shape of the vocal tract; denotes place of articulation

glottal replacement phonological process in which consonants are replaced by the glottal stop

grave refers to speech sounds made at the very front (/p/, /b/, /m/) or the very back (/k/, /g/, /ŋ/) of the oral cavity; denotes distinctive feature

haptic tactile-kinesthetic sensation

high refers to sounds made with the body of the tongue elevated above the neutral position; denotes distinctive feature

homonym word that sounds the same as another word, but has a different meaning

homorganic two phones produced at the same place of articulation

hypernasal tone excessive nasal resonance during phonation

instructional objective written statement describing the desired behavior, the conditions under which the behavior should occur, and the degree of accuracy of the behavior; synonymous with *behavioral objective*

intelligibility degree to which speech is understood by others

interauditory discrimination client's comparison of his own auditory image of the target sound with someone else's production (usually the clinician's) during the discrimination phase of sensory perceptual training

interrupted refers to speech sounds in which the airstream is completely blocked at some point during production; denotes distinctive feature

intervocalic between two vowels

intra-auditory discrimination client's comparison of his auditory image of the target sound with his own production during the discrimination phase of sensory perceptual training

intraoral breath pressure buildup of air within the oral cavity. This air pressure creates the force necessary for the expulsion of air for plosive sounds.

jargon prespeech behavior characterized by connected syllables produced with adult-like intonation patterns

kinesthetic sense of position or movement of articulatory structures

labiodental refers to speech sounds made with the lower lip and upper teeth; denotes place of articulation

lateral refers to speech sounds in which the midline is constricted so that the air escapes around the sides of the tongue; denotes distinctive feature

lax refers to speech sounds made with relatively less muscle tension and shorter duration; denotes distinctive feature

linguadental refers to speech sounds made with the tongue touching or moving close to the teeth; denotes place of articulation

lingual refers to speech sounds made with the tongue as one of the articulators; denotes place of articulation

linguistics the study of language

liquid consonant for which the articulators make only partial, frictionless approximation (/r/ and /l/); also called *semivowel*

liquid simplification phonological process in which liquids are produced as glides; also called *gliding of liquids*

logarithmic graph graph that uses equal intervals to record rate of response

low refers to sounds made with the tongue lowered; denotes distinctive feature

maintenance in articulation training, retention of correct production of a target sound or pattern after the course of therapy is complete

malocclusion abnormal relationship between the upper and lower teeth

manner of articulation the way the breath stream is modified to produce a speech sound; e.g., fricative or stop

marked the value of a feature (usually the plus value) that presumably makes a sound more difficult to produce

meaningful context in articulation training, a speech production that resembles one used in real communication

melodic intonation therapy therapy approach for aphasia that uses exaggerated intonation patterns to help the patient produce fluent speech

metalinguistics the branch of linguistics that deals with the ability to think and talk about language

metathesis transposition of two adjacent sounds, e.g., /æks/ for *ask*

migration phonological process in which a sound is moved to another position in the word

minimal pair two different words (i.e., different meanings) that differ by only one phoneme or one distinctive feature

morpheme smallest unit of language that has meaning

morphophonemics study of the rules that govern the production of sounds in combinations of morphemes. These rules relate phonological rules and syntactic rules.

motor control system central nervous system motor encoding system involved in the planning of articulation

motor execution system parts of the nervous, muscular, and skeletal systems involved in the production of speech sounds

multisyllabic words words with more than one syllable

nasal consonant in which the air resonates in the nasopharynx while the oral cavity is blocked. The velopharyngeal port is open making nasal resonance possible for the sounds /m, n, ŋ/.

nasal resonance modification of the glottal tone resulting from the coupling of the nasal tract with the vocal tract when the velum is lowered

neuro-developmental treatment (NDT) involves early intervention for the treatment of cerebral palsy. This method was developed by Berta Bobath (1967).

neurogenic originating within the nervous system

obstruent consonant produced by creating airstream turbulence within the oral cavity. Obstruents include voiced and voiceless stops, fricatives, and affricates.

occlusion relationship between the upper and lower teeth

open syllable syllable that ends in a vowel, not terminated by a consonant, e.g., "to, saw, lie," etc.

oral apraxia inability to perform oral vegetative movements such as blowing, chewing, protruding the tongue, or licking the lips voluntarily upon request

organic articulation disorders disorders that arise from physical anomalies affecting structure or function of the mechanisms of speech

oronasal fistula small opening in the hard palate

palatal refers to speech sounds that are made with the body of the tongue touching or moving close to the hard palate; denotes place of articulation

palatogram impressions made by the tongue during speech sound production on an artificial palate that is covered with chalk or powder and inserted into the mouth

paraphasia articulatory error resulting from difficulty with phonological and grammatical rules; also called *paraphasic error*

paresis partial paralysis or muscular weakness

pharyngeal fricative friction sound created by constriction of the airstream between the tongue and pharyngeal wall or by constriction of the pharynx

pharyngeal plosive sound created by the explosive release of a complete constriction between the tongue and pharyngeal wall

phonation the production of voice by the vibration of the vocal folds

phone speech sound segment identified as a member of a particular phoneme or representing a specific phoneme

phoneme group of phones that are perceived as belonging to the same sound category. The set of phonemes are considered to constitute the discrete speech units of a language.

phonetic environment the other speech sounds surrounding a given phoneme within a word or syllable

phonetic feature attributes of a sound that can be expressed in acoustic or physiological terms

phonetics the branch of phonology that deals with individual speech sounds, their production, and their representation by written symbols

phonological knowledge information that is an underlying representation of a phonological/articulation unit

phonological pattern standard adult speech pattern of a linguistic community

phonological process patterned modification of speech sound production away from the standard adult production. Phonological processes usually simplify syllable structures or phoneme classes.

phonology the study of linguistic rules governing the sound system of the language, including speech sounds, speech sound production, and the combination of sounds in meaningful utterances

phonotactics rules for allowable sound combinations in syllables

place of articulation the location of the vocal tract constriction for production of a speech sound

positive reinforcer stimulus that immediately follows a response and increases the rate of the response

posterior primary place of articulation in back of oral cavity or in glottal area

postvocalic following the vowel in a syllable

pragmatics the use of language in society

preparatory set voluntary and/or reflexive preparation of an organism to respond in a particular way to anticipated stimuli. In speech, preparatory set may include the combined respiratory, phonatory, and articulatory systems. In articulation, anticipation of upcoming sounds results in alteration of articulatory postures and movements.

prevocalic preceding the vowel in a syllable

production training phase of articulation training designed to elicit and establish a new sound pattern that will replace the client's error pattern

programmed instruction instructional procedure in which the author has written a systematic set of instructions to be presented to the client. Feedback regarding the accuracy of the responses to these instructions is provided.

prompt   exact model of the correct response

punisher   stimulus that immediately follows a response and results in a decrease in the rate of the response

reduplicated babbling   prespeech behavior characterized by combinations of identical or similar syllables

reduplication   phonological process in which different syllables are produced similarly

response cost   immediate removal of a previously acquired reinforcer following an incorrect response

retroflex   refers to sound made with the tip of the tongue curled back; denotes distinctive feature

round   refers to speech sounds made with the lips rounded; denotes distinctive feature

rule   statement that describes some aspect of the language. Phonological rules describe the sound system of the language.

schedule of reinforcement   schedule clinician experimenter devises to determine how frequently a reinforcer will be provided following the correct response

schemata   structured memories of related perceptual, conceptual, social, emotional, and physical information derived from interactions with the environment. Existing schemata are used to process and organize new information.

script   schemata for a series of actions or event. These generalized episodes or routine activities form the basis for semantic knowledge and the ability to participate appropriately in old and new situations.

secondary reinforcer   stimulus that has been paired with a primary reinforcer (conditioned) and acquires the same or similar effect upon rate of response as the primary reinforcer

semantics   meaning in language

semivowel   speech sound made by a movement from one vocal tract shape to another in a manner similar to diphthongs. Although semivowels are resonants, they

are considered to be consonants because they initiate syllables. Also called *liquids* or *glides*.

sensory perceptual training   technique used in articulation training that emphasizes the development of an auditory model to serve as an internal standard against which comparison of speech sound production can be made

shaping   establishing a target behavior (speech sound) by reinforcing successively closer approximations to the target until correct production is achieved

sibilant   fricative with a high frequency hissing quality (/s, z, ʃ, ʒ/)

sonorant   refers to speech sounds that allow the airstream to pass unimpeded through the oral or nasal cavity; denotes distinctive feature. Phonemes include vowels, nasals, glides, and liquids.

speech   dynamic neuromuscular process of producing sounds for transmitting verbal messages

speech sound discrimination   identification of a sound or a comparison between two sounds. Usually the listener is asked to name a sound or indicate whether two sounds are the same or different.

stabilization   phase of articulation training designed to develop the client's ability to produce the target sound easily and quickly

stimulability   ability of a client to correctly produce a target phoneme by imitating the clinician's exaggerated model

stimulus generalization   occurrence of a response, once it is conditioned to a specific stimulus, in the presence of stimuli that are similar

stop   manner of articulation characterized by complete stoppage of the airstream

stopping   phonological process in which stops are substituted for continuants

stridency deletion   phonological process in which the stridency associated with fricative or affricate sounds is deleted. The resulting sound will usually be a stop or glide. Stridency deletion cannot occur alone without some other modification of the sound.

strident   refers to speech sounds in which noise is produced by forceful airflow striking the back of the teeth (sibilants and /f/ and /v/); denotes distinctive feature

submucous cleft   cleft of the soft or hard palate in which the surface mucosal tissues are connected, while the underlying bone or muscle tissues are separated

substitution processes phonological processes that modify the characteristics of a phoneme resulting in the substitution of one phoneme for another.

syllable speech unit consisting of one vowel. The consonants that may surround this vowel are determined by phonotactic rules.

syllable reduction phonological process in which a syllable in a multisyllabic word is deleted

syllable structure process phonological process that modifies the shape of a syllable. Examples include omission or addition of a phoneme or eliminating the syllable altogether.

syntax rules of language that govern the arrangement and sequence of words according to the meaning relationships among them

systematic phonetic level abstract phonetic information that provides direction for the motor control system in articulation

target behavior desired response the clinician wishes to obtain

target pattern adult sound class, syllable shape, or syllable sequence that is the focus of treatment

target phoneme error phoneme that is the principal focus of treatment. The phoneme may represent a target pattern and thus be used to facilitate the development of the pattern.

tense refers to sounds made with a relatively greater degree of muscle tension and longer duration; denotes distinctive feature

time out removal of a subject from conditions in which the subject could receive positive reinforcement

transfer extension of learned behavior from the original setting (i.e., treatment) to other settings

unaspirated stop made without an audible burst of air accompanying the opening of the closure

underlying phonological form an abstract representation from which the actual production can be derived by application of phonological rules

variable ratio schedule of reinforcement reinforcers provided following an average (not fixed) number of correct responses. For example, on a variable ratio schedule of 3, the client might receive a reinforcer after 2 correct responses, another reinforcer after 4 correct responses, another after 1 correct response, another after 4 responses, etc. The average number of reinforcers is one per 3 correct responses.

variegated babbling prespeech behavior characterized by connected syllables produced with adult-like intonation patterns; also called *jargon*

velar refers to sounds made by the back of the tongue touching or moving close to the soft palate (velum); denotes place of articulation

velopharyngeal closure movement of the velum and pharynx to close off or separate the nasal cavity from the oral cavity, thus directing airflow through the mouth rather than through the nose

velopharyngeal incompetence inability to achieve adequate separation of the nasal cavity from the oral cavity by action of the velum and the pharynx when the structures appear normal. Excessive nasal resonance may result.

vocable prespeech utterance produced with a phonetically consistent form in a given context. A vocable is not a true word because it is not based on an adult word.

vocalic referring to vowels

vocalization 1. phonological process in which consonants (usually glides or liquids) are produced as vowels; also called *vowelization*. 2. nonverbal utterance

voice onset time the difference in time between the release of a stop and the onset of voicing

voiced refers to speech sounds in which the vocal folds vibrate; denotes distinctive feature

voiceless sounds in which the vocal folds do not vibrate

voicing phonological process in which voicing is added to voiceless sounds

vowel speech sound made with an open vocal tract. Vowels constitute syllables and are therefore also termed syllabics

Name Index

Subject Index

NANCY ACRA CREAGHEAD received her B.A. from Denison University, her M.S. from Purdue University, and her Ph.D. from the University of Cincinnati, where she is presently Professor of Communication Disorders and Program Director. Dr. Creaghead has worked as a speech pathologist and as coordinator of speech services for the Cincinnati Speech and Hearing Center. She has been active in the American Speech-Language-Hearing Association and the Ohio Speech and Hearing Association, and is a past president of the Southwestern Ohio Speech-Language-Hearing Association. Dr. Creaghead has authored or coauthored numerous articles and gives frequent invited lectures on language disability, normal language development, and the development and assessment of pragmatic skills. She has received fellowships from the Vocational Rehabilitation Administration and Kappa Kappa Gamma, was awarded the Southwestern Ohio Speech-Language-Hearing Association Honors of the Association in 1981, and is a fellow of the American Speech-Language-Hearing Association.

PARLEY W. NEWMAN is Chair of the Department of Educational Psychology at Brigham Young University, where he has also served as coordinator of special education, chairman of the Department of Speech and Dramatic Arts, and professor of speech pathology. For six years he was associate secretary of the American Speech and Hearing Association, where he chaired ASHA's committees on ethical practice and organization structure. Dr. Newman received his Ph.D. from the University of Iowa and his B.S. and M.S. from Utah State University. He is the author of numerous articles on speech pathology and professional affairs and has served as associate editor of *ASHA,* a journal of the American Speech and Hearing Association, and as an editorial consultant for the *Journal of Speech and Hearing Disorders*. He is a member and past president of the Utah Speech and Hearing Association and a fellow of the American Speech-Language-Hearing Association. In 1971 Dr. Newman received the Master Teacher Award from Associated Students of Brigham Young University and in 1965 the Presidental Citation to the Division of Handicapped Children and Youth of the U.S. Office of Education.

WAYNE A. SECORD received his B.S. and M.A. degrees from The Ohio State University and his doctorate degree from the University of Cincinnati. He is currently an Associate Professor of Communication Disorders at Bowling Green State University, where he serves as Department Chair. Dr. Secord has authored or coauthored a number of articles, books, tests, and intervention programs on assessment and treatment of speech and language disorders, and is a frequent conference/workshop speaker. He is the founder and managing editor of *Hearsay,* the journal of the Ohio Speech and Hearing Association. More recently, Dr. Secord coauthored *CELF-R: Clinical Evaluation of Language Fundamentals* (Semel, Wiig, & Secord 1987) and *TLC-E: Test of Language Competence—Expanded* (Wiig & Secord, 1988), a test of metalinguistic abilities in school-age children and adolescents. Dr. Secord also serves as both an author and consultant for The Psychological Corporation.

DOROTHY H. AIR received her B.S. and M.S. from Marquette University and her Ph.D. from the University of Cincinnati, where she is currently Associate Director of Audiology and Speech Pathology in the Medical Center. Before joining the staff at the University of Cincinnati, Dr. Air set up the speech pathology and audiology program at the Veterans Administration Hospital in Downey, Illinois, and served for several years as its director. Her professional memberships include the American Speech-Language-Hearing Association, the Ohio Speech and Hearing Association, and the Aphasiology Association of Ohio. She has served as chairman of the continuing education committees of both the Ohio Speech and Hearing Association and the Ohio Council of Speech and Hearing Executives. Dr. Air has given many presentations and workshops on auditory function, language disorders, and aphasia, and has been a lecturer for several Cincinnati hospitals.

STEPHEN E. BLACHE received his B.A. and M.A. from the University of Massachusetts and his Ph.D. from Ohio University. He is currently Professor of Communication Disorders and Sciences at Southern Illinois University at Carbondale, where he has also served as director of the articulation program. Dr. Blache is the author of a book, *The Acquisition of Distinctive Features,* and of a number of articles and book reviews. His memberships in professional associations include the American Speech-Language-Hearing Association and the Illinois Speech-Language-Hearing Association. He has served as associate editor of the *Journal of Speech and Hearing Research* and as an editorial consultant for the *Illinois Speech-Language-Hearing Journal.* Dr. Blache's current research projects include elaborations of the Blache Phonemic Inventory, which is a computerized system designed to simplify articulatory diagnosis, record keeping, and therapy planning. He has been identified by the American Council on Rural Special Education as one of the six national leaders in software design in speech/language pathology.

DORIS P. BRADLEY is currently a Professor of Speech and Hearing Sciences and chairperson of the Department of Speech and Hearing Sciences at the University of Southern Mississippi. She received her B.S. from the University of Southern Mississippi, her M.A. from the University of Florida, and her Ph.D. from the University of Pittsburgh. For five years, she was the head of clinical services at the Institute of Logopedics, Wichita State University. Dr. Bradley has authored or coauthored numerous articles on articulation disorders and therapy. She serves on the editorial board for the Autistic Society of America and is a member of the professional advisory board and chairman of the publications committee. A member of numerous professional societies, Dr. Bradley has been especially active in the American Speech-Language-Hearing Association and the American Cleft Palate Association.

BARBARA WILLIAMS HODSON is a Professor in the Department of Communicative Disorders and Sciences at Wichita State University, Wichita, Kansas. She received her B.S., M.S., and Ph.D. from the University of Illinois, where she was an Assistant Professor of Speech and Hearing Science. Dr. Hodson has served as a speech pathologist in preschools and public schools in California, Illinois, and Iowa; tested concept development of preschoolers for the Illinois Office of Public Information; and established a speech-language program for the Rock Island Model Cities Early Childhood Project. She is the author of three books and numerous articles. Dr. Hodson has served as a visiting professor or guest lecturer at a number of universities and colleges and presented numerous lectures and demonstrations. She received the California Speech-Language-Hearing Association Outstanding Achievement Award in 1986 and the American Speech-Language-Hearing Foundation Clinical Achievement Award in 1987.

GORDON MORRIS LOW is a Professor Emeritus of Communication Disorders in the Department of Educational Psychology at Brigham Young University, where he served for a number of years as director of the Communication Disorders Center. He was formerly a professor of special education and codirector of the Communicative Disorders Clinic at San Francisco State College. Dr. Low received his B.S. and M.S. from the University of Utah and his Ph.D. from the University of Minnesota. He is a member of the American Speech and Hearing Association and a past president of the Utah Speech and Hearing Association and the Utah Federation of the Council for Exceptional Children. He has been active in public education, serving as president of the Provo City Board of Education and the Utah School Board Association. Dr. Low has coauthored a number of articles in the area of communication disorders, and with Mildred T. Ravsten has written the book *Resource Education for Children Having Communication-Learning Dysfunctions*.

DONALD E. MOWRER received his B.A. and M.A. in speech pathology from Florida State University and his doctorate from the College of Education at Arizona State University, where he is a Professor in the Department of Speech. After receiving his master's degree, he was employed as an itinerant speech correctionist by four rural school districts in Ohio and served as director of a Junior League speech clinic in Georgia. He worked in Arizona as a part-time public school correctionist and taught remedial reading at the high-school level. Dr. Mowrer's area of emphasis has been in the application of behavioral engineering strategies to the management of children's speech. He has many publications on behavioral principles and applications. He is a fellow of the American Speech-Language-Hearing Association.

JEAN R. NEILS, who received her B.S. from Pennsylvania State University and her M.A. and Ph.D. from Case Western Reserve University, is currently an Assistant Professor in the Department of Communication at the University of Cincinnati. She provided speech-language diagnostics and therapy at the Cincinnati V.A. Medical Center, where she continues to serve as a consultant. She managed special therapy programs at the Society for Crippled Children and the Cleveland Hearing Speech Center. Dr. Neil is coauthor of a therapy manual for aphasics (Neils, Weisiger, & Martin, *Language for Living*) and a number of articles.

MILDRED T. RAVSTEN received her B.A. and M.C.H. in speech pathology from Brigham Young University, where she is currently an Assistant Professor of Educational Psychology and a member of the core faculty of the Comprehensive Clinic. She served for a number of years as a consultant on speech and language development and disorders for the Bureau of Indian Affairs, the Ute Tribe Headstart Program, and the Uintah and Vernal school districts in Utah, and has worked as speech therapist and teacher. Ms. Ravsten is a member of the American Speech-Language-Hearing Association and of the Utah Speech-Language-Hearing Association. She coauthored *Resource Education for Children Having Communicative-Learning Dysfunctions* with Gordon M. Low, and is currently engaged in research on the effectiveness of training procedures and skills assessment for clinicians and on the training of parents as facilitators of language development.

RICHARD E. SHINE is Professor of Speech Pathology at East Carolina University. He was an assistant professor in the Department of Speech Pathology at Pennsylvania State University and earlier served with the Weld County (Colorado) Crippled Children's Speech and Hearing Clinic and the Scott County (Iowa) Board of Education as speech pathologist, speech and hearing clinician, and coordinator of these services. Dr. Shine received his B.A. and M.A. from the University of Northern Colorado and his Ed.D. from Pennsylvania State University. He has served since 1971 as an associate editor of *Language, Speech and Hearing Services in the Schools,* a publication of the American Speech-Language-Hearing Association. He was a consultant for the Purdue Speaker Telephone Continuing Education Project. His publications include early work with E. T. McDonald on phonetic profiles and articulatory abilities of kindergarten and first-grade children. He coauthored with J. Proust a book, *Clinical Treatment Manual: Articulatory Production Training: A Programmed Sensory-Motor Approach.*

HARRIS WINITZ, who received his B.A. from the University of Vermont and his M.A. and Ph.D. from the University of Iowa, is currently a Professor of Speech Science and Psychology at the University of Missouri–Kansas City. Over a span of almost 30 years, Dr. Winitz has published numerous articles in the areas of phonetics, psycholinguistics, and articulation; his current research focuses on the relationship between auditory perception and articulation. He is also the author of several widely used textbooks, including *Articulatory Acquisition and Behavior* and *Phonetics: A Manual for Listening*. In 1981, he chaired, organized, and edited the proceedings of a major conference on native and second language acquisition sponsored by the New York Academy of Sciences. Dr. Winitz has served as editor of *Human Communication and Its Disorders: A Review* and as associate editor of the *Journal of Psycholinguistic Research* and the *Journal of Speech and Hearing Disorders*. He is a fellow of the American Speech-Language-Hearing Association.

ANN STACE WOOD is a clinical speech and language pathologist in private practice in Cincinnati. She received her B.A. in English and speech from Miami University and her M.A. and Ph.D. in speech pathology from the University of Cincinnati. In addition to her private practice, Dr. Wood is a part-time instructor in aphasia at the University of Cincinnati and an adjunct affiliate staff member at the Jewish Hospital. She serves as a consultant for Doherty School, Clermont County Senior Services, and the Veterans Administration Hospital in Cincinnati. Her professional memberships include the American Speech-Language-Hearing Association, the Ohio Speech and Hearing Association, the Aphasiology Association of Ohio, and the American Academy of Private Practice in Speech Pathology and Audiology.

WE VALUE YOUR OPINION—PLEASE SHARE IT WITH US

Merrill Publishing and our authors are most interested in your reactions to this textbook. Did it serve you well in the course? If it did, what aspects of the text were most helpful? If not, what didn't you like about it? Your comments will help us to write and develop better textbooks. We value your opinions and thank you for your help.

Text Title _____ Edition _____

Author(s) _____

Your Name (optional) _____

Address _____

City _____ State _____ Zip _____

School _____

Course Title _____

Instructor's Name _____

Your Major _____

Your Class Rank _____ Freshman _____ Sophomore _____ Junior _____ Senior

_____ Graduate Student

Were you required to take this course? _____ Required _____ Elective

Length of Course? _____ Quarter _____ Semester

1. Overall, how does this text compare to other texts you've used?

_____ Superior _____ Better Than Most _____ Average _____ Poor

2. Please rate the text in the following areas:

	Superior	Better Than Most	Average	Poor
Author's Writing Style	_____	_____	_____	_____
Readability	_____	_____	_____	_____
Organization	_____	_____	_____	_____
Accuracy	_____	_____	_____	_____
Layout and Design	_____	_____	_____	_____
Illustrations/Photos/Tables	_____	_____	_____	_____
Examples	_____	_____	_____	_____
Problems/Exercises	_____	_____	_____	_____
Topic Selection	_____	_____	_____	_____
Currentness of Coverage	_____	_____	_____	_____
Explanation of Difficult Concepts	_____	_____	_____	_____
Match-up with Course Coverage	_____	_____	_____	_____
Applications to Real Life	_____	_____	_____	_____

3. Circle those chapters you especially liked:
   1   2   3   4   5   6   7   8   9   10   11   12   13   14   15   16   17   18   19   20
   What was your favorite chapter? _____
   Comments:

4. Circle those chapters you liked least:
   1   2   3   4   5   6   7   8   9   10   11   12   13   14   15   16   17   18   19   20
   What was your least favorite chapter? _____
   Comments:

5. List any chapters your instructor did not assign. _____

6. What topics did your instructor discuss that were not covered in the text?_____

   _____

7. Were you required to buy this book? _____ Yes   _____ No

   Did you buy this book new or used? _____ New   _____ Used

   If used, how much did you pay? _____

   Do you plan to keep or sell this book? _____ Keep   _____ Sell

   If you plan to sell the book, how much do you expect to receive? _____

   Should the instructor continue to assign this book? _____ Yes   _____ No

8. Please list any other learning materials you purchased to help you in this course (e.g., study guide, lab manual).

   _____

9. What did you like most about this text? _____

   _____

10. What did you like least about this text? _____

    _____

11. General comments:

    May we quote you in our advertising? _____ Yes   _____ No

    Please mail to: Boyd Lane
                      College Division, Research Department
                      Box 508
                      1300 Alum Creek Drive
                      Columbus, Ohio 43216

    Thank you!